Knowledge Translation in Nursing and Healthcare

Knowledge Translation in Nursing and Healthcare

A Roadmap to Evidence-informed Practice

Margaret B. Harrison, BN, MHA, PhD
Professor Emerita, School of Nursing
Queen's University
Kingston, Canada

Ian D. Graham, PhD, FCAHS, FNYAM, FRSC
Professor, School of Epidemiology and Public Health
University of Ottawa
Ottawa, Canada
Senior Scientist
Centre for Practice-Changing Research
The Ottawa Hospital Research Institute
Ottawa, Canada

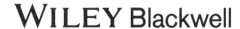
WILEY Blackwell

Registered Office
John Wiley & Sons, Inc., 111 River Street, Hoboken, NJ 07030, USA

Editorial Office
9600 Garsington Road, Oxford, OX4 2DQ, UK

For details of our global editorial offices, customer services, and more information about Wiley products visit us at www.wiley.com.

Wiley also publishes its books in a variety of electronic formats and by print-on-demand. Some content that appears in standard print versions of this book may not be available in other formats.

Library of Congress Cataloging-in-Publication Data

Names: Harrison, Margaret B., author. | Graham, Ian D., author.
Title: Knowledge translation in nursing and healthcare : a roadmap to evidence-informed practice / Margaret B. Harrison, Ian D. Graham.
Description: Hoboken, NJ : Wiley-Blackwell, 2020. | Includes bibliographical references and index.
Identifiers: LCCN 2020033427 (print) | LCCN 2020033428 (ebook) | ISBN 9780813811857 (paperback) | ISBN 9781119123330 (adobe pdf) | ISBN 9781119123323 (epub)
Subjects: MESH: Evidence-Based Nursing | Translational Medical Research
Classification: LCC RT41 (print) | LCC RT41 (ebook) | NLM WY 100.7 | DDC 610.73–dc23
LC record available at https://lccn.loc.gov/2020033427
LC ebook record available at https://lccn.loc.gov/2020033428

Cover Design: NA
Cover Image: © lvcandy/Getty Images

Set in 9.5/12.5pt STIXTwoText by SPi Global, Pondicherry, India

SKY10025058_022221

Finishing this book in the Year of the Nurse and Midwife (2020) and it being released in the Year of Health and Care workers, we dedicate this book to the many nurses, other healthcare providers, and patients who have invited us in to facilitate and study implementation. They provided us with world class living implementation laboratories. We owe them so much for providing the opportunity to study implementation processes in the real world and to develop models and frameworks to facilitate evidence-informed practice. They provided us with opportunities to acquire hands-on experience and tacit implementation knowledge which ultimately allowed us to cultivate and hone our implementation craft and science.

and to

Marjorie and Fern

Contents

About the Authors

Margaret B. Harrison
Professor Emerita
Queen's University, Kingston, Ontario, Canada

After many years of practice Margaret returned to school to pursue research in nursing. Her PhD (Nursing) from McMaster University concentrated on continuity of care for complex populations and using guideline recommendations as a foundation for multi-interventions within randomized controlled trials. This interest began in the early 1990s at the Children's Hospital of Eastern Ontario where, in her professional practice and research role, she was challenged by senior administration to improve specific quality of care issues, e.g. central line care, preparation of repeatedly hospitalized children. In working with care teams, the dialogue always began with a critical review of external evidence to formulate a new local approach based on best available evidence. This approach continued in her role as Nurse Specialist Research and Evaluation at the Ottawa Hospital, a large teaching facility, working closely with the quality portfolio to conduct implementation studies driven by quality/risk issues, e.g. pressure injury prevention and management practices, transitional care of patients with heart failure. During this time, the term "knowledge translation" became formalized and began to emerge as a distinct research paradigm. Margaret undertook regional community work to assist in care improvement for the population with chronic wounds beginning a long series of nursing research initiatives. Then based at Queen's University, Kingston, Ontario (2000–2014), she was Scientific Director, Senior Scientist with the Practice and Research in Nursing (PRN) Group, a unique practice–academic partnership dedicated to producing and using evidence for practice. She established and led the Queen's Joanna Briggs Collaboration where research is synthesized in a rigorous manner for practice use. During that time Margaret received the Queen's Basmajian Medal for research, published 137 peer reviewed papers, and first authored CAN-IMPLEMENT©: Planning for Best-Practice Implementation (2014). She was awarded a Sigma Theta Tau Writing Award as lead author for "Roadmap for a Research-Practice Partnership to Implement Evidence" (Worldviews 2012). As Professor Emerita, Margaret continues this work voluntarily with community partners.

Ian D. Graham, PhD, FCAHS, FNYAM, FRSC

Professor, School of Epidemiology and Public Health
University of Ottawa, Ottawa, Canada
Senior Scientist
Centre for Practice-Changing Research
The Ottawa Hospital Research Institute, Ottawa, Canada

Ian's PhD in medical sociology from McGill University focused on understanding how historically, the obstetrical practice of episiotomy rose to became a routine practice in North America by the 1950s, was questioned by women and midwives in the 1970s and 1980s and lost its status as a routine procedure by the 1990s. During his postdoctoral studies, Ian continued to focus on identifying and understanding factors influencing professional practice and the role evidence could play in changing practice. Upon being appointed to the Ottawa Hospital Research Institute and working with nursing and medical colleagues, he began shifting attention to finding ways to apply social science theory and methods to facilitate the uptake of evidence informed practice (known now as knowledge translation and implementation science). The origins of all the knowledge translation models and frameworks he has developed can be traced back to collaborations with practitioners at the point of care and the desire to find rigorous and collaborative ways for them to leverage external evidence by aligning it with their local context. From 2006–2012 he served as Vice-President of the Knowledge Translation and Public Outreach at the Canadian Institutes of Health Research, Canada's premier health research funder. There he brought in CIHR's first citizen engagement in research framework and open access policy, and funding opportunities to support knowledge translation and engagement of patients and others as research partners. One of his current research foci is on understanding the role of research co-production in the uptake of research findings. He has published over 300 peer reviewed articles and is co-editor of Turning Knowledge into Action: Practical Guidance on How to Do Integrated Knowledge Translation Research (2014), Knowledge Translation in Health Care (2013, 2nd edition) and Evaluating the Impact of Implementing Evidence-based Practice (2010) and co-author of CAN-IMPLEMENT©: Planning for Best-Practice Implementation (2014). He has twice been awarded a Queen Elizabeth II Jubilee Medal (2002, 2012) for contributions to research.

Acknowledgments

The writing of this book has been its own journey. In fact, some of the chapters were drafted during a transatlantic writing retreat aboard the Queen Victoria in her peaceful library. Other chapters were worked while on business trips and academic leave to Australia and the UK. Most of the book, however, was written on the unceded territory of the Algonquin Nation and we honor the Elders and Knowledge Keepers, both past and present.

Our trusty Research Coordinator Meg Carley, BSc guided us through the final phase of this work making great enhancements not only to chapter format but improving our rudimentary schemas and tables – often hand drawn. Meg also skillfully managed the references – her penchant for detail and organization were invaluable. Joan van den Hoek, BNSc took the mental vision we had of the Roadmap and created the graphic for this book.

We would like to thank Christine Cassidy, RN, BScN, PhD; Jed Duff, RN, BN, PhD; and Jo Logan, BScN, PhD for generously reading early drafts of chapters and providing insightful comments and suggestions that have greatly improved the chapters. We are particularly indebted to Sandy Dunn, RN, MScN, PhD for carefully reviewing all the chapters with a critical eye and always offering words of encouragement. Elizabeth Dogherty's RN, BNSc, MNSc, PhD work has enlightened the field and us about implementation facilitation at the point-of-care. Wendy Gifford, RN, BScN, PhD, generously provided material for the Chapter 4 Appendix on implementation leadership. Janet Squires, RN, BN, MN, PhD graciously permitted us to include a TDF interview guide from one of her studies. Melissa Demery Varin RN, BScN, MScN shared literature she had synthesized on feasibility and pilot testing. We are grateful to Peter C. Wyer, MD for discussion about the differences and similarities between quality improvement and knowledge translation and letting us build on his figure comparing the two. We would also like to express our appreciation to Jennifer Meyers, MD for our discussions on the complementarity of quality improvement tools and the Knowledge to Action Cycle. Not withstanding all the excellent advice, we received, any errors and omissions are ours alone.

We appreciate the support from Wiley Blackwell colleagues over the time in writing this book. In particular, we thank our managing editor Louise Barnetson and our publisher Magenta Styles who has been steadfast in her ongoing support and this greatly encouraged us. Thank you.

Some of the material for the leg ulcer case presented in Chapter 2 was previously published in Graham et al. A community-research alliance to improve chronic wound care. *Healthcare Policy* 2007; 2(4):58–64.

Finally, John and Dawn, our spouses, and our families, have been very supportive and patient with us as we have labored over this book. We cannot thank them enough. We will not however, miss them asking, "Is *that* book done yet?"

Foreword

A quick Internet search will show you that many books have been written about evidence-based practice, so why should you be interested in *this* book? There are several good answers to this question, read on.

The proliferation of products that collate and synthesize evidence to offer best practice recommendations has increased exponentially over the last two decades. Yet there is often a disconnect between what is recommended and what happens in practice. Why? It is partly because evidence does not get moved, intact, from one place to another. It cannot. Research is rarely the only piece of the evidence jigsaw that practitioners draw on in their practice, and there needs to be a good fit between evidence and context for it to have a chance of making a difference. There are many factors at play, which need to be considered and negotiated, and this is rarely straightforward. Therefore, if evidence is to get transformed to inform practice, this requires purposeful action. This is why you should pick up this book.

The authors of this book have brought together research, theory and their accumulated expertise and wisdom from decades of practice-based knowledge translation work to provide a map and compass to help those in roles that facilitate evidence-informed care navigate the way. As a "Roadmap to Evidence-Informed Practice" this book provides a comprehensive and systematic approach, drawing on practical examples, offering tips and tools, and reflecting on lessons learnt. As such, it provides a resource for the implementer to focus on solutions rather than get overwhelmed by the challenges.

The book is organized around the Roadmap Framework that Drs Graham and Harrison have developed from their extensive research and practice in the field. The framework includes three overarching phases: issue identification and clarification, build solutions, and field test, and implement, evaluate, sustain, which provides a logical and systematic way of walking the reader through activities required at each stage. A focus on research and evaluation activities at each stage also supports capacity and capability building for professional practice and research awareness. The content is grounded in nursing practice examples, which translates theory and research into concrete implementation actions. It is a book that you can dip in and out of, or read sequentially. The result is an invaluable and accessible "how to" of implementation.

Another notable feature of this book is the thread of collaboration and partnership that runs through it. Translating evidence to inform practice is not an individual practitioner or provider effort. The relationship between knowing and doing is bounded within the health and care systems people work in. Social and interactional aspects of knowledge translation have been receiving increasing attention. The idea that there are two homogenous communities where one produces knowledge and the other uses it, is rightly, becoming outdated. Therefore, it is refreshing to see how the authors weave in a focus on collaboration and partnership working as a pathway to best practice implementation through co-producing knowledge and practice.

As leaders in the field, these authors have created a roadmap that is authoritative, comprehensive, and useful. What they have managed to achieve is a rare balance of theory and research combined with the practical. This book should be a "go to" for those implementing evidence-informed nursing and healthcare practice.

Jo Rycroft-Malone, RN, BSc(Hons), MSc, PhD,
Professor of Health Research
Dean, Faculty of Health & Medicine, Lancaster University, UK
Director, National Institute for Health Research Health Services & Delivery Research
Programme

As I read through this new book by Margaret Harrison and Ian Graham entitled "Knowledge Translation in Nursing and Healthcare: A Roadmap to Evidence-Informed Practice," I reflected on my years of clinical practice as well as some major implementation projects in healthcare that I have been involved in over the years.

I completed my Doctorate in Nursing (with a focus on Knowledge Translation (KT) and Shared Decision Making) following many years of clinical experience in tertiary neonatal intensive care. During my career I have had the privilege of working as a clinician at the point of care, as an educator and consultant to support practice change, and as a KT Specialist and researcher to develop and evaluate different strategies to improve uptake of best practice.

One of the major initiatives I was involved in was a collaboration between a provincial data registry group, a research team of implementation science and clinical experts, and healthcare organizations providing maternal newborn services in Ontario. The aim of the project was to develop and implement an electronic audit and feedback system across the province, and then evaluate the effect on clinical practice for selected performance indicators. The results of this project were very promising with evidence of improved rates for four of six performance indicators of perinatal care over 30 months post implementation. A number of barriers and enablers were identified, and we learned many lessons from this project both with respect to the design of effective audit and feedback, and about contextual and individual factors that enabled or blocked change. For example, leadership support for effective change was critical, as were professional attitudes to the change and staff motivation, trust in the data and credibility of the evidence, the availability of essential resources, and collaborative inter-professional relationships.

Reading this new book by two internationally recognized experts in the field of implementation of change in healthcare, I appreciate the successes and failures of our project even more now. Evidence-based guidelines or data signaling an evidence-practice gap do not automatically trigger practice change, even if the evidence is sound and the data are trustworthy. In my years of clinical practice prior to this initiative I have witnessed quality improvement initiatives where limited strategies were used to support practice change (e.g. staff education or the development and communication of a new policy or procedure). Inevitably, this was insufficient to address the full scope of barriers that existed and as a result implementation was incomplete and practice improvement, if any, was limited – wasting time, effort, resources, and money. Successful practice change in healthcare requires a multi-level, multi-pronged approach informed by current evidence and tailored to address the existing barriers to change within the specific context of care.

This new book provides a comprehensive roadmap to guide you through the planning process for successful implementation of sustained practice change in your organization. This is an extremely interesting, well written resource that is a pleasure to read. It is a rich source of information based on the authors' years of experience in the field and informed by a wide range of theories and scientific evidence. This book also demonstrates the complexity of the change process, what it takes to successfully implement new practices and the commitment of time and resources required to carry out each phase. It is full of real-life examples, tools, tips, references, and a step-by-step approach to help guide you along your journey. This book is a tremendous resource for nurses as well as other healthcare professionals. I wholeheartedly recommend that you read this book and take advantage of the wealth of knowledge contained within to help guide your implementation projects. Enjoy!

Sandra Dunn RN PhD
KT Specialist, BORN Ontario
Adjunct Professor, University of Ottawa, School of Nursing
Senior Research Associate, Ottawa Hospital Research Institute

Praise for Knowledge Translation in Nursing and Healthcare

Changing behavior using theory and evidence can be a daunting challenge – Drs. Harrison and Graham have risen to this challenge by providing us with a thoughtful and pragmatic "Roadmap" to guide our implementation activities from planning to sustainability. These authors have integrated the science and practice of implementation into a user-friendly "Roadmap" to optimize our success as implementers on the clinical frontline.

Dr. Sharon E. Straus, HBSc, MSc, MD, FRCP (C)
Professor, Dept. of Medicine, University of Toronto
Physician-in-Chief, St. Michael's Hospital
Director, KT Program, St. Michael's Hospital

"This is exactly what I've been looking for, something practical to use to teach KT and evidence implementation."

Professor Jed Duff RN PhD FACORN,
Professor and Chair of Nursing, Metro North Hospital and Health Service and Queensland University of Technology
Royal Brisbane & Women's Hospital, Nursing & Midwifery Research Centre, Herston, Queensland 4029

As a healthcare leader with many years of experience in the practice environment and within accreditation, this book offers you a way for moving best practice into the healthcare environment, that is relevant and in touch with your reality. With a focus on improved outcomes for both care recipients and the providers, the approach outlined in this guide is easy to follow and simplifies the pathway to enabling implementation of best practice.

In the complex world within which healthcare is provided, these authors demonstrate their deep understanding of your reality and provide you with this valuable guide. Enjoy the journey guided by The Roadmap!

Wendy Nicklin RN, BN, MSc(A), CHE, FACHE FISQ,ua, UCD.D
Former Vice President of Clinical Services, Chief Nurse Executive, The Ottawa Hospital, subsequently President and CEO of Accreditation Canada, President (Board Chair) of International Society for Quality in Health Care (ISQUA)

Drs. Harrison and Graham are global leaders in knowledge translation and implementation science. Their book provides a practical and science-based approach to move evidence from the page to the hands of the knowledge user where it makes a difference.

Lisa Hopp PhD RN FAAN
Dean and Professor
Director, Indiana Center for Evidence Based Nursing Practice
Purdue University Northwest, Hammond IN

This book is full of outstanding practical advice, based on solid research and real world experiences, on how to best overcome barriers in the implementation of evidence-based care. It should be a staple resource for enhancing the quality and safety of healthcare.

Bernadette Mazurek Melnyk, PhD, APRN-CNP, FAANP, FNAP, FAAN
Vice President for Health Promotion, University Chief Wellness Officer
Dean and Professor, College of Nursing
Executive Director, the Helene Fuld Health Trust National Institute for Evidence-based Practice in Nursing and Healthcare
The Ohio State University and safety of healthcare.

Glossary Terms (Alphabetical): Related to the Implementation of Evidence-Informed Practice

Adapt: to modify or make suitable for one's purpose.

Adherence: following the evidence (e.g. guideline) recommendations.

Adopt: to take up, follow or use.

Barriers Assessment: a process for identifying barriers and drivers to a specific a practice or behavior.

Best Practices: maintaining or improving effective and efficient care based on best available evidence.

Call-to-Action: the point when a practice issue emerges as a problem to be dealt with, when quality or risk data indicate it as a problem, or new evidence emerges that should change practice.

Capacity Building: a process that builds on local existing skills and knowledge, fostering a sense of ownership and empowerment.

Conceptual knowledge use: using knowledge to change the way users think about issues including changes in understanding, attitude, or intentions.

Continuity of care approach: a coordinated and integrated process of care, creating linkages across settings, between providers, with recipients of health care that facilitates the transition of care from sector, institution, agency, or individual to another over time.

Critical appraisal: the process of carefully and systematically assessing the outcome of research (evidence) to judge its trustworthiness, value, and relevance in a particular context.

Customization: the action of modifying a best practice recommendation to optimize its fit with a particular context.

Delphi consensus method: a method used to facilitate a group coming to consensus on something.

Dissemination: identifying the appropriate receivers and users of knowledge (the audience) and tailoring the message and medium to the audience.

Environmental scan: process that systematically surveys and interprets relevant information and data to identify barriers and drivers, assist in planning, and evaluating an implementation.

Evidence-based Nursing: integration of the best evidence available, nursing expertise, and the values and preferences of the individuals, families, and communities who are served. https://www.sigmanursing.org/why-sigma/about-sigma/position-statements-and-resource-papers/evidence-based-nursing-position-statement

Evidence-Informed Practice (EIP): in addition to best available evidence, EIP involves the integration of practice skills, expertise, and experience as well as context knowledge, (local environment and evidence about the population), information on the resources available, patient preferences, as well as assessing local skills and expertise.

Evidence-practice gap: the gap between current practice and best practice. Also known as the know-do gap.

Expenditure review: understanding the costs associated with the current and the new practice.

Experimental study design: participants are allocated to the different groups in an experiment. Experimental study designs include randomized control trials, cluster randomized control trials, and stepped-wedge cluster randomized trials.

Facilitation: to make something possible or easier. With evidence implementation, facilitation can be internal, external, or partnered and carried out either by an individual or a group.

Facilitator: person or group specifically assigned to facilitate the evidence-informed practice.

Fidelity: the degree of accuracy with which something is implemented.

Field test: field tests are undertaken to: (i) determine whether the implementation strategies can be delivered with fidelity, (ii) collect preliminary data on whether the strategies are working as expected, and (iii) assess acceptance of (and satisfaction with) the strategies to the potential adopters of best practice and other stakeholders.

Formative evaluation: evaluation undertaken for learning during the implementation process. Conducted to ensure that an implementation program/initiative is feasible, appropriate, and acceptable before it is fully implemented and to improve it before it is launched.

Guideline adaptation: comprises identifying the practice topic; constituting the evaluation and adaptation group; searching, appraising, and adapting guideline(s) for local use; seeking feedback and peer review of the locally adapted guideline(s); and updating of the local guideline(s).

Hybrid study design: with evidence implementation a study design that simultaneously permits determining the effectiveness of a best practice and the implementation strategies used.

Impact: the outcomes resulting from adherence to best practice (e.g. health outcomes, provider outcomes, health system outcomes).

Impact evaluation: used to determine impact of the implementation on health and other outcomes of interest.

Implementation: efforts undertaken to activate evidence into practice, i.e. the practice of knowledge translation.

Implementation mapping: a process for selecting implementation strategies to address implementation barriers to achieve implementation objectives.

Implementation science: the study of the determinants of knowledge use and effective methods of promoting the uptake of knowledge including (but not limited to) evaluating implementation outcomes.

Indicator: a measure of something (e.g. knowledge use, process, performance, impact)

Instrumental knowledge use: the concrete application of knowledge.

Integrated knowledge translation: interaction between decision-makers and researchers that results in mutual learning through the process of co-planning, co-producing, disseminating, and applying existing or new research in decision-making. It involves bidirectional communication, mutual learning, and co-creation of change by relevant stakeholders.

Intervention mapping: is a process that guides the design of interventions and implementation strategies.

Knowledge, Attitude, Practice (KAP) survey: a method to assess the barriers and drivers to implementation.

Knowledge synthesis: the contextualization and integration of research findings of individual research studies within the larger body of knowledge on the topic. A synthesis must be reproducible and transparent in its methods, using quantitative and/or qualitative methods. https://cihr-irsc.gc.ca/e/41382.html.

Knowledge translation: a dynamic and iterative process that includes synthesis, dissemination, exchange and ethically-sound application of knowledge to improve health, provide more effective health services and products and strengthen the health care system. https://cihr-irsc.gc.ca/e/29418.html.

Knowledge use: ways in which knowledge informs decision making. The three types of knowledge use are conceptual, instrumental and symbolic.

Knowledge user: individuals, groups or organizations that use the results of research or best practices to make decisions or apply research or best practices.

Meta-analysis: statistical analysis that combines the results of multiple scientific studies. https://en.wikipedia.org/wiki/Meta-analysis.

Nominal Group Technique (NGT): a structured method for group brainstorming that encourages contributions from everyone and facilitates quick agreement on the relative importance of issues, problems, or solutions https://asq.org/quality-resources/nominal-group-technique.

Observational study design: observational studies are ones where researchers observe the effect of an intervention or implementation without trying to change who is or is not exposed to it. Observational study designs include cohort studies and case control studies.

Outcome/effectiveness evaluation: evaluations designed to measure the effect (or effectiveness) of the implementation process by assessing the uptake or adherence to the prescribed best practice. This type of evaluation can fall under the category of summative evaluation.

Population profile study: an enquiry where the population of interest is described in terms of socio-demographic, circumstance of living and other key factors.

Practice Audit: a tool to assess care and outcomes from what is documented in the health care record and includes chart audit, audit-and-feedback etc. A way to discover what you are doing right and what might be improved.

Practice Guideline: statements that include recommendations intended to optimize care that are informed by a systematic review of evidence and an assessment of the benefits and harms of alternative care options.

Process/implementation evaluation: determines whether interventions/best practices have been implemented as intended and resulted in certain outputs. It is also a means of understanding how complex interventions work in the field of implementation science.

Program Evaluation: the systematic collection of information about the activities, characteristics, and outcomes of programs, for use by people to reduce uncertainties, improve effectiveness, and make decisions. https://www.atsdr.cdc.gov/communityengagement/pce_program_evaluation.html#:~:text=Program%20evaluation%20can%20be%20defined,39).

Quality improvement: In health care, it is the framework used to systematically improve the ways care is delivered to individuals. Processes have characteristics that can be measured, analyzed, improved, and controlled. https://www.ahrq.gov/ncepcr/tools/pf-handbook/mod4.html.

Quasi experimental study design: involves the manipulation of an independent variable without the random assignment of participants to conditions or orders of conditions. Among the important types are nonequivalent groups designs, pretest-posttest, and interrupted time-series designs. https://opentextbc.ca/researchmethods/chapter/quasi-experimental-research.

Reliability: refers to the consistency of a measure-the extent to which a measure gives the same value each time it used on the same conditions with the same participants.

Sample: this is a portion of a larger group for used to collect information for needs assessment and/or the evaluation.

Scalability: the ability increase the size or amount of implementation.

Scope of practice: is the range of healthcare tasks, decisions or activities of a qualified, licensed healthcare professional (e.g. doctor, nurse practitioner, nurse, pharmacist) allowed by law and the country/state/provincial/territorial licensing authority governing that profession. https://www.cmpa-acpm.ca/serve/docs/ela/goodpracticesguide/pages/teams/Healthcare_teams/scopes_of_practice-e.html.

Social constructivist learning theory: people are shaped by their experiences and interactions.

Spread: the process of encouraging the use of a best practice by others or in different settings

Stakeholder analysis: a process of identifying individuals or groups according to their levels of influence and support for change

Stakeholders: anyone or group with an interest in or affected by the implementation of best practice. Knowledge users are an important type of stakeholder.

Standard: defines the performance expectations of an organization.

Strategic alliance: Agreement among individuals or groups to focus on a specific issue or concern, often in the context of initiating collective action.

Summative evaluation: used for judging the worth or merit of what is being implemented after implementation has occurred. Outcome/effectiveness evaluations and impact evaluations are summative evaluations.

Sustainability: the ongoing or continued use of best practice after the initial implementation.

Sustainability strategies: strategies to promote the ongoing use of best practices.

Symbolic knowledge use: the use of research/ knowledge as a political or persuasive tool. Using knowledge to persuade others.

Systematic review: type of literature review that uses systematic methods to collect secondary data, critically appraise research studies, and synthesize findings qualitatively or quantitatively. https://en.wikipedia.org/wiki/Systematic_review

Taxonomy: classification system.

Usability testing: evaluating a best practice, implementation or sustainability strategy by testing it with representative users.

Utilization-focused evaluation: A type of evaluation specifically designed to generate information that stakeholders can use in their decision-making about a program or implementation.

Validity: refers to how accurately a method measures what it is intended to measure.

1

Introduction

Introduction

Using research evidence in day-to-day practice is a lofty and much touted goal found in mission statements of health care organizations and in nursing and other health professionals' associations. Incidentally it began in Florence Nightingale's time with her use of statistics to demonstrate mortality related to the context of care in hospital versus home deliveries for women (Nightingale 1871). Her many frustrations in trying to change policy and practices based on documented evidence have been well studied (McDonald 2001). Those were different times and there were roadblocks related to being a woman, as well as the control of the medical powers of the era. Yet, the reality nearly a century and a half later, is that the effective uptake of research in practice and policy continues to elude us. This is despite modern health care systems, large-scale investment in research including implementation science, development of international groups committed to synthesizing evidence, and in more recent decades, bodies dedicated to guideline development and translating evidence into practice recommendations.

Good quality evidence that is synthesized and then transformed into recommendations for practice provides the basis for evidence-informed practice (EIP). On the surface this seems like a simple enough task for practitioners and clinical managers to action, but why is it so difficult to do when the evidence that should be applied at the point-of-care is now widely available?

As nurses well know, the point-of-care environment is tremendously complex and dynamic with multiple internal and external influences. These complexities face the "simple" task of using evidence housed in a single evidence-informed recommendation, or even more complicated, a guideline consisting of multiple, sometimes dozens of recommendations. For example, consider the one recommendation commonly found in most guidelines, for a daily head-to-toe skin assessment for pressure injury prevention with complex patients. Factors at play include the patient's condition, nurse's time, team workload, ward environments, availability of a second set of hands for turning, other unscheduled admissions, more urgent duties related to attending to high-tech equipment, patient/family considerations, the nurse's skill and knowledge of risk scales, as well as organizational documentation and referral procedures in the presence of unacceptable risk. On the surface a straightforward task, yet in the field, away from the guideline expert table it involves a quagmire of challenges.

Our journey implementing evidence at the point-of-care in healthcare settings started in the midst of the "best" practices movement in the late 1990s to the early 2000s. Our implementation work brings together the theory and research of Knowledge Translation (KT) with our *actual experience* with initiatives across sectors encompassing community nursing and hospital practice and transitional issues. Much of this work addresses system aspects as well as point-of-care practice issues. We have learned how to activate good quality evidence efficiently and effectively. For nurses and others that we worked with, evidence was viewed as a "means to an end" in improving the quality and efficiency of care and patient health outcomes. For them, and for us, the beginning step was basing practice and health services reorganization on the best available external evidence while considering "local" evidence about the context where implementation was to occur. The journey often included research processes such as environmental scanning to understand the available resources (or lack thereof), or undertaking a prevalence, incidence and population profile enquiry to determine the magnitude of the health issue (i.e. the evidence-practice gap) and determining patients' characteristics and their preferences. For successful uptake, collecting data about the local context is absolutely essential in order to align the external best practice evidence with the local context and population(s).

At the time, knowledge tools such as high-quality guidelines or other evidence-informed protocols were becoming plentiful - the quest was to use them to guide day-to-day practice. Without fail, there was a sense that "we can do better" and maybe even be more efficient. Improvement in patient outcomes was foremost, but outcomes for practitioners themselves and the settings in which they practiced were also important. Thus, another underlying motivation was to improve professional practice and satisfaction with the care nurses delivered and accomplish it in the most cost-efficient manner. Believe it or not, this is possible as you will see in some of our examples.

The mantras of the day, "best practices," "research-based practice," "evidence-based practice" and "evidence-informed practice" were being integrated in quality portfolios and mission statements at the organizational level of hospitals and home nursing agencies, as well as at the team level across the continuum of care. It was during this time as researchers that we were actively involved with groups striving to meet this mandate and finding ourselves engaged in the day-to-day practice of settings. In this way we *discovered* how teams move forward with this mission, how they built strategic alliances, engaged decisions-makers, and understood the range and types of reorganization necessary to deliver evidence-informed care. At the time there was a lack of implementation tools for our practitioner colleagues to support the transformation. They typically found it exceedingly complex to successfully align and activate external evidence with their local context.

After being approached to help, we began developing frameworks and tools to bring structure to the evidence-to-practice process. We referred to it as the *knowledge to action* process (Graham et al. 2006), since it is almost always about more than research evidence. This is a point to ponder. The external evidence available from the research literature, syntheses, and knowledge tools such as guidelines, is a starting point. But much more goes into the process of implementing them that includes what we refer to as "local evidence." This is about the population and context, the experiential knowledge, and ethical knowing about the context. All of these contribute to best practices and their implementation and must be taken into consideration for success.

The purpose of this book is to build on the current state of implementation knowledge by integrating theory and empirical knowledge with experiential knowledge that we have gained in facilitating implementation of evidence in practice settings. It is intended to create a "how to" for nurses and others wanting to, or being responsible for, facilitating the uptake of evidence in practice or de-implementation of ineffective practices (Hanrahan et al. 2015; Montini and Graham 2015; Niven et al. 2015; Helfrich et al. 2018; Rietbergen et al. 2020). Our aim is to provide a practical resource for those wishing to put into service best practices at the point-of-care. The specific objectives for the book are to:

1) Outline a general planning framework that activates knowledge (research, evidence) in practice settings.
2) Provide an action plan with strategies to engage the necessary alliances for decision-making, methodological, and practical support.
3) Describe in operational terms, strategies to move knowledge into action and to sustain the change.
4) In Call Out boxes we offer examples from implementation efforts (successful and not so successful) to illustrate the process.

Activating Evidence in Practice

Evidence-based nursing or practice is described as "integration of the best evidence available, nursing expertise, and the values and preferences of the individuals, families and communities who are served" (Sigma Theta Tau International 2005–2007 Research and Scholarship Advisory Committee 2008). As DiCenso et al. (2005, p. 9) argued some time ago, evidence-based nursing is focused on more than empirical knowing. Drawn from Carper (1978) four ways of knowing (empirical, personal, ethical and aesthetic) as a foundation, Dicenso et al. (2005) also articulate the importance of clinical experience and knowledge, patient preferences and values, and resource implications for EIP in nursing. Melnyk and Fineout-Overholt (2011, pp. 5-6) describe an approach that is evidence-based as the merging of science and art where clinical judgment and reasoning, internal (or local) evidence, and the evaluation of healthcare resources combine for evidence-based practice.

We heartily agree with these authors that *research evidence* is a part of a larger knowledge base and thus prefer the term EIP as it denotes the concept more accurately. Consideration of practice skills, expertise, and experience as well as context knowledge, (local environment and evidence about the population), information on the resources available, patient preferences, as well as assessing local skills and expertise, are vital in activating new knowledge. In our journey with numerous groups we learned how to identify and tailor external research evidence and importantly generate locally relevant evidence. The key is to determine and optimize the "fit" and articulation with the best external evidence. Local evidence is about the context, the professional practice, and the target population(s). Using this information, the task then shifts to tailoring strategies to support implementation in a setting and ultimately evaluating its impact. For effective implementation, the external evidence needs to be aligned with the local circumstances. This is an additional process to simply having good evidence available such as a quality guideline.

Knowledge to Action

The process by which evidence informs practice has been referred to by many terms over the years: knowledge utilization, knowledge transfer, dissemination, research translation, knowledge mobilization, implementation, and KT (Graham et al. 2006). This key concept is defined as a dynamic and iterative process that includes synthesis, dissemination, exchange and ethically-sound application of knowledge to improve health, provide more effective health services and products and strengthen the health care system (Canadian Institutes of Health Research 2016). Each aspect is germane in activating evidence in practice settings.

Synthesis is the integration of research findings from individual research studies within the larger body of knowledge on the topic. There may be dozens of studies on a particular topic, some with contrary findings – often not useful in this form for practitioners. Syntheses are a rigorous, transparent method of pooling findings from quantitative, qualitative or mixed-method studies to produce more conclusive results. This is especially true if there are several small studies, not properly powered, to answer a question.

Dissemination involves identifying the appropriate receivers and users of knowledge (the audience) and tailoring the message and medium to the audience. This can be done in several ways: summaries for or briefings to staff, educational sessions with patients, practitioners and/or policy makers, or working with knowledge users in developing and executing a dissemination plan and dissemination tools.

Knowledge *exchange* refers to the interaction between the typical knowledge user and the researcher, resulting in mutual learning. It is about the engagement between those wanting to implement an evidence-based practice and those tasked with actually implementing it. According to the Canadian Foundation for Healthcare Improvement (CFHI) "Knowledge exchange is collaborative problem-solving between researchers and decision-makers that happens through linkage and exchange (Canadian Foundation for Healthcare Improvement 2019). Effective knowledge exchange involves interaction between decision-makers and researchers and results in mutual learning through the process of planning, producing, disseminating, and applying existing or new research in decision-making." In other words, it is about bidirectional communication, mutual learning, and co-creation of change by relevant stakeholders. The term "integrated knowledge translation" is sometimes also used to refer to this concept of co-production and will be discussed in greater detail in Chapter 3.

Finally, application of knowledge is about the process that results in adoption of an evidence informed practice. It involves the process of implementation including all the strategies to facilitate and promote uptake of the evidence and the active work needed to embed the evidence in the setting while taking account of both population and environment characteristics. "Ethically-sound" application refers to the need to ensure that the approaches to application are consistent with ethical principles and norms, social values, as well as legal and other regulatory frameworks of the setting or context. A strategy considered widely acceptable in one context or jurisdiction to encourage uptake of an evidence-based practice (e.g. making the use of EIPs a condition of employment) might not be considered an appropriate approach in a different context. Another way that ethics comes into implementation efforts relates to implementation opportunity costs. By this we mean that there will always be more best practices that could be implemented than any organization has the capacity and resources to implement. Implementation always comes at a cost (e.g. people's time, cost of equipment, etc.). Having to choose between which best practices to implement may mean that some patients who may not be offered best practices are being denied effective care – a significant ethical dilemma for health care practitioners and their organizations. Considering the ethical application of best practices necessarily includes making potentially difficult decisions about which best practice to prioritize and what this may mean to those not receiving them.

The widely used Canadian Institutes of Health Research definition of KT (cited above) goes on to state that this implementation process takes place within a complex system of interactions in the practice setting which may vary in intensity, complexity, and level of engagement depending on the nature of the evidence to be implemented as well as the needs of particular knowledge users. The point here is that implementation results from the interactions and engagement of multiple stakeholders who are part of a complex system. Taken all together, KT is essentially about making users aware of knowledge and facilitating the use of it to improve health and health care systems; closing the gap between what we know and what we do (moving knowledge into action) and *transforming* evidence into practice.

Evidence-Informed Practice Is a Quality Factor

Since the early 1990s there has been an increasing emphasis on basing practice on best available evidence to provide appropriate, cost-effective, and efficient health care in order to ensure best possible quality of care and outcomes for patients. In the early 2000s several important reports propelled quality and patient safety to the forefront of healthcare delivery in North America and elsewhere. These include, but are not limited to, the landmark US report, *To Err is Human: Building a Safer Health System* (Institute of Medicine 2000), the Canadian report, *Building A Safer System: A National Integrated Strategy for Improving Patient Safety in Canadian Health Care* (National Steering Committee on Patient Safety 2002), and Crossing the Quality Chasm: A New Health System for the 21st Century (Institute of Medicine 2001). A key element in this report is to uphold that care is *knowledge-based*. In other words, practice consistently follows the latest best practices. Thus, developing an evidence-informed approach is a critical element to organizational quality processes. This movement has been spurred by several converging factors including a notable variation in health-care delivery across settings. For example, studies from the USA, the Netherlands and Australia have demonstrated that nearly 50% of patients may not be getting care known to be effective and as many as 25% may be receiving care that is not beneficial or even harmful (Schuster et al. 1998; Seddon et al. 2001; McGlynn et al. 2003; Korenstein et al. 2012; Runciman et al. 2012; Morgan et al. 2016). National databases such as Canadian Institute for Health Information (CIHI) recently contained numerous examples of inadequate and/or unnecessary care practices in Canada (Canadian Institute for Health Information 2017). Other factors included increased public awareness of quality and risks, credible professional bodies producing high quality guidelines that translated evidence into a more useable form for practice, and an increased accountability of professionals to provide quality patient care and reduce risks to the public.

This major focus within quality and practice portfolios in hospitals and other healthcare settings is the emphasis on "best" practices. By definition, "best" practices are based on the use of best available evidence. Many healthcare credentialing and accreditation bodies, such as Accreditation Canada or Magnet Hospitals Recognition, explicitly link service based standards to evidence whereby they require organizations to select and evaluate guidelines and best-practices, for their own services (Accreditation Canada 2019; American Nurses Credentialing Center 2019). The growing emphasis on quality care and it becoming something embedded in accreditation surveys, provides more stimulus to efficiently implement and sustain best practices.

The linkage and overlay of KT activity with quality processes is often implicit and, in our view, should be more explicitly recognized, resourced, and supported by organizations. This would be instrumental in legitimizing the extraordinary time and effort typically required to mobilize knowledge in a setting. It is timely for professionals in quality and practice portfolios and students entering the health care environment to embrace this as an essential part of their practice, i.e. developing the skills and enacting KT within their organizations.

Academic efforts, i.e. the science of KT (also known as implementation science), to date have largely focused on the theoretical and explanatory aspects of KT and evidence-based practice. KT science also referred to as implementation science, is the study of the determinants of knowledge use and effective methods of promoting the uptake of knowledge including (but not limited to) evaluating implementation outcomes. "Knowledge translation" or "implementation" specifically refers to activities undertaken to move evidence into practice, i.e. the practice of KT.

This giant leap to transform "knowledge to action" is what this book begins to tackle in support of those facilitating evidence-informed care in settings at the point-of-care. This work sometimes falls to formal facilitators but more often is embedded in existing roles in health settings: those in professional development/practice portfolios, Clinical Nurse Specialists (CNS), Advanced Practice Nurses (APN), Nurse Practitioners (NP), educators, quality coordinators, nurse managers and clinicians. These roles are often relied upon or are explicitly responsible through their function and core competencies for promoting and implementing EIP in their settings. Importantly for College registered professionals (e.g. nurses, physical therapists, etc.), basing practice on best available evidence is an explicit element of professional licensure. Nurses, as the largest group of care providers, play a major role in virtually all health sectors, thus the EIP endeavor has significant implications for health systems and the discipline. For instance, NP and CNS roles bridge sectors of health care for management of people with long term/chronic conditions such as heart failure, diabetes, mental health conditions, or cancer. Use of EIP is critical not only for improved processes of care and patient outcomes within a care sector such as hospital but also contributing to consistent care and continuity of care across health sectors.

Organization of the Book

The structure of each chapter includes an accessible, brief discussion of relevant theories or frameworks, current evidence, methods, cautions, and lessons learned. Practice exemplars serve to ground discussion throughout the book: pressure injury prevention in acute care, transition of care for people with heart failure (hospital to home), and community leg ulcer care (delivered at home and nurse-led clinics). Each of these examples arose from projects we were involved in and came about because of care and quality issues. These exemplars are provided in callout boxes and threaded throughout the chapters for illustration.

Let us talk about how you might use this book. One could read chapters sequentially from start to finish; or jump around if working on a project and are past the initial phases/ stages. The chapters are designed from the major phases of implementation: issue identification and clarification, solution building and solution implementation, evaluation, and sustainment. Each phase is then comprised of numerous stages with identified actions. Many of the chapters include a description of a reasonable approach for the specific stage for those in practice settings where it may not be feasible or practical to engage in more extensive process of change. As well as there often being a description of what a more detailed process might consist of for those wanting more information. Field examples are included for illustration as well as links to tips and tools.

The following outlines the chapters in the book.

Preface

Glossary of Terms

Chapter 1: Introduction

Chapter 2: Perspectives from the Field

Chapter 3: Guiding Theories, Models, and Frameworks

Chapter 4: A Roadmap to Implementing Best Practice

Phase I: Issue Identification and Clarification

Chapter 5: The Call-to-Action

Chapter 6: Find the Best Practice Evidence

Chapter 7: Assemble Local Evidence on Context and Current Practices

Phase II: Build Solutions and Field Test

Chapter 8: Customize Best Practices to the Local Context

Chapter 9: Discover Barriers and Drivers to Best Practice Implementation

Chapter 10: Implementation Strategies: What Do We Know Works?

Chapter 11: Tailor Implementation Strategies

Chapter 12: Field Test, Plan Evaluation and Prepare to Launch

Phase III: Implement, Evaluate, and Sustain

Chapter 13: Launch and Evaluate

Chapter 14: Sustain the Gains

Chapter 15: Reflections: Is It Worth it?

In the next chapter we present a synopsis of two of the examples we use throughout the book as illustrations of implementation journeys. No doubt you will be able to relate to many of the challenges!

References

Accreditation Canada (2019). *Accreditation Canada*, [Online], Available: https://accreditation.ca [July 26, 2019].

American Nurses Credentialing Center (2019). *ANCC Magnet Recognition Program* © [Online], Available: http://www.nursecredentialing.org/Magnet [July 26, 2019].

Canadian Foundation for Healthcare Improvement (2019). *Glossary of Knowledge Exchange Terms*, [Online], Available: http://www.cfhi-fcass.ca/PublicationsAndResources/ResourcesAndTools/GlossaryKnowledgeExchange.aspx [July 26, 2019].

Canadian Institute for Health Information (2017). *Unnecessary Care in Canada*, Ottawa, ON. Available at: https://www.cihi.ca/sites/default/files/document/choosing-wisely-baseline-report-en-web.pdf.

Canadian Institutes of Health Research (2016). *Knowledge Translation*, [Online], Available: http://www.cihr-irsc.gc.ca/e/29418.html [July 26, 2019].

Carper, B. (1978). Fundamental patterns of knowing in nursing. *Advances in Nursing Science* 1: 13–24.

DiCenso, A., Guyatt, G., and Ciliska, D. (2005). *Evidence-Based Nursing: A Guide to Clinical Practice*. St. Louis, MO: Elsevier Health Sciences.

Graham, I.D., Logan, J., Harrison, M.B. et al. (2006). Lost in knowledge translation: time for a map? *The Journal of Continuing Education in the Health Professions* 26: 13–24.

Hanrahan, K., Wagner, M., Matthews, G. et al. (2015). Sacred cow gone to pasture: a systematic evaluation and integration of evidence-based practice. *Worldviews on Evidence-Based Nursing* 12: 3–11.

Helfrich, C.D., Rose, A.J., Hartmann, C.W. et al. (2018). How the dual process model of human cognition can inform efforts to de-implement ineffective and harmful clinical practices: a preliminary model of unlearning and substitution. *Journal of Evaluation in Clinical Practice* 24: 198–205.

Institute of Medicine (2000). *To Err Is Human: Building a Safer Health System*. Washington, DC: The National Academies Press.

Institute of Medicine (2001). *Crossing the Quality Chasm: A New Health System for the 21st Century*. Washington: National Academies Press.

Korenstein, D., Falk, R., Howell, E.A. et al. (2012). Overuse of health care services in the United States: an understudied problem. *Archives of Internal Medicine* 172: 171–178.

McDonald, L. (2001). Florence Nightingale and the early origins of evidence-based nursing. *Evidence-Based Nursing* 4: 68–69.

McGlynn, E.A., Asch, S.M., Adams, J. et al. (2003). The quality of health care delivered to adults in the United States. *The New England Journal of Medicine* 348: 2635–2645.

Melnyk, B.M. and Fineout-Overholt, E. (2011). *Evidence-Based Practice in Nursing & Healthcare: A Guide to Best Practice*. Philadelphia: Wolters Kluwer/Lippincott Williams & Wilkins Health.

Montini, T. and Graham, I.D. (2015). "Entrenched practices and other biases": unpacking the historical, economic, professional, and social resistance to de-implementation. *Implementation Science* 10: 24.

Morgan, D.J., Dhruva, S.S., Wright, S.M., and Korenstein, D. (2016). 2016 update on medical overuse: a systematic review. *JAMA Internal Medicine* 176: 1687–1692.

National Steering Committee on Patient Safety (2002). *Building a Safer System: A National Integrated Strategy for Improving Patient Safety in Canadian Health Care*. Royal College of the Physicians & Surgeons of Canada.

Nightingale, F. (1871). *Introductory Notes on Lying-in Institutions*. London: Longmans, Green.

Niven, D.J., Mrklas, K.J., Holodinsky, J.K. et al. (2015). Towards understanding the de-adoption of low-value clinical practices: a scoping review. *BMC Medicine* 13: 255.

Rietbergen, T., Spoon, D., Brunsveld-Reinders, A.H. et al. (2020). Effects of de-implementation strategies aimed at reducing low-value nursing procedures: a systematic review and meta-analysis. *Implementation Science* 15: 38.

Runciman, W.B., Hunt, T.D., Hannaford, N.A. et al. (2012). CareTrack: assessing the appropriateness of health care delivery in Australia. *The Medical Journal of Australia* 197: 100–105.

Schuster, M.A., McGlynn, E.A., and Brook, R.H. (1998). How good is the quality of health care in the United States? *The Milbank Quarterly* 76: 517–563, 509.

Seddon, M.E., Marshall, M.N., Campbell, S.M., and Roland, M.O. (2001). Systematic review of studies of quality of clinical care in general practice in the UK, Australia and New Zealand. *Quality in Health Care* 10: 152–158.

Sigma Theta Tau International 2005–2007 Research and Scholarship Advisory Committee (2008). Sigma theta tau international position statement on evidence-based practice February 2007 summary. *Worldviews on Evidence-Based Nursing* 5: 57–59.

2

Perspectives from the Field

Improving Care Through Evidence-Informed Practice

Introduction

Partnerships focused on best practice implementation have led to major improvements in the quality of care for people with complex conditions. Two cases will be highlighted in this chapter: care of people with leg ulcers and those with congestive heart failure. The synthesis of both external and local evidence played a key role in the development and implementation of the evidence-informed approaches and provided the critical context to support reorganization of the existing care and service delivery models that produced demonstrable benefits for patients and health services. The cases illustrate that, with a collaborative partnership approach along with a systematic and transparent enquiry process, best practice evidence can be aligned with the local context and implemented. Being transparent allows replication with another practice issue and greatly supports practice and policy changes.

Case 1: Improving Community-Based Chronic Wound Care

The Home Care Authority in a region of approximately 750 000 people, became concerned about the growing demand for community care of chronic wounds, their burgeoning wound-care supply budgets, as well as a shortage of nurses. To begin to tackle this, the Home Care Authority partnered with a not-for-profit community nursing agency and a team of health services researchers from Queen's University and the University of Ottawa (us!). The intent was to address their mutual concerns about care of individuals with leg ulcers. As a strategic alliance the focus was to improve both the quality of care and health outcomes for individuals with leg ulcers and the efficiency of the community care.

Leg ulcers are a chronic, debilitating, costly, and neglected condition. During implementation of best practice for this population, the practice partners discovered that the annual regional expenditures for 192 individuals in one small health care district was $1.3 million for their leg ulcer care. This group of individuals accounted for only 6% of all home care clients yet consumed 20% of the total supply budget. Thus, the Call-to-Action was started.

At the time, good evidence was available for best practices for conservative management of this chronic problem. Strong evidence, from numerous randomized controlled trials, demonstrated that a thorough initial assessment and application of compression bandages

Knowledge Translation in Nursing and Healthcare: A Roadmap to Evidence-informed Practice, First Edition. Margaret B. Harrison and Ian D. Graham.

provides a very effective treatment for healing venous leg ulcers (Cullum et al. 2001). This has been further strengthened in recent years (O'Meara et al. 2012; Nelson and Bell-Syer 2014; Nelson and Adderley 2016).

This best practice initiative involved both the community and tertiary sectors and was financially supported in part by a number of parties: the Home Care Authority, start-up funds the researchers had competed for, and eventually a health services research grant to evaluate the effectiveness of home versus community clinic care for leg ulcers.

The Knowledge Translation Initiative

The partnership was formed with a common vision of developing a pragmatic, evidence-informed approach to bring about practice and service changes. We approached the research as a collaborative and participatory endeavor. The partnership went through several phases, each with a varying degree of knowledge translation activity. Sometimes occurring simultaneously and often influencing each other. The partnership activity included:

- The identification of the delivery of leg ulcer care as an important organizational issue by the home care authority, community nursing agency managers, and policy makers.
- Reviewing the literature on the effectiveness of leg ulcer care (clinically) as well as the effectiveness of service delivery models and identifying best practices compiled in knowledge tools such as guidelines or other protocols.
- Conducting a regional prevalence and profiling study, environmental scan and practice audit with the home care authority and the nursing agency to determine the magnitude of the problem and current practice (Harrison et al. 2001; Friedberg et al. 2002; Graham et al. 2003b).
- Conducting surveys of care providers to determine provider concerns and issues (Graham et al. 2001, 2003c).
- Engaging the Community Care board with evidence from both the literature and locally derived data to support their decision-making.
- Forming an interdisciplinary group of providers (and researchers), which systematically reviewed the quality and utility of existing practice guideline recommendations and adapted them for local use by creating an evidence-based leg ulcer care protocol (Graham et al. 2000, 2002, 2005).
- Managers, policy makers, and researchers coming together to redesign a service delivery model that would support best practice (a dedicated regional nurse-led leg ulcer team to provide care in home and clinic settings).
- Managers finding innovative ways to overcome organizational inertia and financial and structural barriers to make the redesign happen.
- Researchers, with the support of the agencies, creating opportunities for nurses to advance their wound care knowledge and skills through an exchange program in the United Kingdom.
- Conducting a pre–post study of the impact of the implementation of the evidence-based protocol (Friedberg et al. 2002; Harrison et al. 2005).
- Using the opportunity to prepare a grant proposal to seek peer-reviewed research funding to coalesce researcher–policy maker synergies.

- Securing research funding to conduct a randomized controlled trial of the effectiveness of the service model redesign and later to evaluate the effectiveness and efficiency of types of high compression bandaging (Harrison et al. 2011; Pham et al. 2012).

Results of the Knowledge Translation Experience

Qualitative feedback indicated that the partnership process had positive effects for all involved. Several nurses engaged in the implementation became interested in furthering their education and returned to school for courses and in some cases completed advanced degrees (Lorimer et al. 2003a, b; Nemeth et al. 2003a, b, 2004; Lorimer 2004; Buchanan 2010). A review of clients' health records indicated that the quality of care improved (Lorimer 2004). The results of the pre–post implementation evaluation indicated that the proportion of leg ulcers healed within three months increased to 56% from 23% following introduction of the evidence-informed protocol, coupled with significant reductions in nursing visits and supply costs (Harrison et al. 2005). The randomized controlled trial evaluation of the effectiveness of home versus clinic care included one year of follow-up (Harrison et al. 2008). The results revealed that the organization of care, not the setting where care is delivered, influenced healing rates. In other words, delivering best practices was the key and the factors we uncovered were: having a system that supported delivery of evidence-informed care (e.g. time for nurses to conduct assessments and develop a care plan), having a dedicated and trained nurse team, and ongoing outcome assessment of wound healing through the quality processes.

Perhaps most importantly, arrangements were made to ensure the leg ulcer service would continue to serve the region once the research study ended. The methodology used to evaluate and adapt existing guidelines (Graham et al. 2003a) has been adopted by the nursing agency to develop protocols for other conditions.

The end result of this partnership, however, was the restructuring and reorganization of service delivery to support the provision of evidence-informed leg ulcer care. This required a major organizational commitment from service providers, as it involved altering staffing and remuneration arrangements and procuring additional provider education and training.

The partnership was labor intensive for the researchers. The research team was regularly and actively engaged in the day-to-day ups and downs of the service and, at times, took on an active role as implementation facilitators. The researchers, who were perceived as credible and neutral, often worked between the home care authority and the nursing agency to assist in negotiating change. This direct contact helped to create the common understanding and trust needed for the partnership to succeed. While continually renegotiating and establishing trust with new personnel can be frustrating, having access to policy makers and being able to influence decision-making is ultimately very rewarding.

We have also found that one successful implementation journey can subsequently lead to other journeys. During the leg ulcer project nurses identified the need for evidence on the different types of available high compression for community care of these wounds. At the time there was no conclusive research on this, thus with the support of our clinical partners and others, we mounted a randomized clinical trial of the two most commonly used bandaging systems and received a national peer reviewed grant for the study. The information assisted the nursing agency and home care authority in terms of choosing bandaging systems for their region. (Harrison et al. 2011).

Making Research Evidence Work for Policy Makers

As researchers, we had to develop methods of synthesizing and presenting external and local evidence that was useful, user friendly and timely for policy makers. We also had to gain consensus on the value of "quick but good" research methods to meet the needs of the policy makers for immediate answers, while respecting researchers' concerns that the evidence be derived using rigorous methods.

In our experience, a critical success factor for the adoption of the evidence-based protocol was the synthesis of external and local data. The external evidence from the literature provided the practice direction for the care that "ought" to be delivered – in other words a benchmark. This was a key credibility factor. It was a lever to convince authorities of the need for change. However, the local data about current practice, the organization of care and the population in care, provided the critical contextual information. Without it, the external evidence could not have been aligned locally to enable the delivery of effective and efficient care.

A Note on Funding

External peer-reviewed research funding can be used to leverage change within organizations that value research. The downside is that it can also hold things up when a proposal resubmission to granting agencies and peer review is required when work cannot proceed without the external funding.

Conclusions and Implications

The initiative was driven by a common goal of improving care and making service delivery more efficient and effective, using the best available evidence as the foundation. It demonstrates how policy making can become more evidence-informed when researchers and policy makers adopt a collaborative partnership approach, and how this approach can increase appreciation of each other's worlds and perspectives, build trust, encourage learning from each other, and provide new opportunities to use research to improve decision-making. It can be very rewarding when a visible difference is made to a population receiving care, and when that change creates additional successes.

The initiative also revealed that it is possible to develop systematic, transparent, and relatively quick research processes (e.g. the Practice Guideline Evaluation and Adaptation Cycle) that can support policy making (MacLeod et al. 2002; Graham and Harrison 2005). The protocol was updated (Graham et al. 2005) and formed the basis of an implementation study in three other health care regions. The protocol was adopted in two regions but not the third. This was because organizational changes necessary to support delivery of the protocol were not made at the third site.

Case 2: Improving Transition from Hospital to Home

In this second example, the partnership was formed because nurses on a medical service in a large teaching hospital were concerned that the discharge process for the population with congestive heart failure (CHF) was lacking since there seemed to be a significant number readmitted in a relatively short period. Hospital to home transition for people with chronic and ongoing health issues can be challenging as health care systems are often not well linked to coordinate this transition.

In many health care systems, heart failure is the most common discharge diagnosis. People with heart failure present as a complex group with frequent exacerbations and are often hospitalized for issues in managing their care and condition. Following hospital discharge they need to transition back home and resume their care themselves. At the time of implementation evidence-informed recommendations were contained in quality guidelines about the hospital to home transition for those with CHF (Johnstone et al. 1994; Hunt et al. 2001; Liu et al. 2001; Remme et al. 2001; Liu et al. 2003). However, these recommendations can be difficult to enact during the discharge process which can often be hurried and busy. With CHF being a common discharge and readmission diagnosis, it was recognized locally as a priority for improved transition in our region. Working with hospitals, home care authorities, and specialized clinics we supported the implementation of evidence-informed care aimed at improving this transition to self-care for individuals with CHF. Thus, the Call-to-Action was initiated with a common vision of developing a pragmatic, evidence-informed approach to bringing about practice and service changes for this population.

The Knowledge Translation Initiative

Again, the approach was a collaborative and participatory endeavor with the hospitals connecting with the home care providers. The partnership went through several phases: first to understand the readmission data, then to assess the issues from the perspective of the hospital and the home care authority and community nursing agencies, and finally to develop a cross sector response that was evidence-informed. These phases occurred simultaneously and often affected each other. The activities of the partnership included:

- The identification of the discharge and readmission of patients with heart failure as an important organizational issue by both the hospital and community nursing agencies.
- Reviewing the literature on the effectiveness of hospital to home transition for those with heart failure and identifying best practices compiled in knowledge tools such as guidelines or other protocols (Harrison et al. 1998; Toman et al. 2001).
- Conducting a review of available hospital and community data profiling the population.
- One-day workshop with community and hospital nurses to share the population data analyses and determine the day-to-day magnitude of the problem and current practice.
- Using their experience and the evidence from both the literature and locally derived data to support the development of an improved discharge process.
- Regional home care authority, home nursing, and hospital managers and policy makers coming together to redesign the service delivery model to support best practice (enhanced communication across care sectors, telephone follow-up on discharge, take home self-management booklet, designated number of home care visits).
- Managers finding innovative ways to overcome cross sector organizational, financial, and structural barriers to make the redesign happen.
- Conducting a study of the impact of the implementation of the evidence-informed transition (Harrison et al. 2002).
- Securing research funding to conduct an implementation study in 10 sites (Harrison et al. 2007).

In the beginning the initiative was supported by local funds but eventually morphed into funded research to evaluate the transitional approach (Harrison et al. 2002, 2007). At times, the initiatives served as momentum for funding as local work progressed. Other times the external funding served as a lever to keep things on track when other local initiatives were prioritized by local players over the CHF project.

In summary, this best practice initiative involved building the evidence base both from the external research and the evidence of the local context. The external evidence at the time consisted of eight recommendations related to hospital-to-home transition (Konstam et al. 1994). Following that the effort shifted to understanding the needs of the patients and family and the practice environments in both the hospital and home settings. After consultation and local data analyses, clinical and health services changes were required to deliver an evidenced-informed approach which involved nursing supportive care for CHF self-management and improved linkage between hospital and home care nurses. No new resources were added but rather the processes of care and discharge were tweaked to address the identified issues.

Results of the Knowledge Translation Experience

The implementation of evidence-informed transitional care resulted in improved quality of life and function for individuals with CHF and fewer visits to the emergency room (Harrison et al. 2002). The evidence-informed self-management guide was widely used in a 10-site implementation endeavor and had similar improvements in quality of life measures (Harrison et al. 2007).

Conclusions and Implications of the CHF Case

The initiative was driven by data and nursing concern that readmissions were occurring too quickly after a hospital discharge for patients with CHF. Initial data on the readmission came from the quality portfolio and conversations with point-of-care nurses highlighted some of the granular issues. This led to a search for evidence and guidelines on transitioning care for this population to improve care and make service delivery more efficient and effective. The collaboration with organizational level quality managers and the actual experiences of staff was key to designing a better approach. This was more efficient and effective, using the best available evidence as the foundation. It demonstrates how decision-makers can become more evidence-informed and nurses, in this case, can appreciate population data about a concern. Sharing perspectives resulted in trust, encouraged learning from each other, and provided new opportunities to use research to improve decision-making. The quality data seemed less esoteric and the on-the-ground experience contributed practically to solution building.

The CHF transition initiative showed how it was possible to develop practical, hands-on tools from the external evidence. Other sites requested the self-management guide and participated in a 10-site implementation study (Harrison et al. 2007). Subsequently the copyright of the self-management guide was transferred to the Canadian Heart and Stroke Foundation where it was made available nation-wide and regularly updated by clinical experts (Heart and Stroke Foundation 2015).

Overarching Conclusions and Lessons Learned from the Wound Care and Transitional Care Implementations

We encountered some major challenges throughout the implementation of the best practice, but we also learned important lessons. One of the biggest challenges was policy maker/manager partners changing with reorganizations, requiring the need to continuously develop and foster relationships with new partners. This was further compounded because we were working in multiple sectors which added to the number of players that needed to be involved.

Lessons Learned from the Two Cases

We learned central lessons from our experiences with both implementation initiatives that we believe can be considered fundamental principles and are applicable to most implementation efforts:

- Form local partnerships that focus on the problem and improving care (do not focus exclusively on the players or organizations).
- Include all stakeholders in the problem clarification and solution building activity.
- Understand the decision-making levels required for needed changes.
- Gather local evidence from multiple perspectives to fully appreciate the issues, which are often multi-level (and multi-sectoral) (e.g. clinical and health service and policy level; community, acute, long-term care).
- Align external evidence with the local context which typically requires data and information collection to fully appreciate the local environment and population.
- Use of external evidence brings a level of objectivity and neutrality, i.e. not one partner's complaint or idea on how to fix it, also the use of quality guidelines from respected guideline developers (national associations or government programs) can bring credibility to the process.
- Creative approaches are required to build the local approach to fit the context. Local assessment of facilitating factors and barriers guides the tailoring of implementation interventions and strategies.
- Linkage with evaluation/research/program development expertise can be very helpful (this can be mutually beneficial because of research opportunities).
- Sustaining the best practice changes should be worked on from the outset not at the end of an implementation.

In this chapter we shared the knowledge we gained from our experiences implementing evidence-informed practice with two complex populations – people with heart failure and those with chronic wounds. They represented multi-sector encounters and occurred following identification that neither group was receiving best practices based on evidence.

We trust this Perspectives from the Field chapter has provided a sampling of how we work with groups on implementation. In the next chapter we present a review of the theories, models, and frameworks that have guided our work. This is followed by a chapter that introduces an implementation framework we call Roadmap, which has evolved from our work with practice settings to improve the use of evidence-informed practice.

References

Buchanan, M. (2010). *The Impact of Clinical Factors and Sociodemographic Variables on Health-Related Quality of Life in Venous Leg Ulceration.* Masters dissertation, Queen's University, Kingston, Ont.

Cullum, N., Nelson, E.A., Fletcher, A.W., and Sheldon, T.A. (2001). Compression for venous leg ulcers. *Cochrane Database of Systematic Reviews* (2): CD000265. https://doi.org/10.1002/14651858.CD000265.

Friedberg, E.H., Harrison, M.B., and Graham, I.D. (2002). Current home care expenditures for persons with leg ulcers. *Journal of Wound, Ostomy, and Continence Nursing* 29: 186–192. https://doi.org/10.1067/mjw.2002.125137.

Graham, I.D. and Harrison, M.B. (2005). Evaluation and adaptation of clinical practice guidelines. *Evidence-Based Nursing* 8: 68–72. https://doi.org/10.1136/ebn.8.3.68.

Graham, I.D., Lorimer, K., Harrison, M.B. et al. (2000). Evaluating the quality and content of international clinical practice guidelines for leg ulcers: preparing for Canadian adaptation. *Canadian Association of Enterostomal Therapy Journal* 19: 15–31.

Graham, I.D., Harrison, M.B., Moffat, C., and Franks, P. (2001). Leg ulcer care: nursing attitudes and knowledge. *The Canadian Nurse* 97: 19–24.

Graham, I.D., Harrison, M.B., Brouwers, M. et al. (2002). Facilitating the use of evidence in practice: evaluating and adapting clinical practice guidelines for local use by health care organizations. *Journal of Obstetric, Gynecologic, and Neonatal Nursing* 31: 599–611. https://doi.org/10.1111/j.1552-6909.2002.tb00086.x.

Graham, I.D., Harrison, M.B., and Brouwers, M. (2003a). Evaluating and adapting practice guidelines for local use: a conceptual framework. In: *Clinical Governance in Practice* (eds. S. Pickering and J. Thompson), 213–229. London: Harcourt.

Graham, I.D., Harrison, M.B., Nelson, E.A. et al. (2003b). Prevalence of lower-limb ulceration: a systematic review of prevalence studies. *Advances in Skin & Wound Care* 16: 305–316. https://doi.org/10.1097/00129334-200311000-00013.

Graham, I.D., Harrison, M.B., Shafey, M., and Keast, D. (2003c). Knowledge and attitudes regarding care of leg ulcers. Survey of family physicians. *Canadian Family Physician* 49: 896–902. https://www.cfp.ca/content/49/7/896.long.

Graham, I.D., Harrison, M.B., Lorimer, K. et al. (2005). Adapting national and international leg ulcer practice guidelines for local use: the Ontario leg ulcer community care protocol. *Advances in Skin & Wound Care* 18: 307–318. https://doi.org/10.1097/00129334-200507000-00011.

Harrison, M.B., Toman, C., and Logan, J. (1998). Hospital to home evidence-based education for CHF. *The Canadian Nurse* 94: 36–42.

Harrison, M.B., Graham, I.D., Friedberg, E. et al. (2001). Regional planning study. Assessing the population with leg and foot ulcers. *The Canadian Nurse* 97: 18–23.

Harrison, M.B., Browne, G.B., Roberts, J. et al. (2002). Quality of life of individuals with heart failure: a randomized trial of the effectiveness of two models of hospital-to-home transition. *Medical Care* 40: 271–282. https://doi.org/10.1097/00005650-200204000-00003.

Harrison, M.B., Graham, I.D., Lorimer, K. et al. (2005). Leg-ulcer care in the community, before and after implementation of an evidence-based service. *Canadian Medical Association Journal* 172: 1447–1452. https://doi.org/10.1503/cmaj.1041441.

Harrison, M.B., Graham, I.D., Logan, J. et al. (2007). Evidence to practice: pre-post-implementation study of a patient/provider resource for self-management with heart failure. *International Journal of Evidence-Based Healthcare* 5: 92–101. https://doi.org/10.1111/j.1479-6988.2007.00057.x.

Harrison, M.B., Graham, I.D., Lorimer, K. et al. (2008). Nurse clinic versus home delivery of evidence-based community leg ulcer care: a randomized health services trial. *BMC Health Services Research* 8: 243. https://doi.org/10.1186/1472-6963-8-243.

Harrison, M.B., VanDenKerkhof, E.G., Hopman, W.M. et al. (2011). The Canadian bandaging trial: evidence-informed leg ulcer care and the effectiveness of two compression technologies. *BMC Nursing* 10: 20. https://doi.org/10.1186/1472-6955-10-20.

Heart and Stroke Foundation (2015). *Managing Heart Failure*, [Online], Available: https://www.heartandstroke.ca/-/media/pdf-files/canada/health-information-catalogue/en-managing-heart-failure-v3.ashx Accessed May 29, 2020.

Hunt, S.A., Baker, D.W., Chin, M.H. et al. (2001). ACC/AHA guidelines for the evaluation and management of chronic heart failure in the adult: executive summary a report of the American College of Cardiology/American Heart Association Task Force on Practice Guidelines. *Circulation* 104: 2996–3007. https://doi.org/10.1161/hc4901.102568.

Johnstone, D.E., Abdulla, A., Arnold, J.M. et al. (1994). Diagnosis and management of heart failure. Canadian Cardiovascular Society. *The Canadian Journal of Cardiology* 10: 613–631, 635-54.

Konstam, M., Dracup, K., Baker, D. et al. (1994). *Evaluation and Care of Patients with Left Ventricular Systolic Dysfunction*, Clinical Practice Guideline 11, AHCPR Publication No. 94–0612. Rockville, MD: US Department of Health & Human Services Agency for Health Care Policy and Research.

Liu, P., Arnold, M., Belenkie, I. et al. (2001). The 2001 Canadian Cardiovascular Society consensus guideline update for the management and prevention of heart failure. *The Canadian Journal of Cardiology* 17 (Suppl E): 5E–25E.

Liu, P., Arnold, J.M., Belenkie, I. et al. (2003). The 2002/3 Canadian Cardiovascular Society consensus guideline update for the diagnosis and management of heart failure. *The Canadian Journal of Cardiology* 19: 347–356.

Lorimer, K. (2004). Continuity through best practice: design and implementation of a nurse-led community leg-ulcer service. *The Canadian Journal of Nursing Research* 36: 105–112.

Lorimer, K.R., Harrison, M.B., Graham, I.D. et al. (2003a). Assessing venous ulcer population characteristics and practices in a home care community. *Ostomy/Wound Management* 49: 32–34, 38–40, 42–3. https://www.o-wm.com/content/assessing-venous-ulcer-population-characteristics-and-practices-a-home-care-community.

Lorimer, K.R., Harrison, M.B., Graham, I.D. et al. (2003b). Venous leg ulcer care: how evidence-based is nursing practice? *Journal of Wound, Ostomy, and Continence Nursing* 30: 132–142. https://doi.org/10.1067/mjw.2003.122.

MacLeod, F.E., Harrison, M.B., and Graham, I.D. (2002). The process of developing best practice guidelines for nurses in Ontario: risk assessment and prevention of pressure ulcers. *Ostomy/Wound Management* 48: 30–32, 34–38.

Nelson, E.A. and Adderley, U. (2016). Venous leg ulcers. *BMJ Clinical Evidence* 2016 https://www.ncbi.nlm.nih.gov/pmc/articles/PMC4714578/.

Nelson, E.A. and Bell-Syer, S.E. (2014). Compression for preventing recurrence of venous ulcers. *Cochrane Database of Systematic Reviews* (9): CD002303. https://doi.org/10.1002/14651858.CD002303.pub3.

Nemeth, K.A., Graham, I.D., and Harrison, M.B. (2003a). The measurement of leg ulcer pain: identification and appraisal of pain assessment tools. *Advances in Skin & Wound Care* 16: 260–267. https://doi.org/10.1097/00129334-200309000-00017.

Nemeth, K.A., Harrison, M.B., Graham, I.D., and Burke, S. (2003b). Pain in pure and mixed aetiology venous leg ulcers: a three-phase point prevalence study. *Journal of Wound Care* 12: 336–340. https://doi.org/10.12968/jowc.2003.12.9.26532.

Nemeth, K.A., Harrison, M.B., Graham, I.D., and Burke, S. (2004). Understanding venous leg ulcer pain: results of a longitudinal study. *Ostomy/Wound Management* 50: 34–46.

O'Meara, S., Cullum, N., Nelson, E.A., and Dumville, J.C. (2012). Compression for venous leg ulcers. *Cochrane Database of Systematic Reviews* (11): CD000265. https://doi.org/10.1002/14651858.CD000265.pub3, https://www.ncbi.nlm.nih.gov/pmc/articles/PMC7068175/.

Pham, B., Harrison, M.B., Chen, M.H., and Carley, M.E. (2012). Cost-effectiveness of compression technologies for evidence-informed leg ulcer care: results from the Canadian Bandaging Trial. *BMC Health Services Research* 12: 346. https://doi.org/10.1186/1472-6963-12-346.

Remme, W.J., Swedberg, K., Cleland, J. et al. (2001). European Society of Cardiology task force for the diagnosis and treatment of chronic heart failure: comprehensive guidelines for the diagnosis and treatment of chronic heart failure. *European Heart Journal* 22: 1527–1560. https://doi.org/10.1053/euhj.2001.2783.

Toman, C., Harrison, M.B., and Logan, J. (2001). Clinical practice guidelines: necessary but not sufficient for evidence-based patient education and counseling. *Patient Education and Counseling* 42: 279–287.

3

Guiding Theories, Models, and Frameworks

Knowledge translation (KT) is a growing field of enquiry and as with all new fields there is a growing body of literature – both theoretical and research based. In the area of implementing evidence you may find macro or grand theory (very broad theory encompassing a wide range of phenomena) useful. At other times, mid-range, or point-of-care theory (more limited in scope, less abstract, addresses specific phenomena and reflects practice) may be particularly relevant. At other times, micro or situation-specific theory, also referred to as prescriptive theory (the narrowest range of interest and focus on specific phenomena that reflect clinical practice, limited to specific populations of field of practice) may be called for. In this chapter we will decipher theories, models, and frameworks and describe ones we have found particularly relevant.

What follows are several sources that list implementation theories, models, and frameworks (TMF). Given the growing number of theories, we do not survey all the relevant theories related to knowledge translation. For more information on implementation and knowledge translation terms see Curran's paper (Curran 2020). We do, however summarize the theories, models, and frameworks that have specifically influenced our approach and ones that we have found useful in nursing and/or multi-disciplinary initiatives. We also describe how they led us to develop point-of-care methods and approaches. A key message is that there is no need to feel intimidated or anxious about implementation theories, models, or frameworks. They are simply conceptual tools that can assist in approaching planning for, implementing, evaluating and sustaining change.

Introduction

In working with numerous groups, we have realized that many people suffer from what we refer to as TAS – "Theory Averse Syndrome" and FAS – "Framework Averse Syndrome." These individuals often feel anxious about using TMFs, may not appreciate their value, or may just want to get on with implementation and not want to get bogged down with theory. Others may not realize fundamental theories exist or appreciate how they can inform practice. The usefulness of conceptual models comes from the organization they provide for thinking, observing, and interpreting what is seen. They provide a systematic structure and a rationale for activities – as one author puts it "clarity out of chaos" (Damschroder 2020).

Knowledge Translation in Nursing and Healthcare: A Roadmap to Evidence-informed Practice, First Edition. Margaret B. Harrison and Ian D. Graham.

A recent paper by Australian colleagues, entitled, "There is nothing so practical as a good theory: a pragmatic guide for selecting theoretical approaches for implementation projects" expounds on the value of using theory and should be a required reading (Lynch et al. 2018). These authors offer five key questions to help in selecting a theoretical approach:

- Who? Are you looking at individuals, groups, or wider settings?
- When? Are you planning, conducting, or evaluating?
- Why? What is your aim and what do you need to understand?
- How? What data will be available to use?
- What? What resources do you have to support you?

They also describe how theory can support a project at different stages. For example, before the project starts, theory can inform planning an implementation strategy, anticipating barriers, or engaging stakeholders. During implementation, theory can be used to: identify how to introduce and embed new ways of working, make explicit the mechanisms of action, or track and explore process of change. After the project, theory can be used to: identify data that should be collected to evaluate success, understand what happened and why, or inform the approach for reporting evaluation outcomes. The paper illustrates the learnings with six commonly used implementation theoretical approaches.

A few words on definitions is in order before proceeding. Lynch et al. (2018) offer the following definitions that we find helpful. A *framework* lists the basic structure and components underlying a system or concept. A *model* is a simplified representation of a system or concept with specified assumptions. A *theory* may be explanatory or predictive and underpins hypothesis and assumptions. In the implementation literature the terms theory, model, and framework are often used interchangeably which can cause confusion. Trainees and implementation scientists are often preoccupied with using the "correct" label for theories, models, and frameworks. However, in the real word it is not as straightforward as that, as the authors of these things often do not follow any labeling convention. For example, some implementation "theories" on closer examination may not meet the definition above and are probably better classified as a model or even a framework. Similarly, some "models" are probably better labeled as frameworks and vice versa. Our advice is to not get bogged down with the labels and call "the thing" whatever the authors call it. For simplicity here we will use the abbreviation TMF to refer to theories, models, and frameworks.

Finally, Nilsen (2015) published a taxonomy intended to distinguish between different categories of TMFs in implementation science. The goal for the taxonomy was to facilitate appropriate selection and application of relevant theories to promote uptake of evidence-based practice. The taxonomy comprises five categories of TMF which he labeled: process models (planned action), determinants frameworks (barriers and facilitators), classic theories, implementation theories, and evaluation frameworks. He notes that essentially the three overarching goals of implementation theories, models and frameworks are to either: describe and/or guide the process of translating research into practice (process models); understand and/or explain what influences implementation outcomes (determinant frameworks, classic theories, implementation theories); or evaluate implementation (evaluation frameworks). Many find this classification helpful in thinking about the different purposes of theories, models, and frameworks.

The take-home message here should be there is no need to feel intimidated or anxious about implementation theories, models, or frameworks. They can be used to guide implementation planning (e.g. to increase understanding of barriers and drivers to better select implementation strategies), to develop an understanding about the implementation process, or to guide evaluation of implementation initiatives. You get to decide what TMF you may want to use for what purpose.

Finding Theories, Models, and Frameworks

Before describing the TMFs we have used (some of which we have developed), we will identify some syntheses that are excellent sources when seeking to identify potential implementation TMF to use.

A thoughtful comparative analysis of implementation models and frameworks can be found in Jo Rycroft-Malone and Tracey Bucknall's 2010 book, "Models and Frameworks for Implementing Evidence-based Practice" (Rycroft-Malone and Bucknall 2010).

One of the first major reviews was published by Tabak et al. (2012) and focused on theories and frameworks (which the authors refer to as models) of dissemination and implementation. This review identified 61 models published before 2011 and categorized them by: the flexibility to be used broadly or operationally; whether the focus is on dissemination and/or implementation activities; and the level at which the model operates (system, community, organization, and individual). Models that addressed policy activities are also noted. Interestingly this review failed to identify the Knowledge to Action Cycle which we will describe shortly. The models reported in this review were subsequently used to assess their citation networks to determine the role of these models in the development of implementation science (Skolarus et al. 2017).

Several syntheses of implementation TMF were published in 2013 in the first text on knowledge translation science and practice. These syntheses covered: planned action theories (Graham et al. 2013), cognitive psychology theories of change in provider behavior (Hutchinson and Estabrooks 2013a), educational theories (Hutchinson and Estabrooks 2013b), organizational theories (Denis and Lehoux 2013) and quality improvement theories (Sales 2013).

More recently, Lisa Strifler and colleagues conducted a systematic review of knowledge translation TMF used to guide dissemination or implementation of evidence-based interventions targeted at prevention and/or management of cancer or other chronic diseases (Strifler et al. 2018). They searched databases from 2000 to 2016 and identified 596 studies reporting on the use of 159 KT TMF. Each model, theory, or framework (60%) was used in only one study. Twenty-six were used across the full implementation spectrum (from planning/design to sustainability/scalability). Few were used to inform dissemination and sustainability/scalability activities. The TMF in the studies focused on multiple levels. This review revealed that all TMF were used at least at the individual-level (practitioner/patient behavior change), 48% were used for organization-level, 33% at community-level, and 17% were used for system-level change.

Three recently published implementation science texts are good sources of synthesized information on implementation TMF (Greenhalgh 2017; Nilsen and Birken 2020; Wensing et al. 2020). Still others have synthesized implementation science frameworks and application to global health gaps. Villalobos Dintrans et al. (2019) found that common elements of the frameworks they examined included: diagnosis, intervention provider/system, intervention, recipient, environment, and evaluation.

A useful interactive database of implementation TMF can be found on the Canadian National Collaborating Centre for Methods and Tools website (National Collaborating Centre for Methods and Tools 2016). The database allows users to view and select from implementation models. The models can be sorted, filtered, and compared by defining characteristics, which include: type of construct(s) models use (e.g. reach, adoption, readiness, feasibility), focus on dissemination and/or implementation activities, flexibility of model constructs (five-point scale from broad [1] to operational [5]), socio-ecological levels at which models operate (e.g. individual, organization, community, system, policy), field of study in which the models originate (e.g. public health, clinical healthcare settings, strategic management, any domain), number of times publications have been cited, and rating by users.

It is important to remember that there are many theories, models and frameworks relevant to implementation that derive from different disciplines: psychology, sociology, communications, education, management and health to name a few. Implementation theories, models, and frameworks often focus on different aspects of change although common elements often include the evidence and practice to be implemented, those doing the implementing, aspects of the context that affect the implementors and implementation, and the strategies to promote implementation. Selecting a TMF should always be guided by "fit for purpose" considerations.

Our Approach to Theories, Models, and Frameworks

Our approach has always been organic; when something was needed, we would review and appraise the literature and if nothing useful was found we experimented with approaches. Thus, we developed several models and frameworks while working with care settings to better understand and manage implementation. Before describing these models and frameworks it may be helpful to understand our philosophy related to implementation.

Although our main role was as researchers, the approach to implementation brought us to care settings (hospital and community settings) in a collaborative venture. You may find a partnership with your local university, college, or research centre helpful with some aspects of implementation. We found ourselves working with individuals and groups outside of our academic environment all the time. We drew on different fields including sociology, and sociological theory became important – not surprising since one of us (IDG) is a health sociologist.

At a philosophical (high level) we accept the tenets of social constructivist learning theory that people are shaped by their experiences and interactions. This sociological theory of knowledge stresses the importance of social interactions in the construction of knowledge. Thomas et al. (2014) nicely describe this tradition, better than we could paraphrase it, so we provide the quote in its entirety:

> Constructivism is based on three assumptions about learning (Driscoll 1994; Slavin 1994; Savery and Duffy 1995; Steffe and Gale 1995; Gredler 1997). First, learning is a result of the individual's interaction with the environment. Knowledge is constructed as the learner makes sense of their experiences in the world. The

content of learning is not independent of how the learning is acquired; what a learner comes to understand is a function of the context of learning, the goals of the learner, and the activity the learner is involved in. Second, cognitive dissonance, or the uncomfortable tension that comes from holding two conflicting thoughts at the same time, is the stimulus for learning. It serves as a driving force that compels the mind to acquire new thoughts or to modify existing beliefs in order to reduce the amount of dissonance (conflict). Cognitive dissonance ultimately determines the organization and nature of what is learned (Festinger 1957). Third, the social environment plays a critical role in the development of knowledge. Other individuals in the environment may attempt to test the learner's understanding and provide alternative views against which the learner questions the viability of his knowledge. Constructivism supports the acquisition of cognitive processing strategies, self-regulation, and problem solving through socially constructed learning opportunities (Glasersfeld 1995; Savery and Duffy 1995; Steffe and Gale 1995; Gredler 1997), all of which are critical skills for evidence-based knowledge uptake and implementation in clinical practice. (Thomas et al. 2011)

Adopting a social constructivist approach to implementation means privileging social interaction and adaptation of research evidence by taking the local context and culture into account (Graham and Tetroe 2010).

On to More Practical Background

Let us turn now to some of the pragmatic frameworks and models that we have used to underpin our implementation work over the past two decades. Early on we developed the Ottawa Model of Research Use (OMRU) (Figure 3.1) (Logan and Graham 1998; Graham and Logan 2004; Logan and Graham 2010). This is what is known as a "planned action model" meaning it was designed to prescribe, rather than simply describe action steps, to guide implementation of best practice. The key elements of the model are the innovation (best practice) to be implemented, the potential adopters (e.g. nurses, unit managers, patients), and the practice environment (setting and context). These three elements were selected because of the evidence showing that potential adopters' perceptions of the innovation influences their willingness to adopt it, attributes of the potential adopters (e.g. knowledge, attitudes, intentions, skills) affect their willingness and ability to adopt it, and the practice environment/setting or context in which the implementation takes place (e.g. structural factors, cultural and social factors, patient factors, economic factors – to name some of the main ones) also influences uptake.

The model directs those interested in bringing about change to assess the innovation, potential adopters, and practice environment for possible barriers and facilitators. Based on the results of this assessment the next step is to select implementation strategies to address the identified barriers and take advantage of the facilitating factors that exist. Implementation strategies are things like education, audit and feedback, and guideline adaptation to the context. The implementation strategies are to be differentiated from the evidence-informed practice interventions contained in the guideline (e.g. an assessment for risk).

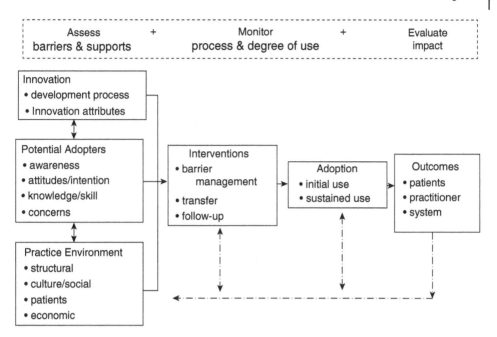

Figure 3.1 The Ottawa Model of Research Use. *Source:* Graham, I. D. & Logan J. (2004) Knowledge transfer and continuity of care research, (p. 94). Canadian Journal of Nursing Research, 36(2), 89–103. Licenced under CC BY 4.0

With the OMRU model, implementation strategies are divided into three categories: barrier management, transfer, and follow up. The effect of the implementation strategies needs to be monitored over time to ensure all potential adopters are being exposed to the implementation strategies, and if it is found they are not working as expected in bringing about the desired change in practice, the approach needs to be modified or changed. To know if all is going as planned, adoption of the innovation (which can be thought of as initial use and sustained or ongoing use) then needs to be monitored. Finally, the outcomes/impact of uptake must be evaluated as there may be effects on patients and their health status, practitioners, and/or the health system.

The usefulness of the OMRU rests in its breaking down the complex social and scientific process of implementation into discrete and achievable phases while providing an overview of the entire process. The guidance for assessing the innovation, potential adopters, and the practice setting, monitoring the implementation intervention and adoption, and evaluating outcomes along with the focus on feedback loops, distinguishes the framework as a planned action model by identifying the elements that need to be attended to, to achieve success. Some have noted the similarities with the model's Assess, Monitor, and Evaluate (AME) functions with the nursing process. Ultimately, the OMRU offers a rigorous and systematic process for bringing about implementation.

Quality: Structure, Process, Outcome

Avedis Donabedian's influential conceptual model (1966) for the quality of healthcare, whereby one considers structure, process, and outcomes, has underpinned a great deal of our thinking about the health care settings we found ourselves working in (Donabedian 2005). It was first described in 1966 and has been further developed, critiqued and adapted by many. The seemingly simple breakdown of healthcare into these three elements can be misleading. In following Donabedian's model, one must remember he considered them a way of thinking about problems – a sort of a deconstruction map rather than, an all-encompassing directive. As anyone who works in the practice environment knows, the complexity across and between these three elements is daunting when attempting to make changes. We have found that this rubric of quality fits well with a systematic approach to evidence-informed practice.

The Knowledge-to-Action (K2A) Framework

Wanting to better understand the critical ingredients that promote successful implementation, we undertook a theory analysis of planned action models. This essentially involved conducting a synthesis of common elements in over 30 planned action theories and resulted in the K2A Cycle (Graham et al. 2006, 2007; Straus et al. 2013a). In keeping with our general approach, the K2A framework adopts a social constructivist perspective and privileges social interaction and adaptation of research evidence by emphasizing the importance of local culture and context. The framework depicts two major processes: knowledge creation and planned action (see Figure 3.2). The two processes can be undertaken in isolation by different groups (e.g. researchers produce evidence and clinicians implement it) or they can be undertaken using an integrated knowledge translation (IKT) approach where the producers and users of the evidence work collaboratively across both processes. This co-production of knowledge understandably has added benefits.

Figure 3.2 The knowledge to action cycle (application). *Source:* Reproduced with permission from Straus et al. (2013b). This edition first published 2013 © 2013 by John Wiley & Sons.

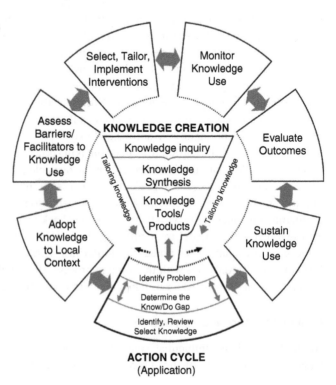

Knowledge creation involves three stages to tailor and refine information for use: knowledge inquiry (e.g. primary studies), knowledge synthesis (e.g. a body of work, meta-analysis), and creation of knowledge tools or products (e.g. guidelines). Recognition of a gap in care may serve as an important stimulus for action. Distilled knowledge is applied or set in motion when a care issue is identified (either because there are concerns about patients or the care provided) or when new knowledge (best practices) becomes known. This trigger prompts a cycle of activity, sequentially or concurrently, requiring users to:

1) Identify and clarify the practice problem or issue(s) to be addressed.
2) Identify, review, and select the knowledge (i.e. knowledge synthesis or knowledge product such as a guideline) that provides a solution to the identified problem.
3) Adapt or customize the knowledge (solution) to the local context (i.e. practice and system).
4) Assess local determinants of knowledge use (i.e. barriers and facilitating factors).
5) Select, tailor, and implement strategies to promote knowledge use (i.e. implement the change).
6) Monitor the uptake.
7) Evaluate the impact of using the knowledge.
8) Sustain knowledge use.

The Knowledge to Action Cycle (Figure 3.2) illustrates the iterative, dynamic, and complex process that is knowledge creation and application. Knowledge creation and application are interconnected with fluid boundaries. It is important to note that different activities can occur simultaneously and not necessarily as a linear route.

As an overarching model or framework, at each phase of the K2A cycle, other theories (e.g. psychological, sociological, educational, organizational theories, etc.) may be relevant and useful to consider. A detailed summary of many of these theories may be found in Straus et al. (2013a) in their Section 4 chapters.

Many have used the K2A cycle. A recent citation analysis of dissemination and implementation research frameworks revealed the K2A cycle was the most frequently cited framework in their analysis of 62 frameworks (Skolarus et al. 2017) and ranks the 13th most frequently cited medical education article of all time published across all journals in the Web of Knowledge (Azer 2015). The use of the framework reported in the literature has also been subjected to citation analysis (Field et al. 2014). The K2A cycle became one of the most frequently mentioned KT articles in citation indices. The K2A cycle is the basis of the book, Knowledge Translation in Health Care: Moving from Evidence to Practice, now in its second edition (Straus et al. 2013a). The book describes the phases of knowledge creation and action, and the current evidence and research gaps related to each phase. There are also chapters synthesizing planned action theories, cognitive psychology theories of change, educational theories, organizational theories, and quality improvement theories. The last two sections of the book focus on evaluation of knowledge to action and ethical issues related to implementation and implementation science. We suggest consulting this book for a more detailed discussion of the evidence base for implementation (including implementation strategies).

Initially as our guide, the K2A cycle provided a theoretical grounding to track our processes and our developing implementation methods. However, it was not long before it had another interesting use; people in the throes of implementation highlighted using it to explain to managers and decision-makers the process they were undertaking locally. They noted that they found it extremely valuable as it emphasized, and in some cases legitimized, the required time and effort in the movement to best practice. Importantly they could position where their local implementation had progressed to at any specific point in time when reporting.

As we began developing expertise in knowledge translation, practitioners and managers at the point-of-care began approaching us to help them bring about the implementation of best practices. We quickly realized that practice settings often could not take a practice guideline off the proverbial shelf and implement it as is. Reasons for this include: multiple guidelines on the same topic from which to choose, some with similar, differing or even contradictory recommendations; not finding a credible guideline; guideline scope being overwhelming (from assessment to prevention and management of a health topic); and the recommendations from a potential guideline not being applicable or feasible to implement in the local context (e.g. a northern or rural setting with less resources available).

Tackling the Guideline Quagmire: The Practice Guideline Evaluation and Adaptation Cycle

At the time, there were also few published processes for helping clinical groups think through these issues, so working with homecare nurses around best practices for venous leg ulcers we developed the Practice Guideline Evaluation and Adaptation Cycle (PGEAC) (Figure 3.3) (Graham et al. 2002, 2003, 2005; Graham and Harrison 2005). This "simple" 10-step process guides groups through the key steps of what we called guideline adaptation that essentially comprises identifying the clinical topic; constituting the evaluation and adaptation group;

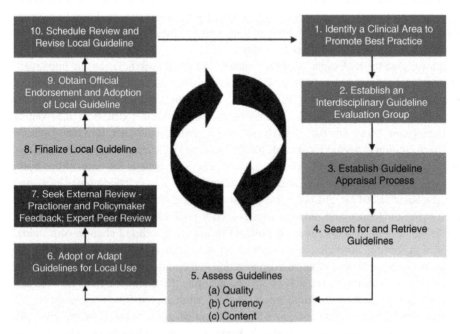

Figure 3.3 Practice guidelines evaluation and adaptation cycle. *Source:* Reproduced with permission from Graham et al. (2005). Available at: https://journals.lww.com/aswcjournal/Abstract/2005/07000/Adapting_National_and_International_Leg_Ulcer.11.aspx

searching, appraising and adapting guideline(s) for local use; seeking feedback and peer review of the locally adapted guideline(s); and updating of the local guideline(s). The process of course can be anything but 'simple'. Updating a guideline follows a similar process.

With the PGEAC, guideline adaptation is considered a "means to an end" (i.e. local implementation having primacy over simply producing an adapted protocol). Critical to this tradition is the engagement of all the relevant local interprofessional stakeholders or end users in the adaptation process of the best practices. This leads to co-creation of the customized best practices. The co-creation resulting from the group working collectively through the adaptation process not surprisingly can lead to improved acceptance of the recommendations (buy-in) and adherence to them. The PGEAC offers a systematic and transparent process for groups to follow and by focusing attention on the evidence, promotes collaboration, and helps to minimize power differentials between professional groups. Active involvement of the targeted guideline end-users in this process has been shown to lead to significant changes in practice (Ray-Coquard et al. 2002; Harrison et al. 2005, 2013a).

The International ADAPTE Process

We subsequently joined forces in 2005 with a team from France and Quebec as founding members of the ADAPTE Collaboration (Guidelines International Network 2017). As a group of guideline developers, researchers, implementers, and guideline users we collaborated to enhance use of research evidence through more efficient development and implementation of guidelines (Straus et al. 2013a; Guidelines International Network 2017). Following development of the ADAPTE manual, worksheets, tools, and templates (ADAPTE Collaboration 2009), the group turned copyright of the ADAPTE material over to the Guidelines International Network (Harrison et al. 2010; Guidelines International Network 2017). The ADAPTE process consists of three phases and 24 steps (Figure 3.4). Users' perceptions of the ADAPTE process have been surveyed but the process was not formally field tested prior to its release (Fervers et al. 2011). More recent articles continue to reveal the use of the ADAPTE process to adapt guidelines produced in another jurisdiction (e.g. the World Health Organization, the European Union, or guidelines from professional bodies in other countries), to create a national guideline (Gupta et al. 2009; Han and Choi-Kwon 2011; Howell et al. 2013; Kristiansen et al. 2014; Larenas-Linnemann et al. 2014) or to adapt guidelines for local implementation (Kis et al. 2010; Pantoja et al. 2011; Burgers et al. 2012). A recurrent theme that applies to this framework is the systematic and transparent nature of the process which is participatory.

CAN-IMPLEMENT

We started a field study of the ADAPTE methodology in spring 2007 with multiple groups across Canada intent on implementing best practices (Harrison et al. 2013a) that led to our adaptation and expansion of the ADAPTE process. The new process is known as CAN-IMPLEMENT (Harrison et al. 2013b, 2014). Differing from the ADAPTE process, CAN-IMPLEMENT, as denoted by the name, was designed exclusively for groups wishing to implement best practices but unsure about how to go about it. It maps onto the phases of the K2A framework but also includes other steps that emerged while we were working with the implementation groups.

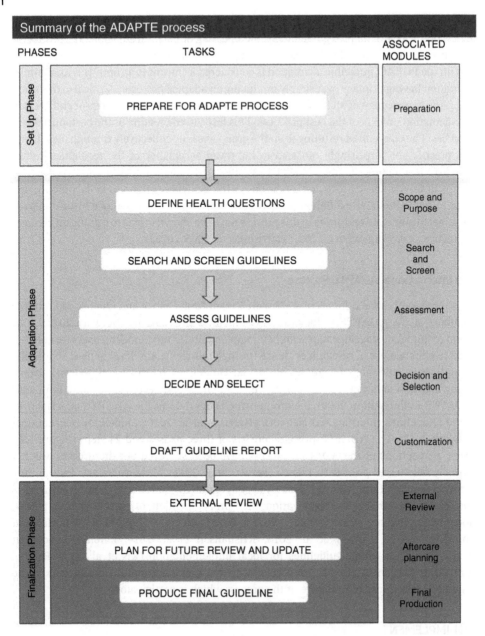

Figure 3.4 Summary of the ADAPTE process. *Source:* B Fervers, JS Burgers, R Voellinger, M Brouwers, GP Browman, ID Graham, MB Harrison, J Latreille, N Mlika-Cabane, L Paquet, L Zitzelsberger, B Burnand, The ADAPTE Collaboration, (2011). Guideline adaptation: an approach to enhance efficiency in guideline development and improve utilisation, BMJ Qual Saf 2011;20:228e236 © 2011 British medical journal.

In short, CAN-IMPLEMENT is a systematic and participatory approach for planning for implementation, including evaluating and adapting available guidelines to local context while ensuring the integrity of the evidence of the source guidelines. CAN-IMPLEMENT

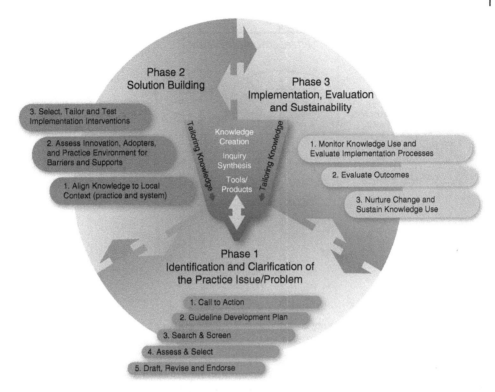

Figure 3.5 CAN-IMPLEMENT. *Source:* Reprinted with permission from Harrison et al. (2014). Available at: https://www.nursingcenter.com/journalarticle?article_id=1713163

includes three phases and 11 steps (Figure 3.5). The CAN-IMPLEMENT is a quick reference guide/manual and resource toolkit that became the foundation of a book (Harrison et al. 2014). Additionally, there is a detailed library sciences supplement providing direction on how to locate best practices (Ross-White et al. 2014). Most of the steps of CAN-IMPLEMENT are relevant to chapters in this book and often provide greater detail on how to undertake the key aspects of implementation. We consider CAN-IMPLEMENT (Harrison et al. 2014) along with Knowledge Translation in Health Care (Straus et al. 2013a) as key resources for planning and effecting implementation.

The usefulness of CAN-IMPLEMENT relates to the real-world nature of the approach with many tools and tips that evolved from the actual experience of people implementing guidelines. Practical examples are included.

Thinking Inside and Outside of the Box – Other Frameworks

Transitions

We have also developed or used some content specific frameworks along with the knowledge translation ones described earlier to help us identify specific areas needing greater attention while implementing best practices. For example, the Inter-sectoral Continuity of Care (ICC) framework (Figure 3.6) (Harrison et al. 1999) is a health services planning and evaluation approach focusing on the components of continuity of care (e.g. linkages, care activities,

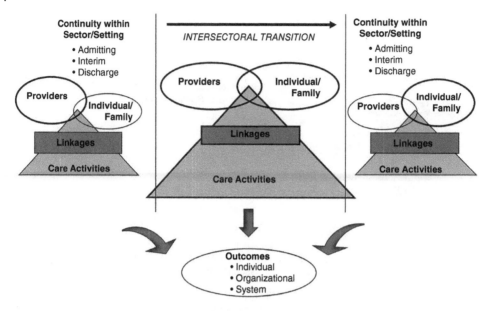

Figure 3.6 Inter-sectoral continuity of care framework. *Source:* Reprinted with permission from Harrison (1998). © by Margaret B. Harrison, January 1998.

providers) and the transitions either along a condition trajectory (diagnosis to treatment) or between sectors (e.g. hospital-home-long term care). This framework clarifies the types of inter-sector linkages that will improve the families' experiences during transitions. It also focuses attention on the important balance between professional and family provided care.

We found that the ICC focus on transitions is a key element in terms of the factors in maintaining evidence-informed practice as individuals shift from one setting of care to another or along the illness trajectory. During any transition, it can guide the conversation as to the care activities (direct and indirect), the involved providers and the linkage needed to maintain the provision of evidence-informed practice.

Supportive Care

Another mid-range or practice framework that has often been helpful in focusing attention on the needs of people requiring health care is a Supportive Care Framework. Originally this framework was developed for use with individuals dealing with cancer (Fitch 1994; Fitch et al. 2008). It focuses on the provision of supportive care across the trajectory from pre-diagnosis to active treatment then supportive care and palliation. However, the tenets of the framework apply not only to the population with cancer but also many other long term, chronic, and or complex populations (Harrison and MacIsaac 2008). The needs categories include physical, informational, emotional, psychological, social, spiritual, and practical.

The Supportive Care Framework provides a frame of reference for implementation from a patient and family perspective on receiving evidence-informed supportive care. Using this framework provides added insurance that the changes you are making with care are based on the evidence and will be truly person-centered.

The Roadmap for Knowledge Implementation

Our most recent implementation framework (Roadmap) and the one that is the overarching framework for this book, is a practical approach in eliciting and using the needed local, contextual information (Harrison and Graham 2012). As we observed groups undertaking implementation, we found common themes in terms of the process. The Roadmap framework encompasses the phases of the K2A Cycle and elements of the CAN-IMPLEMENT process and integrates them into three broad phases, each consisting of multiple stages. Roadmap details the journey from knowledge creation to implementation providing concrete actions on how practitioners, patients and families, policy makers and where necessary, researchers, build on local knowledge and evidence to bring external evidence to bear. Generally, Roadmap makes explicit the mutually supporting and interconnected cycles of activity supporting implementation. The external evidence (from guidelines and the literature) serves as a *foundation* providing leverage in designing (or redesigning) that must be "fitted" or "aligned" to local resources, populations, and context. Implementation typically consists of three major phases of *linked* enquiry and implementation activity:

i) Phase I: Issue Identification and Clarification
ii) Phase II: Build Solutions and Field Test
iii) Phase III: Implement, Evaluate and Sustain

Implementation activity with practitioners and decision-makers is iterative to effectively plan for evidence-informed services, and to reveal the major supports and barriers at practice, health services, population, and decision-making levels. A key factor is a proactive, incremental, and iterative technique of using and producing evidence where appropriate. The next chapter will describe Roadmap Phases and the various stages of activity in more detail.

Working Together as Patients, Practitioners, Decision-Makers and Researchers: Guiding Principles and Assumptions

Several guiding principles and assumptions underlie our approach to evidence activation. Our approach is "solutions-focused" rather than "problem-based." While it is essential to understand the challenges and barriers to implementation, the ultimate goal is to overcome these obstacles and build on facilitators and successes. A solutions-based approach is about collaboration, teamwork, inquisitiveness, and innovativeness. It also requires motivation, prioritization, and commitment. Additionally, it is about framing implementation efforts as solutions to evidence-practice gaps, which takes everyone's thinking beyond simply describing the gaps and focusing on deficits.

Research as a Means to an End

As we have already suggested, our view (and that of most practitioners) of research is that it should be considered as a "means" rather than an "end," in and of itself. Many researchers and others think the fundamental goal of research is to produce the findings – not necessarily to have the findings used in the real world. Similarly, many guideline developers focus on developing the guideline and its release rather than on its implementation which may be because it is often considered beyond their ability to influence. In both these examples, research is considered to be the primary goal. There is little doubt research should be the starting point for all implementation efforts. Research is needed to determine what evidence-informed practice should look like. We also argue that knowledge synthesis, i.e. the use of all studies available on a given topic, is the best source of evidence on the effectiveness of clinical interventions. However, simply knowing what evidence is available for practice will very seldom result in the use of that research.

External evidence/research can be a source of information on the effectiveness of implementation strategies. It may provide useful information in helping to select which implementation strategies to consider using in a specific context. Local evidence about patient needs and preferences, patient populations, the evidence-practice gap, potential barriers to implementation, use of the best practices and their impact is also critical for successful implementation. Data on these factors are essential for effective implementation planning. In our models and frameworks, we advocate combining local evidence and external research to understand context and to better plan for implementation – making research a means to an implementation end.

Engagement

As is probably obvious by now, we place a great emphasis on engagement of all relevant stakeholders, which in the context of implementation in health care is often about interprofessional work and team building. To be explicit, we would include the individuals and the family and their care givers as part of that team.

We find it useful to distinguish between the broad category of stakeholders (everyone who is directly (i.e. affected by) or indirectly (i.e. interested in) involved in implementing best practice) and knowledge users (those who have the capacity to act on research findings) (Jull et al. 2019). Knowledge users are particularly important stakeholders who need to play a central role in all implementation initiatives given they are the ones who will ultimately make the decision to adopt the best practice.

In fact, we support the concept known as IKT (Canadian Institutes of Health Research 2016; Gagliardi et al. 2016; Kothari et al. 2017; Graham et al. 2018) which is an approach to implementation and its application involves engaging those who may use or benefit from the research findings (knowledge users) in decision-making during the research process. Research conducted this way is intended to address the research needs and questions of the knowledge users, treat knowledge users as equal partners by reducing power differentials between the producers of research and knowledge users. Similar concepts include co-production or co-creation of knowledge, engaged scholarship, participatory research, and community based research, to name just a few (Graham and Tetroe 2009; Graham et al. 2019; Nguyen et al. 2020). For a description of team-based IKT see the paper by Keefe and colleagues (Keefe et al. 2020).

Changing the approach to research has been proposed by research funding agencies and others to accelerate the uptake of research findings into practice by engaging stakeholders and potential users of research findings. By engaging knowledge users in the research process from identifying and refining the research question through deciding on the methodology, being involved in data collection and tools development, and interpreting the findings, the resulting research is more relevant, useful, and more likely to be applied. Stakeholders become partners in the research enterprise and involved in decision making about the research – not to be confused with individuals who become research participants who are the focus of research. The IKT approach is essentially grounded in the Two-Communities theory (Caplan 1979; Dunn 1980). The theory suggests that an important reason that research is not taken up into policy is because academics (researchers) and policy makers form separate communities that work in silos and are poorly connected with each other and each community has its own language, operates under different rules, contexts and timelines, and is motivated by different reward systems. For example, researchers usually value things like controlling or minimizing the effect of context, methodological rigor, statistical significance, generalizability of findings and the need for ongoing research. They usually privilege empirical evidence over other types of knowledge. They also like the freedom of pursuing their own curiosity driven research questions. On the other hand, those who would use research findings (decision makers) may place greater emphasis on context, work under conditions of uncertainty, need to make decisions under time pressures and value other forms of evidence in addition to evidence from empirical research. You can see how this idea also applies to researchers and practitioners.

Because of these differences, the Two-Communities' theory posits that research may not be used because it is not perceived to be relevant or timely by those who could use it. Getting researchers and knowledge users working together and breaking down the silos and cultures is then thought to improve the communication between the groups making it more likely that researchers develop better appreciation of the context under which knowledge users are working and knowledge users come to appreciate the scientific method (i.e. there is mutual learning from each other which leads to better research). Because the research is conducted in a co-created way to directly address the issues of importance to the knowledge users, they are more likely to apply the findings when they become available. When the findings are applied, the resulting impact becomes evident. We acknowledge one important limitation of this theory – that there are not two communities (researchers and policy makers) but the researcher community (which is not itself homogeneous) and multiple decision maker communities (e.g. practitioners and within this category multiple disciplines and specialties), health system managers, bureaucrats, politicians, patients, the general public, industry, etc.). But in keeping with the theory, our experience has been that these multiple decision makers and knowledge user communities are often isolated from, or poorly engaged with the research community (and often from each other). This contributes to the failure to translate evidence into action. Moreover, knowledge user communities may not be embracing research because they do not perceive the research being conducted to be addressing their needs. For all these reasons we still like the metaphor of the two (multiple) communities.

We also believe this theory generally applies to the implementation of best practice (outside the research context), where different health care professions (e.g. nursing, medicine, rehabilitation, etc.) and groups (e.g. patients, etc.) represent different communities with different cultures, perspectives, and approaches and power. For successful implementation to occur, all the relevant stakeholders (communities) need to be involved in co-creating the local solutions and their implementation. By working together to implement best practices, individuals from different professions and involved groups can learn to collaborate better. One thing we have found is that by focusing on the evidence and learning how to better use it results in more productive discussions and can minimize power differences between professionals.

Additional Resources

In addition to our own research, our approach to implementation has also been informed by the literature on knowledge translation science. Our work complements (and sometimes) builds on excellent resources such as the texts, *Models and Frameworks for Implementing Evidence-based Practice* (Rycroft-Malone and Bucknall 2010), *Clinical Context for Evidence-based Practice* (Kent and McCormack 2010), *Evaluating the Impact of Implementing Evidence-Based Practice* (Bick and Graham 2010), and *Improving Patient Care: The Implementation of Change in Health Care* (Wensing et al. 2020). *Handbook on Implementation Science,* and *How to Implement Evidence-based Healthcare* are also recent informative authoritative texts (Greenhalgh 2017; Nilsen and Birken 2020). *The Registered Nurses' Association of Ontario (RNAO) Implementation Toolkit* is another resource that provides a lot of information on how to plan guideline implementation and is an open access document (Registered Nurses' Association of Ontario 2012). The RNAO toolkit is based on the K2A cycle and we have both been members of the Toolkit writing committee (Registered Nurses' Association of Ontario and Canadian Patient Safety Institute 2020). A recent text on implementation facilitation is Harvey & Kitson's (2015), *Implementing Evidence-Based Practice in Healthcare: A Facilitation Guide.*

The international journals *Implementation Science* and *Implementation Science Communications* are other excellent sources of literature on the science of knowledge translation. They are easy to access given that these journals are open access (BioMed Central Ltd 2019). Nursing journals that often have implementation content are *Worldviews on Evidence-Based Nursing, Nursing Research and Practice, the International Journal of Nursing Practice,* and the *Journal of Continuing Education in the Health Professions.* Lastly, a recent scoping review by Esmail et al. (2020) provides an up to date synopsis for interested readers.

This chapter provides the theoretical background to what lies ahead in the next chapters. If you have managed to get through this chapter without an attack of either Theory Adverse Syndrome or Framework Averse Syndrome, you will be happy to know that you have likely learned enough about theory to get you through the rest of the book. Well almost! A more detailed description of Roadmap is presented in the next chapter followed by a walk-through of the three phases of implementation. The implementation journey begins!

References

ADAPTE Collaboration (2009). *The ADAPTE Process: Resource Toolkit for Guideline Adaptation. Version 2.0,* [Online], Available: https://www.g-i-n.net/document-store/working-groups-documents/adaptation/adapte-resource-toolkit-guideline-adaptation-2-0.pdf (26 July 2019).

Azer, S.A. (2015). The top-cited articles in medical education: a bibliometric analysis. *Academic Medicine: Journal of the Association of American Medical Colleges* 90: 1147–1161. https://doi.org/10.1097/acm.0000000000000780.

Bick, D. and Graham, I.D. (2010). *Evaluating the Impact of Implementing Evidence-Based Practice*. Chichester: Wiley Blackwell.

BioMed Central Ltd (2019). *Implementation Science*, [Online], Available: https://implementationscience.biomedcentral.com (26 July 2019).

Burgers, J.S., Anzueto, A., Black, P.N. et al. (2012). Adaptation, evaluation, and updating of guidelines: article 14 in integrating and coordinating efforts in COPD guideline development. An official ATS/ERS workshop report. *Proceedings of the American Thoracic Society* 9: 304–310. https://doi.org/10.1513/pats.201208-067st.

Canadian Institutes of Health Research (2016). *Knowledge Translation*, [Online], Available: http://www.cihr-irsc.gc.ca/e/29418.html (26 July 2019).

Caplan, N. (1979). The two-communities theory and knowledge utilization. *American Behavioral Scientist* 22: 459–470. https://doi.org/10.1177/000276427902200308.

Curran, G.M. (2020). Implementation science made too simple: a teaching tool. *Implementation Science Communications* 1 https://doi.org/10.1186/s43058-020-00001-z.

Damschroder, L.J. (2020). Clarity out of chaos: use of theory in implementation research. *Psychiatry Research* 283: 112461. https://doi.org/10.1016/j.psychres.2019.06.036.

Denis, J.L. and Lehoux, P. (2013). Organizational theories. In: *Knowledge Translation in Health Care: Moving from Evidence to Practice* (eds. S.E. Straus, J. Tetroe and I.D. Graham), 308–319. Oxford, UK: Wiley Blackwell BMJ Books.

Donabedian, A. (2005). Evaluating the quality of medical care 1966. *The Milbank Quarterly* 83: 691–729. https://doi.org/10.1111/j.1468-0009.2005.00397.x.

Driscoll, M.P. (1994). *Psychology of Learning for Instruction*. Needham, MA: Allyn and Bacon.

Dunn, W. (1980). The two-communities metaphor and models of knowledge use: an exploratory case survey. *Science Communication* 1: 515–536. https://doi.org/10.1177/107554708000100403.

Esmail, R., Hanson, H.M., Holroyd-Leduc, J. et al. (2020). A scoping review of full-spectrum knowledge translation theories, models, and frameworks. *Implementation Science* 15: 11. https://doi.org/10.1186/s13012-020-0964-5.

Fervers, B., Burgers, J.S., Voellinger, R. et al. (2011). Guideline adaptation: an approach to enhance efficiency in guideline development and improve utilisation. *BMJ Quality and Safety* 20: 228–236. https://doi.org/10.1136/bmjqs.2010.043257.

Festinger, L. (1957). *A Theory of Cognitive Dissonance*, 2e. Stanford, CA: Stanford University Press.

Field, B., Booth, A., Ilott, I., and Gerrish, K. (2014). Using the knowledge to action framework in practice: a citation analysis and systematic review. *Implementation Science* 9: 172. https://doi.org/10.1186/s13012-014-0172-2.

Fitch, M.I. (1994). *Providing Supportive Care for Individuals Living with Cancer (Task Force Report)*. Toronto, Canada: Ontario Cancer Treatment and Research Foundation.

Fitch, M.I., Porter, H.B., and Page, B.D. (eds.) (2008). *Supportive Care Framework: A Foundation for Person-Centred Care*. Pembroke: Pappin Communications Ontario.

Gagliardi, A.R., Berta, W., Kothari, A. et al. (2016). Integrated knowledge translation (IKT) in health care: a scoping review. *Implementation Science* 11: 38. https://doi.org/10.1186/s13012-016-0399-1.

Glasersfeld, E.V. (1995). A constructivist approach to teaching. In: *Constructivism in Education* (eds. L.P. Steffe and J.E. Gale), 3–15. Hillside, NJ: Lawrence Erlbaum Associates.

Graham, I.D. and Harrison, M.B. (2005). Evaluation and adaptation of clinical practice guidelines. *Evidence-Based Nursing* 8: 68–72. https://doi.org/10.1136/ebn.8.3.68.

Graham, I.D. and Logan, J. (2004). Innovations in knowledge transfer and continuity of care. *The Canadian Journal of Nursing Research* 36: 89–103.

Graham, I.D. and Tetroe, J.M. (2009). Getting evidence into policy and practice: perspective of a health research funder. *Journal of the Canadian Academy of Child and Adolescent Psychiatry* 18: 46–50. https://www.ncbi.nlm.nih.gov/pmc/articles/PMC2651211/.

Graham, I.D. and Tetroe, J. (2010). The knowledge to action framework. In: *Models and Frameworks for Implementing Evidence-Based Practice: Linking Evidence to Action* (eds. J. Rycroft-Malone and T. Bucknall), 207–222. Oxford, UK: Wiley Blackwell.

Graham, I.D., Harrison, M.B., Brouwers, M. et al. (2002). Facilitating the use of evidence in practice: evaluating and adapting clinical practice guidelines for local use by health care organizations. *Journal of Obstetric, Gynecologic, and Neonatal Nursing* 31: 599–611. https://doi.org/10.1111/j.1552-6909.2002.tb00086.x.

Graham, I.D., Harrison, M.B., and Brouwers, M. (2003). Evaluating and adapting practice guidelines for local use: a conceptual framework. In: *Clinical Governance in Practice* (eds. S. Pickering and J. Thompson), 213–229. London: Harcourt.

Graham, I.D., Harrison, M.B., Lorimer, K. et al. (2005). Adapting national and international leg ulcer practice guidelines for local use: the Ontario Leg Ulcer Community Care Protocol. *Advances in Skin & Wound Care* 18: 307–318. https://doi.org/10.1097/00129334-200507000-00011.

Graham, I.D., Logan, J., Harrison, M.B. et al. (2006). Lost in knowledge translation: time for a map? *The Journal of Continuing Education in the Health Professions* 26: 13–24. https://doi.org/10.1002/chp.47.

Graham, I.D., Tetroe, J., and K.T. Theories Research Group (2007). Some theoretical underpinnings of knowledge translation. *Academic Emergency Medicine* 14: 936–941. https://onlinelibrary.wiley.com/doi/abs/10.1111/j.1553-2712.2007.tb02369.x?sid=nlm%3Apubmed.

Graham, I.D., Tetroe, J., and K.T Theories Group (2013). Planned action theories. In: *Knowledge Translation in Health Care: Moving from Evidence to Practice* (eds. S.E. Straus, J. Tetroe and I.D. Graham), 277–287. Oxford, UK: Wiley Blackwell.

Graham, I.D., Kothari, A., McCutcheon, C., and Integrated Knowledge Translation Research Network Project Leads (2018). Moving knowledge into action for more effective practice, programmes and policy: protocol for a research programme on integrated knowledge translation. *Implementation Science* 13 https://doi.org/10.1186/s13012-017-0700-y.

Graham, I.D., McCutcheon, C., and Kothari, A. (2019). Exploring the frontiers of research co-production: the Integrated Knowledge Translation Research Network concept papers. *Health Research Policy and Systems* 17: 88. https://doi.org/10.1186/s12961-019-0501-7.

Gredler, E.M. (1997). *Learning and Instruction: Theory into Practice*. New Jersey: Merrill.

Greenhalgh, T. (2017). *How to Implement Evidence-Based Healthcare*. Hoboken, NJ: Wiley Blackwell.

Guidelines International Network (2017). *Working Groups / Adaptation*, [Online], Available: http://www.g-i-n.net/working-groups/adaptation (26 July 2019).

Gupta, S., Bhattacharyya, O.K., Brouwers, M.C. et al. (2009). Canadian Thoracic Society: presenting a new process for clinical practice guideline production. *Canadian Respiratory Journal* 16: e62–e68. https://doi.org/10.1155/2009/397818.

Han, J.Y. and Choi-Kwon, S. (2011). Adaptation of evidence-based surgical wound care algorithm. *Journal of Korean Academy of Nursing* 41: 768–779. https://doi.org/10.4040/jkan.2011.41.6.768.

Harrison, M. B. (1998). Continuity of care for complex health populations: Effectiveness and efficiency of two models of hospital to home transfer. Doctor of Philosophy, McMaster University.

Harrison, M.B. and Graham, I.D. (2012). Roadmap for a participatory research-practice partnership to implement evidence. *Worldviews on Evidence-Based Nursing* 9: 210–220. https://doi.org/10.1111/j.1741-6787.2012.00256.x.

Harrison, M.B. and MacIsaac, L. (2008). Use and applicability of the supportive care framework with complex non-cancer populations. In: *Supportive Care Framework: A Foundation for Person-Centred Care* (eds. M.I. Fitch, H.B. Porter and B.D. Page), 71–87. Pembroke: Pappin Communications Ontario.

Harrison, M.B., Browne, G., Roberts, J. et al. (1999). Continuity of care and bridging the inter-sectoral gap: a planning and evaluation framework. *National Academies of Practice Forum: Issues in Interdisciplinary Care* 1: 315–326.

Harrison, M.B., Graham, I.D., Lorimer, K. et al. (2005). Leg-ulcer care in the community, before and after implementation of an evidence-based service. *Canadian Medical Association Journal* 172: 1447–1452. https://doi.org/10.1503/cmaj.1041441.

Harrison, M.B., Legare, F., Graham, I.D., and Fervers, B. (2010). Adapting clinical practice guidelines to local context and assessing barriers to their use. *Canadian Medical Association Journal* 182: E78–E84. https://doi.org/10.1503/cmaj.081232.

Harrison, M.B., Graham, I.D., Fervers, B., and van den Hoek, J. (2013a). Adapting knowledge to local context. In: *Knowledge Translation in Health Care: Moving from Evidence to Practice* (eds. S.E. Straus, J. Tetroe and I.D. Graham), 110–120. Chichester: Wiley.

Harrison, M.B., Graham, I.D., van den Hoek, J. et al. (2013b). Guideline adaptation and implementation planning: a prospective observational study. *Implementation Science* 8: 49. https://doi.org/10.1186/1748-5908-8-49.

Harrison, M.B., van den Hoek, J., and Graham, I.D. (2014). *CAN-IMPLEMENT: Planning for Best-Practice Implementation (Book 20)*. Philadelphia: Lippincott Williams & Wilkins.

Harvey, G. and Kitson, A. (2015). *Implementing Evidence-Based Practice in Healthcare: A Facilitation Guide*. Abingdon: Routledge.

Howell, D., Keller-Olaman, S., Oliver, T.K. et al. (2013). A pan-Canadian practice guideline and algorithm: screening, assessment, and supportive care of adults with cancer-related fatigue. *Current Oncology* 20: e233–e246. https://doi.org/10.3747/co.20.1302.

Hutchinson, A.M. and Estabrooks, C.A. (2013a). Cognitive psychology theories of change in provider behavior. In: *Knowledge Translation in Health Care: Moving from Evidence to Practice* (eds. S.E. Straus, J. Tetroe and I.D. Graham), 288–297. Oxford, UK: Wiley Blackwell BMJ Books.

Hutchinson, A.M. and Estabrooks, C.A. (2013b). Educational theories. In: *Knowledge Translation in Health Care: Moving from Evidence to Practice pp. 298–307* (eds. S.E. Straus, J. Tetroe and I.D. Graham). Oxford, UK: Wiley Blackwell BMJ Books.

Jull, J.E., Davidson, L., Dungan, R. et al. (2019). A review and synthesis of frameworks for engagement in health research to identify concepts of knowledge user engagement. *BMC Medical Research Methodology* 19: 211. https://doi.org/10.1186/s12874-019-0838-1.

Keefe, J., Hande, M.J., Aubrecht, K. et al. (2020). Team-based integrated knowledge translation for enhancing quality of life in long-term care settings: a multi-method, multi-sectoral research design. *International Journal of Health Policy and Management* 9: 138–142. https://doi.org/10.15171/ijhpm.2019.123.

Kent, B. and McCormack, B. (eds.) (2010). *Clinical Context for Evidence-Based Practice.* Chichester: Wiley Blackwell.

Kis, E., Szegesdi, I., Dobos, E. et al. (2010). Quality assessment of clinical practice guidelines for adaptation in burn injury. *Burns* 36: 606–615. https://doi.org/10.1016/j.burns.2009.08.017.

Kothari, A., McCutcheon, C., and Graham, I.D. (2017). Defining integrated knowledge translation and moving forward: a response to recent commentaries. *International Journal of Health Policy and Management* 6: 299–300. https://doi.org/10.15171/ijhpm.2017.15.

Kristiansen, A., Brandt, L., Agoritsas, T. et al. (2014). Adaptation of trustworthy guidelines developed using the GRADE methodology: a novel five-step process. *Chest* 146: 727–734. https://doi.org/10.1378/chest.13-2828.

Larenas-Linnemann, D., Mayorga-Butron, J.L., Sanchez-Gonzalez, A. et al. (2014). ARIA Mexico 2014. Adaptation of the Clinical Practice Guide ARIA 2010 for Mexico. Methodology ADAPTE. *Revista Alergia México* 61 (Suppl 1): S3–S116.

Logan, J. and Graham, I.D. (1998). Toward a comprehensive interdisciplinary model of health care research use. *Science Communication* 20: 227–246. https://doi.org/10.1177/1075547098020002004.

Logan, J. and Graham, I.D. (2010). The Ottawa model of research use. In: *Models and Frameworks for Implementing Evidence-Based Practice: Linking Evidence to Action* (eds. J. Rycroft-Malone and T. Bucknall), 83–108. Oxford: Wiley Blackwell.

Lynch, E.A., Mudge, A., Knowles, S. et al. (2018). "There is nothing so practical as a good theory": a pragmatic guide for selecting theoretical approaches for implementation projects. *BMC Health Services Research* 18: 857. https://doi.org/10.1186/s12913-018-3671-z.

National Collaborating Centre for Methods and Tools (2016). *Implementation frameworks, theories and models: An interactive site for practitioners and researchers*, [Online], Available: https://www.nccmt.ca/knowledge-repositories/search/254 (7 February 2020).

Nguyen, T., Graham, I.D., Mrklas, K.J. et al. (2020). How does integrated knowledge translation (IKT) compare to other collaborative research approaches to generating and translating knowledge? Learning from experts in the field. *Health Research Policy and Systems* 18: 35. https://doi.org/10.1186/s12961-020-0539-6.

Nilsen, P. (2015). Making sense of implementation theories, models and frameworks. *Implementation Science* 10: 53. https://doi.org/10.1186/s13012-015-0242-0.

Nilsen, P. and Birken, S.A. (eds.) (2020). *Handbook on Implementation Science.* Cheltenham, Gloucestershire, UK: Edward Elgar Publishing Limited.

Pantoja, C.T., Ferdinand, O.C., Saldias, P.F. et al. (2011). The adaptation methodology of a guideline for the management of adults with community-acquired pneumonia. *Revista Médica de Chile* 139: 1403–1413. https://scielo.conicyt.cl/scielo.php?script=sci_arttext&pid=S0034-98872011001100003&lng=en&nrm=iso&tlng=en.

Ray-Coquard, I., Philip, T., de, L.G. et al. (2002). A controlled "before-after" study: impact of a clinical guidelines programme and regional cancer network organization on medical practice. *British Journal of Cancer* 86: 313–321. https://doi.org/10.1038/sj.bjc.6600057.

Registered Nurses' Association of Ontario (2012). *Toolkit: Implementation of Best Practice Guidelines*. Toronto, ON: Registered Nurses' Association of Ontario. Available at: https://rnao.ca/sites/rnao-ca/files/RNAO_ToolKit_2012_rev4_FA.pdf.

Registered Nurses' Association of Ontario and Canadian Patient Safety Institute (2020). *Leading Change Toolkit. Expected date of completion: November 2020* Toronto, ON: Registered Nurses' Association of Ontario. Available at: https://rnao.ca/bpg/resources/leading-change-toolkit.

Ross-White, A., Oakley, P., and Lockwood, C. (2014). *Guideline Adaptation: Conducting Systematic, Exhaustive, and Reproducible Searches (Book 19)*. Philadelphia: Lippincott Williams & Wilkins.

Rycroft-Malone, J. and Bucknall, T. (eds.) (2010). *Models and Frameworks for Implementing Evidence-Based Practice: Linking Evidence to Action*. Chichester: Wiley Blackwell.

Sales, A. (2013). Quality improvement. In: *Knowledge Translation in Health Care: Moving from Evidence to Practice* (eds. S.E. Straus, J. Tetroe and I.D. Graham), 320–328. Oxford, UK: Wiley Blackwell BMJ Books.

Savery, J.R. and Duffy, T.M. (1995). Problem based learning: an instructional model and its constructivist framework. *Educational Technology* 35: 31–38. https://doi.org/10.2307/44428296.

Skolarus, T.A., Lehmann, T., Tabak, R.G. et al. (2017). Assessing citation networks for dissemination and implementation research frameworks. *Implementation Science* 12: 97. https://doi.org/10.1186/s13012-017-0628-2.

Slavin, R.E. (1994). *Educational Psychology: Theory and Practice*, 4e. Boston: Allyn and Bacon.

Steffe, L.P. and Gale, J.E. (eds.) (1995). *Constructivism in Education*. Hillside, NJ: Lawrence Erlbaum Associates.

Straus, S., Tetroe, J., and Graham, I.D. (eds.) (2013a). *Knowledge Translation in Health Care. Moving from Evidence to Practice*, 2e. Chichester: Wiley Blackwell.

Straus, S.E., Tetroe, J., and Graham, I.D. (2013b). Knowledge translation: What it is and what it is not. In: *Knowledge Translation in Health Care: Moving from Evidence to Practice*, 2e (eds. S.E. Straus, J. Tetroe and I.D. Graham), 3–13. West Sussex, UK: Wiley.

Strifler, L., Cardoso, R., McGowan, J. et al. (2018). Scoping review identifies significant number of knowledge translation theories, models, and frameworks with limited use. *Journal of Clinical Epidemiology* 100: 92–102. https://doi.org/10.1016/j.jclinepi.2018.04.008.

Tabak, R.G., Khoong, E.C., Chambers, D.A., and Brownson, R.C. (2012). Bridging research and practice: models for dissemination and implementation research. *American Journal of Preventative Medicine* 43: 337–350. https://www.ncbi.nlm.nih.gov/pmc/articles/PMC3592983/.

Thomas, A., Saroyan, A., and Dauphinee, W.D. (2011). Evidence-based practice: a review of theoretical assumptions and effectiveness of teaching and assessment interventions in health professions. *Advances in Health Sciences Education: Theory and Practice* 16: 253–276. https://doi.org/10.1007/s10459-010-9251-6.

Thomas, A., Menon, A., Boruff, J. et al. (2014). Applications of social constructivist learning theories in knowledge translation for healthcare professionals: a scoping review. *Implementation Science* 9: 54. https://doi.org/10.1186/1748-5908-9-54.

Villalobos Dintrans, P., Bossert, T.J., Sherry, J., and Kruk, M.E. (2019). A synthesis of implementation science frameworks and application to global health gaps. *Global Health Research and Policy* 4: 25. https://doi.org/10.1186/s41256-019-0115-1.

Wensing, M., Grol, R., and Grimshaw, J. (2020). *Improving Patient Care: The Implementation of Change in Health Care*, 3e. Wiley Blackwell.

4

A Roadmap for Implementing Best Practice

The Journey to Best Practice

In the last chapter, we described some of the theories and frameworks that we used to guide our implementation work. Many of them are ones we developed while working with practice groups to help advance the implementation process. These frameworks were presented in chronological order to illustrate how our thinking about implementation has evolved over time. The previous chapter introduced the Implementation Roadmap, a comprehensive implementation planning framework, the focus of this book. The Implementation Roadmap process was built on our work in the areas of knowledge to action, adaptation, implementation, our experiences in activating evidence in practice in numerous settings, and our recognition of what were often needed supports for implementing evidence (Harrison and Graham 2012).

The purpose of this chapter is to explain the phases of Implementation Roadmap in sufficient detail to demonstrate how each can contribute to successful implementation. By the end of this chapter you will have enough knowledge about the framework to use it to begin planning how to bring about change in your setting.

The Implementation Road

As we described earlier, the journey moving evidence into practice typically consists of three major phases of implementation activity:

- Issue Identification and Clarification
- Build Solutions and Field Test
- Implement, Evaluate, and Sustain

With each phase, there are numerous activities to be accomplished (Figure 4.1).

Phase I: Issue Identification and Clarification

An implementation initiative may start with new and practice-changing evidence that is now housed in an available guideline. Often though, we found that it resulted from an issue

Knowledge Translation in Nursing and Healthcare: A Roadmap to Evidence-informed Practice, First Edition. Margaret B. Harrison and Ian D. Graham.

or problem uncovered in quality processes or the desire for risk reduction. Sometimes it may even be the expenditures that have gotten out of line and cause a second look. It is then the best available evidence is sought out.

This phase might be thought of as problem deconstruction – it requires your working group to describe the issue to be tackled through implementation of best practices, clearly and explicitly. The issue identification and clarification phase is comprised of two main steps: the call-to-action and determining the extent of the evidence-practice gap.

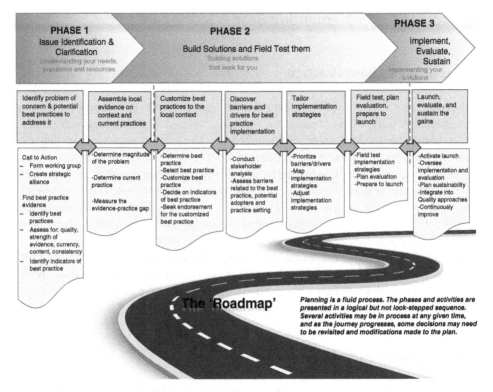

Figure 4.1 The implementation roadmap.

Box 4.1   Raising the Alarm

In one example with best practice for pressure ulcer prevention the unusual increase in flap procedures to repair ulcer damage provided cause for an in-depth look at the incidence and prevalence across an organization.

Within a large medical unit nurses became concerned with repeated admissions of those with heart failure and were questioning the effectiveness of their discharge procedures.

In another example the expenditures for leg ulcer supplies and nursing visits prompted a review of the care and discovery of new evidence for managing this chronic wound.

Box 4.2   Understand the Issue from All Sides

In the beginning the Call-to-Action is exploratory to determine what information is alerting the need for some action and what other information might be available. In the leg ulcer example, it was the district managers who raised the first alarm bell over rising expenditures. Further consultation revealed concern at the point of care with the quality of care and feedback from individuals and families about self-management of this condition.

Local experience, expertise, data on unmet patient needs often raises awareness of the issue providing the momentum for the formation of *a strategic alliance* among stakeholders (for example, providers, patients, managers) within and/or across agencies and settings. Ideally the alliance will have clinical and management expertise as well as representation from an appropriate range of decision-making levels as well as evaluation or research expertise. The inclusion of patients or people with experience with the condition of interest and their caregivers and family can greatly strengthen the strategic alliance. Over time a working group or task force will evolve to lead the implementation activity. There is more on the alliance formation in Chapter 5.

The other step in this phase is determining the evidence-practice gap which entails two components: finding the best practice evidence and assembling the local evidence on the issue and context.

As revealed by the Knowledge to Action cycle, after identifying the issue of concern, sometimes a group starts by collecting the local evidence on the magnitude of the care issue, what is known about the patients and providers, and what current practice is, before looking for best practices for the condition. Other times a group may start by identifying best practice and then focus on what current practice is and how care is provided. Our experience has been that both collecting local evidence and identifying external evidence on best practice can happen simultaneously, to some extent. We usually like to identify what is evidence-informed best practice for the issue or condition quite early on. This information can be used to determine what information about current practice should be collected. Regardless of whether a group starts with identifying the best practice or determining the state of the issue and current practice, the key is that both pieces of information are required to determine the evidence-practice gap. The local evidence about patient and provider populations and current practice provides an understanding of how things are currently working, or how things may not be working.

When wanting to identify best practice, it is good to begin with a critical review and quality assessment of the available practice guidelines to ascertain best obtainable evidence related to the care issue. If guidelines are not available or appropriate, then external evidence synthesized from systematic reviews would be the next source of evidence to consider. If practice guidelines and systematic reviews cannot be used as the source of best available practice, the next step would be to look to the primary research studies, however this is often not feasible or practical for most practice settings. For this reason, the focus of the book is primarily on the implementation of practice guidelines and uses examples of guideline implementation. Chapter 6 describes how to assess the quality and content of practice guidelines as this is essential for determining if the guideline is of adequate quality to warrant being implemented. While we are not going to focus on implementing the results from knowledge syntheses or primary studies, the processes we describe are nevertheless applicable and useful when implementing these knowledge products too.

Next, an environmental assessment conducted locally will determine the extent of the issue, the context and setting in which it occurs, and how care is currently delivered. Information about these considerations is used to develop the foundation for decision-making and planning for any needed changes. Bear in mind that the enquiry during this phase is not focused on the individual but rather the population (e.g. a clinic's group of patients or a regional home care authority's catchment area). This may include practice audits as a gap analyses; an environmental scan to understand the current organization and delivery of care; and knowledge, attitudes, and practice (KAP) surveys with local providers. Chapter 7 delves further into how to determine current practice.

Ultimately, the goal of Phase I is to determine the extent of the evidence-practice gap by comparing what is recognized as best practice to current practice in your setting. If the group considers the gap significant, then this serves as the rationale for action. If the size of the gap is considered acceptable, then no action is required, and the group can move on to another issue of concern. Remember that even small evidence-practice gaps may be deemed by stakeholders to be worthy of action because of the number of people potentially affected or the significance of the impact on those not receiving best practice.

During Phase I a reliable, comprehensive, and *shared* understanding of the issue is created along with exploration of the evidence-informed care needed to address it. By the end of Phase I you will have a lot of information that will help clarify what needs to be done. For example, the call-to-action step will help you figure out exactly what the issue or concern is that the group wants to focus on and who else needs to be involved. You will have collected local evidence on the extent and magnitude of the issue, know the characteristics of the patient population with the condition, have a profile of the healthcare providers serving the population and how care is organized and delivered. You will also know from the external evidence what best practice is to care for this population and the magnitude of the gap between current practice and recommended best practice.

Phase II: Build Solutions and Field Test

In this Phase, the alliance works with the local information focusing on what implementation of "best practice" would entail in their context. There is a proactive exchange to identify and recognize gaps between best available evidence and current practice, and changes that may be needed in the current practice and delivery of care. The approach in Phase II is about customizing and aligning the best practice to the local context, discovering the barriers and drivers (facilitators) to implementing the best practice, and selecting and tailoring implementation strategies. It also involves developing an evaluation plan (including identifying measures of best practice use and impact), and field testing the customized best practice.

During Phase II, the first step is for the group, whose membership might now be modified to include more point-of-care providers, is to re-examine all the potential best practices related to management of the condition of interest. Whereas in Phase I, the group was assessing the quality of best practice, now it must consider the clinical content and utility, acceptability, implementability, and sustainability of the recommendations and make decisions about which guideline or recommendations to adopt and which require some form of customization or adaptation to make them appropriate for implementation (Harrison et al. 2014). Customization may simply involve selecting specific recommendations from multiple best practice guidelines that collectively will best meet the local needs – you can think of this as the mix and match or buffet approach to best practice customization. In other instances, it may involve changing the wording of a recommendation to make it more user friendly. Simultaneously, when groups are working through how to customize best practice, they often begin to also consider how care is currently delivered and how the best practice might need to be aligned to the context. For example, the group might not have access to a high technology diagnostic test recommended be used as part of a guideline, so the group must identify the next best diagnostic test the setting has access to and is feasible to implement. Another example is when the recommendation suggests one type of care provider (e.g. a nurse) should be responsible for a clinical action (e.g. an assessment) and the group realizes that in their setting, the social worker would be a better person to do the assessment. In both examples, the essence of the best practice recommendation was customized to align with the context.

Current delivery of care may need to be modified or aligned to be able to deliver the desired best practice. Consideration of customization and alignment issues provides the insights needed for key players to identify clinical, health services, and/or policy changes (small or large) in order to move forward with evidence-informed care. When the group considers how to customize best practice and how the best practice may need to be aligned with existing processes of care to provide the best practice, this signals that the group is beginning to actively identify and process implementation issues. Best practice customization and alignment involves the group figuring out how to stay true to the intent of recommendations but delivering it in a way that works for the setting. Chapter 8 describes how to customize best practices and think about how best practice can be aligned with the current process of service delivery to be able to successfully implement the best practices.

Once the group has customized the best practice for local use, attention can turn to identifying barriers and drivers to implementation of the adapted best practices. Some factors may be known but others could be more difficult to tease out. Finding out what the barriers and drivers are can be done by surveying stakeholders or conducting interviews or focus groups in the setting with key informants. Chapter 9 describes different approaches and techniques for assessing barriers and drivers to implementation of the best practices.

After the barriers and drivers to implementation have been identified, the next activity is to select implementation strategies and often tailor them to the local context to overcome the barriers to facilitate uptake of the best practices. When mapping implementation strategies to barriers and drivers, it is important to know about the evidence for the effectiveness of implementation strategies, and fortunately there are many systematic reviews that report on this evidence (see Chapter 10). Chapter 11 discusses how to go about selecting and tailoring implementation strategies.

One other important activity during Phase II is for the group to decide how it will determine use or adherence to the best practice recommendations. This represents the knowledge use phase in the Knowledge to Action cycle. All implementation efforts should include monitoring uptake of the best practices and once the best practices have been customized, then it is possible to think about how their use can be measured. The use of the best practices (i.e. new process of care) must be differentiated from the *impact* of using best practices. In other words, when best practices are being used, what difference does it make to patient outcomes, provider outcomes, and health system outcomes? Chapter 12 discusses considerations related to developing an evaluation plan including monitoring best practice use and evaluating its impact. Appendix 12.A presents some of the theory about and approaches to measuring knowledge use and impact.

Field testing the implementation strategies and the best practices is also a key stage of Phase II (Chapter 12). Field testing should be done to ensure that the implementation strategies can be deployed, to determine how they are received by those affected by them, to find out whether there are any fatal flaws with them (e.g. whether a greater dose is needed), and to see whether they appear to promote use of the customized best practices. The intent is to see how the implementation and implementation strategies can be improved. The field test can also be used to pick up any potential issues with the actual recommendations that may have been missed during the customization phase. It is always better to try out the best practice implementation in a small way before launching it organization or system wide. In our experience, despite the best intentions and a thorough approach to implementation, there can be one or a few small (often unexpected) factors that can diminish and even scuttle successful implementation. It is much better to identify these flaws and fix them as part of a field test than to learn about them in the middle of an implementation initiative.

The final stage in this phase is preparing to launch the implementation process. This involves checking the readiness of the implementation strategies, leadership support, the processes and people involved, etc. before going live with the implementation of the best practice. If all is not ready, then it is better to delay and address the outstanding issues than launch and risk the implementation being stalled or worse, aborted.

The purpose of Phase II is to build a solution to ameliorate the identified issue/problem and to field test it. This involves reaching consensus on what best practice for the setting should be, figuring out what barriers/drivers might exist to implementing the best practice and tailoring implementation strategies to overcome the barriers and leverage the drivers, deciding on how to measure successfulness of the implementation efforts, and testing implementation in a small way to determine whether everything is in order to launch the full-scale implementation and evaluation effort.

By the end of the Build Solutions Phase, you will have selected best practices to implement, and adapted the recommendations as needed to your context and figured out how provider practice or the delivery of health services needs to be organized or re-organized to deliver the recommended best practice. You will have learned what factors are drivers or barriers to implementing best practice and how significant they are. You will also have selected and tailored implementation strategies to overcome the barriers and build on the drivers and determined what resources will be needed to deploy the implementation strategies. You will have decided on the indicators and metrics to be used to measure adherence (uptake) of the new best practices and the impact of using the best practices on patient, provider, and health system outcomes. Finally, you will have field tested the implementation strategies, made any course corrections and determined that you are ready to launch the implementation of the best practices.

Phase III: Implement, Evaluate, and Sustain

In the last phase of Roadmap, the focus is on the actual implementation of best practices, evaluating their uptake and impacts (outcomes) and finally attending to what needs to be done to sustain the practice change. In Phase III, the alliance undertakes strategies to implement the best practice, begins to understand how well the implementation has gone, and the impact and benefit of their work by conducting outcome and impact evaluations (Chapter 13). Planning for implementation underpins both Phases I and II and culminates in Phase III with setting those plans into motion and implementing the best practices and determining how well they have been implemented and with what effect.

The evaluation activities in Phase III present the opportunity to assess potential longer-term monitoring and outcome assessment for the setting, for example an outcome measure that could serve as a quality indicator (e.g. monthly pressure ulcer prevalence survey). This Phase can be thought of as encompassing an outcomes evaluation (measuring best practices uptake – also known as knowledge use) and an impact evaluation (measuring the outcomes or impact of using best practices). *Outcomes evaluation* can be used to first reveal the important process-of-care information about delivering the evidence recommendations (e.g. organization of teams to carry-out the needed comprehensive assessment). This sort of evaluation is often carried out as a quality initiative to determine the general fit of the evidence-informed care within clinical routines, timeliness of care, change in resource use etc. As well, it is the initial experience with the feasibility, appropriateness, and sensitivity of outcomes that may later be useful for quality monitoring. Evaluating impact can range from fairly simple approaches such as pre-post audits to full blown research where there is a before and after test of the implementation.

Sustainability

Nurturing change requires proactive work to promote sustainability. Ideally, how to sustain evidence-informed care is considered throughout the journey. While the focus on sustainability appears as a stage at the end of Roadmap, in fact, sustainability issues have to be considered from the very beginning of Phase I. Successful implementation planning involves thinking about whether and how sustainability considerations can be built into the implementation journey. For example, is there a sustainable process for continuously checking the literature for changes in best practice. Do the best practices need to be kept up to date? Are the implementation/sustainability strategies workable (using implementation strategies that are overly complex, expensive, and/or not practical may result in their use being discontinued)? Are the selected measures of best practice use and impact ones that can be sustained after the implementation? If data on best practice use and impact post implementation are not collected there is no way to know whether the change has continued.

To consolidate earlier observations and experience, the final stage of Phase III involves focusing on sustainability issues (Chapter 14). This relates to not only the ongoing use of what initially were the "new" best practices, but also on the impacts achieved by implementation of best practices, and other sustainability issues related to the journey to best practice. This usually involves continuing to collect data on best practice use and impact after the completion of the implementation initiative to know whether the best practice is in fact still being used or whether practice is regressing to past (not best) practice. If the latter, then additional sustainability strategies may be required. These may be more of the same implementation strategies or new strategies. Another barriers assessment may be needed to determine if the already known barriers to the use of best practice persist, or whether new ones have arisen that implementation and sustainability strategies need to target.

By the end of Phase III, the implementation will have been evaluated and you will know how effective and efficient it was and the impact the implementation has had on the outcomes you have chosen. You will also have decided what will need to be done to sustain the ongoing use of the best practices. And if you have been successful you will start the process all over again with the next issue of concern; if you have not achieved your goals, you will revisit the previous steps.

The implementation phase is essentially about putting into action the implementation strategies selected to address the identified barriers. The activities related to this stage are largely leadership for change and implementation facilitation. Of course, these activities are relevant to all stages of Roadmap but become particularly critical during and post implementation.

Navigating Roadmap (Some Obvious and Less Obvious Points)

Because it is about fitting the best external evidence within a given environment (yours), you can see how essential it is for the Roadmap process to be local, interactive, and engaging. It is about customizing best external evidence to the local context when necessary, aligning best practice with the delivery of care to be able to provide the best practice, tailoring implementation strategies to identified barriers, implementing those strategies, and evaluating the effect and paying attention to sustainability of the process and outcomes. This 3-phase approach is about thorough implementation planning and contributes to several important aspects for successful implementation: sustaining a strategic alliance; generating collective consensus about what needs to be done and how, providing a natural avenue for learning about, and fully appreciating the external evidence in relation to the local circumstances; utilizing available supports within the environment; and developing a process to undertake future implementations of evidence-informed practice.

When thinking about Roadmap and how to use it in your setting, there are some assumptions behind our approach that should be made explicit:

- The focus should be on how to influence or bring about change in the group, unit, program, or health system.
- Implementation efforts should be evidence informed.
- Implementation efforts should be pragmatic while being methodologically rigorous to optimize benefit and impact.
- Leadership and facilitation drives and nurtures implementation.
- Implementation does not happen without planning.

While ultimately individual practitioners make decisions with and for patients/families, we are interested in influencing the collective or group to be more evidence informed. This means appreciating the systems and structures where practitioners function and work which can influence individual and group decision-making. Creating systems and processes that make it easy for practitioners to do the right thing, at the right time for the right patient, facilitates evidence implementation. We are not suggesting that focus on psychological determinants of patient and provider decision-making is not important or should not be considered but rather, it should be complemented with more sociological and organizational perspectives on implementation. Even small changes made by members of a group can have large influences on that group.

We strongly value an evidence-informed approach to implementation itself (Grol and Grimshaw 2003). By this, we mean that evidence about implementation should be used to guide implementation. Far too often implementation simply involves practitioners deciding what seems like a good way to facilitate use of evidence-informed practice without any attempt to look at the literature on what is known about effective strategies to bring about implementation. If the expectation is that practice should be evidence-informed, there should be an equally strong expectation that implementation of those practices should be evidence-informed. This is where everyone responsible for implementation should have some understanding of implementation science – which is the study of methods to promote the integration of research findings and evidence into healthcare policy and practice. It seeks to understand the behavior of healthcare professionals and other stakeholders as a key variable in the sustainable uptake, adoption, and implementation of evidence-based interventions (Fogarty International Center-National Institutes of Health 2019). In subsequent chapters, where appropriate, you will see references to what we know from research about effective ways to support implementation of best practice.

At the same time, we believe that evidence-informed implementation efforts should be pragmatic while being methodologically rigorous. For example, due diligence must be done to determine there is sufficiently strong evidence supporting the proposed best practice to justify its implementation into practice. Implementing practices that are not sufficiently evidence-informed run the risk of causing greater harm or expense than benefit. When thinking about the implementation process, you will see how local data and information are required at each phase and stage to inform the implementation plan. We advocate that this data collection should be as sufficiently rigorous as needed to ensure the information is valid and reliable – this should not be meant to imply we are promoting only the use of the most rigorous methods. Some like to argue for being "quick and dirty" in collecting these data. We reject this in favor of the concept of "quick and good." By "good" we mean accurate, reliable, valid, and relevant information that is good enough. In this information gathering the intent should be to balance rigor and what is reasonable and possible to obtain locally.

In some cases, it may be prudent to seek ethics approval to collect the data if the organization considers this sort of data collection beyond what might be done under clinical circumstances or quality improvement initiatives. If the intent is to eventually publish the data, then having Research Ethics Board (REB) approval may also be helpful since some journals will not publish papers unless REB approval has been given. In other cases, collecting these data falls under the quality improvement paradigm of the organization and are exempt from REB review or subject to an expedited review. The key is to understand the difference between what the organization considers research and quality improvement to guide implementation plans and efforts accordingly.

Our experience has been that leadership is a key ingredient for successful evidence activation. Leadership for implementation can come from those in formal positions of authority such as the health system executives, Chief Nursing Officers, Program Directors, and Unit Managers but also from practitioners at the point-of-care such as Advanced Practice Nurses, Clinical Nurse Specialists, educators, staff nurses and unregulated workers. There is a growing body of literature on the role formal leaders can play in bringing about and maintaining change (Gifford et al. 2007, 2013, 2014a, b, 2017; Tistad et al. 2016). Not surprisingly, organizational leaders set strategic directions and can include the use of best practices within the strategic priorities. They can assign individuals to be responsible for implementation and create performance expectations and incentives for the desired actions. They can sanction behavior that does not adhere to best practices. Importantly they have capacity to provide the resources (staff and funding) to support implementation and its sustainability. And finally, they can role model evidence-informed decision making, and be seen to support the implementation of best practices. However, leaders can also be a barrier because they have the power to obstruct especially when there may be competing organizational priorities. They are pivotal in moving change forward or preventing it at all. Gifford et al. (2017) have a useful framework for thinking about how to influence point-of-care and senior managers so that they can encourage and support evidence-informed practice by their staff, which will be discussed further in Appendix 4.A.

In addition, our experience has been that implementation of best practice does not happen without some form of implementation facilitation. Many think that facilitation is an individual who supports, promotes, encourages uptake of best practices. We conceptualize facilitation as a process that maybe undertaken by individuals or teams and is more about what is involved in facilitation than who does it. Appendix 4.A also elaborates on the roles of facilitation in the implementation of evidence.

The value of planning for implementation cannot be overstated. The Roadmap framework breaks down the process into manageable components and identifies what data and actions may be required or helpful to proceed. There is less chance that important steps may be missed by systematically thinking through implementation efforts. Importantly this prompts attention and actions for all involved, and all who may be impacted, to understand the big picture and how they fit into it. The reality is that change usually takes longer than expected. When staff and managers understand where the organization is going (from an implementation perspective) and the role they must play in changes, they are better equipped to participate and meet the expectations set out for them.

One last consideration as researchers, we think it is important to note that in addition to data and information that is available locally from population and administrative sources, there is potential for doing research throughout these phases. It can assist in understanding the population and health environment, ensuring the use of research in selecting best practices and implementation strategies, and measuring best practice use and impact. Not surprisingly along this journey there can be many opportunities for collaborations with researchers during an implementation initiative. You may find that researchers can serve as coaches to facilitate the implementation of evidence informed practice by asking questions, offering suggestions, problem-solving, serving as a "neutral" external voice, advocating to decision-makers, providing methodological and scientific support, and resources through grants to conduct full-scale evaluations. The *modus operandi* for research support is "informed responsiveness," not for researchers to be prescriptive. Harvey and Kitson (2015) have also noted how researchers can serve as external implementation facilitators. The researcher should always be in an assisting role when working *with* a local team not doing it for them. On the other hand, collaboration with researchers is not essential given successful implementation can also occur without researchers' involvement. Decisions about inviting researchers along for the journey should always be about how they can contribute and add value to the process but not necessarily lead it.

Hopefully, this chapter has provided an understanding of the three Phases and stages of Roadmap, and you are ready and excited to get on your way. The next chapters are devoted to each of the stages and tasks in Roadmap and provide the details of what needs to be done and how the activities might be accomplished. Each chapter concludes with a grid style action planning tool to track processes and results called the Action Map (see Tables 4.1–4.3). As well, there is a concrete example from a pressure injury implementation included in the chapters that follow. The Action Map serves as a day-to-day work tool and in-progress plan. Also, the Action Map can be incorporated into an overall Implementation Plan that details your approach. With this overview of Roadmap, it is time to delve into the processes involved with the implementation of evidence-informed practice.

Table 4.1 Phase 1: ACTION MAP for issue identification and clarification.

Call-to-Action *Thinking about clinical issue, get various perspectives from working group*	External Recommendations *Discuss & identify clinical issue, get external evidence (broadly)*	Assemble local evidence about setting, care providers, & population	Current practice *(audit, focus group, observation)*	Gaps *Discrepancy between recommendation and current practice*
Insert key information about issues, potential working group	Insert actual external recommendations	Understand the magnitude of the issue, provider considerations caring for these people	Understand how the issue is currently being managed	Decide whether to address the gap and how
	1.			
	2.			
	3. Etc.			
Sustainability thinking starts here. . .				
Chapter 5	Chapter 6	Chapter 7	Chapter 7	Chapter 7

Table 4.2 Phase 2: ACTION MAP for solution building.

Adopted recommendations *Operationalization of recommendation*	Customize recommendations by aligning them with context to become local best practice intervention *(who, what/how, when/timing)*	Barriers & facilitating factors (drivers)	Implementation Strategies & Field Testing
Guideline/ recommendations selected for local use	Guideline/ recommendations customized for local use	Factors related to each recommendation, context, or potential adopters. *Determine what would aid or prevent implementation*	Implementation strategies are mapped, tailored and field tested.
1.			
2.			
3. etc.			
Sustainability thinking continues here. . .			
Chapter 8	Chapters 8 and 9	Chapters 8 and 9	Chapter 10 (+ appendix), 11, 12

Table 4.3 Phase 3: ACTION MAP for implementing, evaluating and sustaining.

(for reference)	Deploy & monitor implementation strategies *(conduct Process Evaluation)*	Measure outcomes. What is adherence to the best practice? *(Outcomes Evaluation of knowledge use indicators)*	Measure impact *(Impact Evaluation)*
Customized Recommendations	Full-scale implementation of field-tested strategies. Make adjustments to strategies as needed.	Monitor uptake/ adherence of the best practices.	Analyze impact over set period (Impact Evaluation). Develop a report & seek endorsement for ongoing use of best practice.
1.			
2.			
3. Etc.			
Sustainability thinking continues here. . .			
	Chapter 13	Chapter 13	Chapter 13

Appendix 4.A: Leadership for Implementation and Facilitation of Implementation

Leadership for Implementation

It is being increasingly recognized that leaders have an important role to play in promoting the uptake and maintenance of best practice by their subordinates. Wendy Gifford at the University of Ottawa and colleagues recently published a mixed methods systematic review of leadership behaviors related to nurses and allied health professionals' use of research (Gifford et al. 2018). The search yielded 7019 articles of which 31 studies reported in 34 articles were included in the review. The methods used in the studies were qualitative ($n = 19$), cross-sectional survey ($n = 9$), and mixed methods ($n = 3$). Studies were conducted in Canada ($n = 14$), Sweden ($n = 6$), USA ($n = 5$), China ($n = 1$), Mongolia ($n = 1$), the Netherlands ($n = 1$) and in multiple European countries ($n = 1$). All studies included nurses, and six also included allied health professionals. In terms of the quality of the studies, 20 were rated as strong (65%), seven were high-moderate (23%), two (6%) were low-moderate, and only one (3%) was rated as weak.

Twelve leadership behaviors were extracted from the data for point-of-care managers and 10 for senior managers (See Table 4.A.1 below). The findings reveal that managers performed a diverse range of leadership behaviors that encompassed change-oriented, relation-oriented and task-oriented behaviors. The most commonly described behavior was support for the change, which involved demonstrating conceptual and operational commitment to research-based practices.

Table 4.A.1 Leadership behaviors studied in association with research use by clinical staff.

Point-of-care managers' leadership behavior	Quantitative studies (n = 8)	Mixed methods (n = 2)	Qualitative studies (n = 15)	Total no. (n = 26)
Change-oriented leadership behaviors				
• Align with organizational mission/vision	–	–	6	6
• Build coalitions with inter-professional colleagues	–	1	8	9
• Participate in planning implementation strategies	–	1	6	7
• Support the change	4 [2+/2−]	1	13	18
Relation-oriented leadership behaviors				
• Communicate with staff	1 [−]	2	8	11
• Encourage	1 [+]	1	7	9
• Emotionally intelligent leadership	4 [1+/3−]	–	–	4

(Continued)

Table 4.A.1 (Continued)

Point-of-care managers' leadership behavior	Quantitative studies (*n* = 8)	Mixed methods (*n* = 2)	Qualitative studies (*n* = 15)	Total no. (*n* = 26)
Task-oriented leadership behaviors				
● Embed practices in policy	–	–	3	3
● Distribute work fairly	1 [+]	–	–	1
● Monitor indicators	–	1	5	6
● Provide resources	–	1	3	4
● Support learning activities	–	1	6	7
Senior managers' leadership behaviors	Quantitative studies (n = 1)	Mixed methods (n = 1)	Qualitative studies (n = 11)	Total no. (n = 13)
Change-oriented leadership behaviors				
● Align with organizational mission/vision	–	–	5	5
● Build coalitions with inter-professional colleagues	–	–	4	4
● Participate in planning implementation	–	–	2	2
● Support the change	1 [+]	–	7	8
Relation-oriented leadership behaviors				
● Communicate with staff	–	–	3	3
● Encourage	–	–	2	2
Task-oriented leadership behaviors				
● Embed practice in policies	1 [+]	–	3	4
● Monitor indicators	–	–	1	1
● Provide resources	–	1[+]	1	2
● Support learning activities	–	1 [+]	3	4

[+] association statistically significant, *[−]* association not statistically significant
Reprinted with permission under the terms of the Creative Commons Attribution License (http://creativecommons.org/licenses/by/4.0) from Gifford et al. (2018).

Note how the implementation leadership behaviors in Table 4.A.1 are ones working groups are also encouraged to exhibit themselves (as leaders of change) or to promote among organizational leaders when following Roadmap to implement best practice. For example, under *change-oriented leadership behaviors*, we suggest that working groups find ways to align the implementation with organizational mission and or vision and to build coalitions with inter-professional colleagues as well as patients and other stakeholders (the Call to Action stage is all about developing these coalitions). The working group is urged to encourage leaders to participate in planning implementation strategies and to support best practice and its implementation. In terms of *relation-oriented leadership behaviors*, our approach to Roadmap also emphasizes the key role of communicating with staff and other stakeholders and continuously encouraging potential adopters (or leaders) about the change. Roadmap does not explicitly address emotionally intelligent leadership but the participatory and engaged nature to implementation required if following Roadmap does require emotionally intelligent leadership by the working group and other organizational leaders who should be involved. Finally, specific to *task-oriented leadership behaviors*, Roadmap encourages embedding best practices in policy as an implementation strategy, encourages the working group to work with leaders to encourage them to provide resources and support learning activities (and other implementation strategies). Roadmap also highlights the importance of monitoring process/implementation, outcome/effectiveness and impact indicators (several chapters are devoted to the role of evaluation) as the data generated can be used to manage performance and better direct change. The task-oriented leadership behavior of distributing work fairly is not addressed by Roadmap. Although working groups will be challenged to be effective if work is not fairly distributed among working group members. In summary, most of the change-oriented, relation-oriented and task-oriented behaviors for implementation identified by the review apply to either the leadership behaviors of the working group or the organizational leaders with whom the group is working, or both.

During PhD studies, Gifford became intrigued with the role of leadership and research use. Over the past 15 years Dr. Gifford has been developing, revising, refining, and testing what has become known as the Ottawa Model of Implementation Leadership (O-MILe) (Figure 4.A.1), a theoretical model based on leadership theory and empirical research (Gifford et al. 2006, 2013, 2017, 2019; Tistad et al. 2016; Hu et al. 2019a). One of us (IDG) has been part of this interesting journey which explains why our approach to implementation always includes engaging managers and leaders in implementation efforts, the sooner the better.

Originally known as the Gifford model, it was developed in a qualitative grounded theory study that compared and contrasted the activities of nursing leaders in nine health care organizations (hospitals, home care, and long-term care) that successfully or unsuccessfully implemented and sustained the use of evidence-based recommendations from clinical practice guidelines (Gifford et al. 2006). Based on the analysis, leadership for successful implementation involved the following: (i) facilitating staff, (ii) creating a positive climate, and (iii) influencing organizational structures and processes.

The first-generation Gifford model was then integrated with behavioral leadership theory and change theories, and a second-generation model was developed that explicated three meta-categories of effective leadership (Gifford et al. 2008). Supported by decades of research, the three meta-categories of effective leadership are: (i) relations-oriented, (ii) change-oriented, and (iii) task-oriented leadership behaviors (Yukl 2013). Relations-oriented behaviors include supporting, developing skills, and recognizing others and their

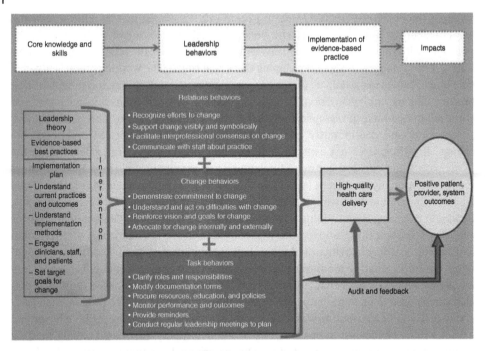

Figure 4.A.1 The O-MILe. *Source:* Reprinted with permission from Gifford et al. (2017). © 2017 Gifford et al. This work is published and licensed by Dove Medical Press Limited.

contributions to increase mutual trust, cooperation among members, and commitment to a unit and organization. Change-oriented behaviors are concerned with integrating a vision, demonstrating commitment, building coalitions to support change, and creating a sense of need. Task-oriented behaviors include planning, clarifying roles, monitoring operations and performance, and efficiently using resources. The leadership process hypothesized in the second-generation model influences individuals, the practice environment, and the organizational infrastructure to address barriers and implement evidence-informed practice.

Based on the second-generation Gifford model, a leadership intervention was developed and piloted in a mixed-methods study with an embedded cluster randomized control trial (Gifford et al. 2013). The purpose of the intervention was to develop a leadership process among frontline managers and clinical leaders to implement evidence-informed nursing care for diabetic foot ulcers. The leadership intervention showed promise, with statistically significant increases in best practice observed in the intervention group. In the intervention, managers and clinical leaders prioritized which practices needed to change based on evidence/practice gaps in care and developed detailed leadership action plans with measurable short-term goals of change. Qualitative data expanded the findings and showed that leaders in the intervention group used more relations- and change-oriented leadership behaviors than leaders in the control group. Specific strategies included communicating more with staff, recognizing efforts, demonstrating commitment, and reinforcing goals for change. These findings were then integrated into the third-generation Gifford leadership model (Gifford et al. 2013). However, results showed there was still a need for further refinement on how to develop implementation leadership.

In 2013, a group of implementation science researchers and organizational decision makers from the US, Sweden, and Canada convened at the University of Ottawa, for a three-day planning meeting to clarify and refine the key components of a leadership intervention for implementing evidence-informed practice (Gifford et al. 2014c). Using principles from the Medical Research Council Complex Interventions Framework (Craig et al. 2008, 2013), tacit knowledge from the experiences of organizational decision makers was synthesized with findings from the broader research on leadership and implementation science to identify components of an intervention for developing implementation leadership that were salient to both researchers and organizational decision makers. Combined with relations, change, and task-oriented leadership behaviors from our previous work, a fourth-generation model was developed and revised as the O-MILe. In addition to specifying the leadership behaviors, the O-MILe identifies the knowledge and skills that are necessary for leaders to conduct the behaviors and facilitate implementation (Gifford et al. 2017). The O-MILe postulates that for successful implementation, front-line leaders require the knowledge of effective leadership practices, site-specific evidence-practice gaps, implementation strategies, and planned change processes, including barriers management. Leaders must additionally have skills to prioritize change, set goals and target outcomes, engage patients and staff, and develop an implementation plan. The knowledge and skills portrayed in the O-MILe are described as the key components of a leadership intervention for participants to develop relations-, change-, and task-oriented leadership behaviors for implementing best practice in health care settings.

Incorporating primary research with theoretical and empirical evidence from leadership and planned action theories, the O-MILe provides a theoretical foundation for developing and operationalizing unit-level leadership to implement best practice in health care settings, identifying both the knowledge and skills required to develop implementation leadership and the specific behaviors required for practice. Concepts within the O-MILe are consistent with research showing that leaders who focus on individualized consideration (Kouzes and Posner 2003), are proactive and present (Aarons et al. 2015), and address barriers to change have a greater capacity for successfully implementing change (Baker et al. 2015), themes also evident in Roadmap.

Concepts within the O-MILe have been conceptually aligned to the items of the Implementation Leadership Scale (ILS), an empirically validated tool for measuring implementation leadership (Aarons et al. 2014). All 12 items of the ILS correspond to at least one O-MILe concept, demonstrating compatibility of the ILS as a measurement tool for the O-MILe constructs (Gifford 2017). Used together, the O-MILe and ILS provide an evidence- and theory-based approach for developing and measuring leadership for implementing evidence-based practices in health care.

We have used the ILS with the O-MILe in a feasibility study to develop implementation leadership knowledge and skills of nurses and supportive care staff to implement evidence-based fall prevention practices in a residential long term care setting in Ontario, Canada (Gifford et al. 2019). The leadership intervention was feasible to deliver and useful to participants with supportive and perseverant leadership items, the highest rated items in the ILS for individual leadership development.

The O-MILe has also been used as the foundation in a leadership intervention for nurse managers to implement evidence based pain management practices in infants and children in a large acute care hospital in Shanghai China (Hu et al. 2019a). The ILS was translated into Chinese through a systematic process which provided a deep understanding of leadership for implementing evidence informed practices in the Chinese nursing context (Hu et al. 2019b).

For each and every phase and stage of Roadmap, it is important to always consider how to engage point of care leaders and managers as well as executives in understanding evidence informed practice, the process of implementation and the role they play or can play in bringing about change. This is particularly important when calls to action are coming from the ground up (as opposed to ones that are from the top down). But even when the call to action is from the top, all leaders may still need to be actively engaged and encouraged to support Roadmap phases. It is our experience that some leaders may not appreciate or have all the implementation support skills to be totally effective as they have not considered leading implementation as one of their roles. The O-MILe offers a relatively simple framework focused on leaders and what they can do to promote best practice use by staff that is extremely complementary to the goals and advice of Roadmap.

Facilitation of Implementation

Facilitation is judged essential for implementation of best practices to occur. Generally, facilitation is described as an enabling process. In our experience, we consider it a challenging and complex activity in the journey to evidence-informed practice. Harvey and Kitson (2015) call it the "active ingredient" in implementation. Facilitation as a process, dynamically engages key stakeholders in implementation in a meaningful manner to advance evidence-informed practice and be part of co-creating it. Because of this engagement and interactional process with stakeholders Berta and colleagues (2015) suggest a more far reaching impact. Facilitation's "promise" is with promotion of higher order learning in organizations, i.e. facilitation with small-scale implementations may lead to organizational learning (Berta et al. 2015). Table 4.A.2 displays some of the definitions used in research and theory papers.

Early written works mainly described an individual as a facilitator, but more recently authors describe the concept as a "role" (Tiberg et al. 2017) or a "role and process" taken on by an individual or group (Dogherty et al. 2010, 2012). In their ground-breaking 1998 paper, Kitson et al. (1998) described facilitation along with the nature of the evidence, and the quality of the context, as necessary elements in their framework to enable successful implementation of evidence. This group further developed the notion of facilitation seeing it as a change agent role involving a range of activities from task-focused ones (e.g. providing practical help, episodic contact) to a broader concept of holistic, wider focus facilitation (e.g. sustaining partnerships, enabling personal development) (Harvey et al. 2002).

Elizabeth Dogherty had a special interest in facilitation and had witnessed a number of failed implementations on the nursing unit. To understand facilitation, we studied a natural experiment of facilitation. First, though, we undertook a systematic review of theory and research papers focused on facilitation (Dogherty et al. 2010). At the time, the review was an update of Harvey's germinal work, and these two were further built on in a review by Cranley et al. (2017). After the review and in working through the Roadmap phases in relation to facilitation, our group concluded that (Dogherty et al. 2010):

- Facilitation is both an individual role as well as a process involving individuals and groups.
- Project management and leadership are important.
- Facilitation must be tailored to the local context, no matter whether a person or group is facilitating.
- Evaluation and linking outcomes to action is key to facilitation i.e. nurses seeing positive effects because of the change to best practice.

In the natural experiment, we followed sites engaged in the implementation of a chosen nursing guideline. We tracked the internal and external facilitation engaged in by these sites as they proceeded with implementation using the three phases of Roadmap. Support was provided by us as requested but essentially the sites were independently implementing their guideline and allowing us to be informed observers. Our intent was to understand the practical approaches they were using and to observe the facilitation strategies they selected and tailored by themselves. It was a mixed method study using case audit, stakeholder interviews and focus groups. The focus groups were intended to fill in some of the blanks on the case audit findings. The participants were most forthcoming and provided helpful real-time data to further refine CAN-IMPLEMENT and add to Roadmap. What we found from this study about facilitation activities falls into the following four major categories:

Table 4.A.2 Examples of facilitation definitions over time.

Author(s)	Definition Statement
Kitson et al. (1998)	"A technique by which one person makes things easier for others" (Kitson et al. 1998, p. 152)
Harvey et al. (2002)	"The process of enabling (making easier the implementation of evidence into practice." (Harvey et al. 2002, p. 579)
Caldwell (2003)	"an internal or external individual or team responsible for initiating, sponsoring, directing, managing or implementing a specific change initiative, project or complete change programme" (Caldwell 2003, p. 139; Lessard et al. 2016)
Stetler et al. (2006)	"A deliberate and valued process of interactive problem solving and support that occurs in the context of a recognized need for improvement and a supportive interpersonal relationship." (Stetler et al. 2006, p. 1)
Dogherty et al. (2010)	Facilitation is described as . . . "supporting and enabling practitioners to improve practice through evidence implementation." (Dogherty et al. 2010, p. 76)
Harvey and Kitson (2015)	". . . to make things easier for others through clarifying what has to be done, how best to do it and how to reflect and learn from that process . . .. without taking responsibility" (Harvey and Kitson 2015, Chapter 5, p. 75)
Lessard et al. (2016)	"Facilitation is an approach used by appointed individuals, which teams can also foster, to build capacity and support practice change. Within organizational contexts. It encompasses a broad array of roles, oriented toward both implementing change and supporting individuals or groups." (Lessard et al. 2016, p. 1)
Cranley et al. (2017)	". . . facilitation as an innovation and its potential to support an integrated, collaborative approach to improving healthcare delivery." (Cranley et al. 2017, p. 1)

1) Planning for change
2) Leading and managing change
3) Monitoring progress and ongoing implementation
4) Evaluating change.

The full quota of 51 activities under these four groupings can be found in Table 4.A.3 (Dogherty et al. 2012, p. 7).

Table 4.A.3 Facilitating done on study sites.

Planning for change

Increasing awareness

1) Highlighting a need for practice change
2) Selecting an area for change relevant to staff/recognized as a priority
3) Stimulating critical inquiry and assisting groups to develop/refine specific clinical practice questions
4) Assisting with/performing a formal/ informal practice audit
5) Interpreting baseline data and providing feedback/insight into performance gaps
6) Emphasizing enhanced patient outcomes as opposed to poor practice as reason for change

Developing a plan

7) Goal-setting and assisting with development of an action plan
8) Helping identify and determine solutions to address potential barriers to evidence-based practice
9) Displaying and generating enthusiasm at the start of the project
10) Thinking ahead in the process

Leading and managing change

Knowledge and data management

11) Knowledge translation/dissemination (assisting with conducting literature searches, obtaining articles, appraising and summarizing the evidence)
12) Helping to interpret the research and apply it in practice
13) Providing resources/tools for change

Project management

14) Identifying a leader
15) Establishing and allocating roles/ delegating responsibilities
16) Advocating for resources and change

Recognizing the importance of context

17) Creating an open, supportive, and trusting environment conducive to change
18) Helping to build in the structures/ processes to support staff and help them overcome obstacles
19) Creating local ownership of change
20) Assisting with adapting evidence to the local context
21) Boundary spanning (addressing organizational systems/culture), managing the different requirements of each discipline/role
22) Tailoring/adapting facilitation services to the local setting

Fostering team-building/group dynamics

23) Relationship building
24) Encouraging effective teamwork
25) Enabling individual and group development
26) Encouraging/ensuring adequate participation
27) Increasing awareness of and helping overcome resistance to change
28) Consensus building (shared decision-making)

Table 4.A.3 (Continued)

Leading and managing change

Increasing awareness	*Developing a plan*
Administrative and project-specific support	
29) Organizing/scheduling meetings	32) General planning
30) Leading/participating in meetings	33) Providing skills training
31) Gathering information and assembling/distributing reports and materials	34) Taking on specific tasks

Monitoring progress and ongoing implementation

Problem solving	*Providing support*
35) Problem solving and addressing specific issues	38) Mentoring and role-modeling evidence-based practice
36) Making changes to the developed plan as necessary	39) Maintaining momentum and enthusiasm
37) Networking	40) Acknowledging ideas and efforts
	41) Providing ongoing support/ reassurance and constructive feedback
Effective communication	42) Empowering group members
46) Providing regular communication (emails, phone calls)	43) Providing advice/guidance/ assistance
47) Keeping group members informed	44) Being available as needed
48) Acting as a liaison	45) Ensuring group remains on task and things are not missed (process/ methodology is followed)

Evaluating change

Assessment

49) Performing/assisting with evaluation
50) Linking evidence implementation to patient outcomes
51) Acknowledging success, recognizing, and celebrating achievements

Reprinted with permission under the terms of the Creative Commons Attribution License (https://creativecommons.org/licenses/by/2.0) from Dogherty et al. (2012).

Activities were performed by both internal or external facilitators or sometimes both. Interestingly activities not previously identified in the theory or research literature were found. See Table 4.A.4 from Dogherty et al. (2012, p. 8).

Practically speaking, some of the most helpful information came directly from the people facilitating when they were asked, "what were the key activities in their efforts implementing evidence-informed practice." They emphasized the patient outcomes rather than poor practice as the reason for change. It was important to have a strong "leader" – . . . "right person with right knowledge. . . someone with street credibility." Helping to overcome resistance to change was important and this started with some awareness there actually was resistance. Communication was considered vital throughout and this meant folks were getting all the

Table 4.A.4 Missing and new elements not previously found in the literature.

Activities for which no documented evidence was found in the case-audit data of being performed by recognized facilitators	New activities identified as performed by recognized facilitators
Interpreting baseline data and providing feedback/insight into performance gaps	Displaying and generating enthusiasm at the start of the project
Creating an open, supportive, and trusting environment conducive to change	Thinking ahead in the process
Linking evidence implementation to patient outcomes	Taking on specific tasks
	Being available as needed
Acknowledging success, recognizing and celebrating achievements	Ensuring group remains on task and things are not missed

appropriate materials in a timely manner. The facilitators told us that both the working group and affiliated stakeholders needed to be kept in the loop especially, because if and when issues arise, facilitators need to be networking to secure support as required. One facilitator described being a cheerleader – it was about the coaching and keeping people motivated to maintain momentum and enthusiasm. Another crucial aspect was ensuring the group remains on task and things are not missed.

In summary, the various explorations we undertook into facilitation that was happening in a natural way, provided extremely valuable information that informed both CAN-IMPLEMENT and Roadmap and were built into our processes. There is nothing like experiential knowledge!

Internal, External, and Partnered Facilitation

Three types of facilitation are described in the implementation literature, internal, external, and partnered (internal and external) facilitation (Cranley et al. 2017). Internal facilitation has occurred informally for a long time in nursing with facilitation of best practices often embedded in the roles of nurse educators, advanced practice nurses, and clinical manager roles for example. Early on, in the 1990s as the evidence-based practice movement was taking hold we saw distinct roles emerge that were focused on evidence to practice facilitation in health care organizations. These roles were known by such titles as knowledge brokers, practice facilitators and research facilitators. Often the internal facilitator role and function are intertwined with the more general practice development role. Recently a US study across 10 hospitals described four characteristics of internal facilitation for evidence implementation: leadership, buy-in, customization, and accountability (Baloh et al. 2018). The facilitation was carried out by an individual, a team or both.

At one point we examined a sample of 28 studies in nursing where a guideline was being implemented and found that although the activities were well recognized as facilitation, they were not necessarily labeled as such (Dogherty et al. 2014). Most of them exhibited evidence of external facilitation by the research team. Stetler et al. (2006) were one of the first groups to examine the external facilitator role in a prospective observational study. In their study of a large healthcare organization, they defined *External facilitation* as facilitation that comes from a change agent outside of the implementation site such as their study team. Further they concluded that external facilitation could be described as a distinct role focused primarily on *problem solving and support* as well as integrating other implementation interventions. We have found that external facilitation can provide some of the expertise that is missing from a working group, e.g. library science searching, data management and analyses. Also, the neutrality of external facilitators can be helpful because they are not part of the setting and able to negotiate things internal facilitators might not be able to do.

As facilitation became more widespread with the best practice movement, either in formal roles or integrated into other health care roles, the combination and partnering of internal and external roles has become more prevalent. There is a belief that partnering the two is the ideal approach. We certainly have found that in our implementation work (Dogherty et al. 2012). This is supported by evidence from a study in the Veterans Affairs (VA) administration in the United States (Kirchner et al. 2014). Kirchner and colleagues study focused on primary care for mental health across multiple sites where some had partnered internal facilitation support and others only had national external support. The study authors concluded that "the addition of a highly partnered internal facilitation strategy to national level support resulted in greater Reach and Adoption of the mandated initiative, thereby increasing patient access to VA mental health care" (Kirchner et al. 2014).

The US Department of Veterans Affairs has produced an implementation facilitation training manual that offers good guidance (Ritchie et al. 2017). The manual has sections on facilitation roles; knowledge, skills and core competencies and characteristics of facilitators; facilitation activities in the pre-implementation, implementation, and sustainability phases; virtual implementation facilitation; and evaluation of the implementation facilitation strategies. Two recent studies have examined facilitation interventions (Harvey et al. 2018; Midboe et al. 2018).

Summary

Facilitation is one of the most interesting and researched aspects of implementation science. There is increasing qualitative and quantitative enquiry of facilitation to fully understand both the how to do it, as well as its effectiveness. Again, as with many aspects of evidence-informed practice, it will be context specific. The facilitation in a large teaching hospital where resources are accessible and plentiful will be different than in a rural mental health clinic. The idea of external facilitation or partnered facilitation may become infinitely more necessary. The descriptive work done by us and others on the facilitation tasks, skills and abilities will hopefully provide guidance in nominating facilitating individuals or teams for your journey to evidence-informed practice.

References

Aarons, G.A., Ehrhart, M.G., and Farahnak, L.R. (2014). The implementation leadership scale (ILS): development of a brief measure of unit level implementation leadership. *Implementation Science* 9: 10. https://doi.org/10.1186/1748-5908-9-45.

Aarons, G.A., Ehrhart, M.G., Farahnak, L.R., and Hurlburt, M.S. (2015). Leadership and organizational change for implementation (LOCI): a randomized mixed method pilot study of a leadership and organization development intervention for evidence-based practice implementation. *Implementation Science* 10: 11. https://doi.org/10.1186/s13012-014-0192-y.

Baker, R., Camosso-Stefinovic, J., Gillies, C. et al. (2015). Tailored interventions to address determinants of practice. *Cochrane Database of Systematic Reviews* (4): CD005470. https://doi.org/10.1002/14651858.CD005470.pub3.

Baloh, J., Zhu, X., and Ward, M.M. (2018). Types of internal facilitation activities in hospitals implementing evidence-based interventions. *Health Care Management Review* 43: 229–237. https://www.ncbi.nlm.nih.gov/pmc/articles/PMC6816731/.

Berta, W., Cranley, L., Dearing, J.W. et al. (2015). Why (we think) facilitation works: insights from organizational learning theory. *Implementation Science* 10: 141. https://doi.org/10.1186/s13012-015-0323-0.

Caldwell, R. (2003). Models of change agency: a fourfold classification. *British Journal of Management* 14: 131–142. https://doi.org/10.1111/1467-8551.00270.

Craig, P., Dieppe, P., Macintyre, S. et al. (2008). Developing and evaluating complex interventions: the new Medical Research Council Guidance. *British Medical Journal* 337: 979–983. https://doi.org/10.1136/bmj.a1655.

Craig, P., Dieppe, P., Macintyre, S. et al. (2013). Developing and evaluating complex interventions: the new medical research council guidance. *International Journal of Nursing Studies* 50: 587–592. https://doi.org/10.1016/j.ijnurstu.2012.09.010.

Cranley, L.A., Cummings, G.G., Profetto-McGrath, J. et al. (2017). Facilitation roles and characteristics associated with research use by healthcare professionals: a scoping review. *BMJ Open* 7: e014384. https://doi.org/10.1136/bmjopen-2016-014384.

Dogherty, E.J., Harrison, M.B., and Graham, I.D. (2010). Facilitation as a role and process in achieving evidence-based practice in nursing: a focused review of concept and meaning. *Worldviews on Evidence-Based Nursing* 7: 76–89. https://doi.org/10.1111/j.1741-6787.2010.00186.x.

Dogherty, E.J., Harrison, M.B., Baker, C., and Graham, I.D. (2012). Following a natural experiment of guideline adaptation and early implementation: a mixed-methods study of facilitation. *Implementation Science* 7: 9. https://doi.org/10.1186/1748-5908-7-9.

Dogherty, E.J., Harrison, M., Graham, I., and Keeping-Burke, L. (2014). Examining the use of facilitation within guideline dissemination and implementation studies in nursing. *International Journal of Evidence-Based Healthcare* 12: 105–127. https://doi.org/10.1097/XEB.0000000000000008.

Fogarty International Center-National Institutes of Health (2019). *Implementation Science Information and Resources*, [Online], Available: https://www.fic.nih.gov/researchtopics/pages/implementationscience.aspx (26 July 2019).

Gifford, W.A. (2017). Ottawa Model of Implementation Leadership and Implementation Leadership Scale: mapping concepts for developing and evaluating theory based leadership interventions. *Journal of Healthcare Leadership* 9: 9. https://doi.org/10.2147/jhl.s125558.

Gifford, W., Davies, B., Edwards, N., and Graham, I. (2006). Leadership strategies to influence the use of clinical practice guidelines. *Nursing Leadership* 19: 72–88. https://doi.org/10.12927/cjnl.2006.18603.

Gifford, W., Davies, B., Edwards, N. et al. (2007). Managerial leadership for nurses' use of research evidence: an integrative review of the literature. *Worldviews on Evidence-Based Nursing* 4: 126–145. https://doi.org/10.1111/j.1741-6787.2007.00095.x.

Gifford, W., Davies, B., Graham, I.D. et al. (2008). A mixed methods pilot study with a cluster randomized control trial to evaluate the impact of a leadership intervention on guideline implementation in home care nursing. *Implementation Science* 3 https://doi.org/10.1186/1748-5908-3-51.

Gifford, W.A., Davies, B.L., Graham, I.D. et al. (2013). Developing leadership capacity for guideline use: a pilot cluster randomized control trial. *Worldviews on Evidence-Based Nursing* 10: 51–65. https://doi.org/10.1111/j.1741-6787.2012.00254.x.

Gifford, W., Lefebre, N., and Davies, B. (2014a). An organizational intervention to influence evidence-informed decision making in home health nursing. *The Journal of Nursing Administration* 44: 395–402. https://doi.org/10.1097/NNA.0000000000000089.

Gifford, W.A., Holyoke, P., Squires, J.E. et al. (2014b). Managerial leadership for research use in nursing and allied health care professions: a narrative synthesis protocol. *Systematic Reviews* 3: 57. https://doi.org/10.1186/2046-4053-3-57.

Gifford, W., Graham, I., Eldh, A. and Lefebre, N. (2014c) 'Theoretical foundations of dissemination and implementation leadership: a conceptual model for leadership development.' Annual Conference on the Science of Dissemination and Implementation: Transforming Health Systems to Optimize Individual and Population Health, Bethesda, MD.

Gifford, W., Graham, I.D., Ehrhart, M.G. et al. (2017). Ottawa model of implementation leadership and implementation leadership scale: mapping concepts for developing and evaluating theory based leadership interventions. *Journal of Healthcare Leadership* 9: 15–23. https://doi.org/10.2147/jhl.s125558.

Gifford, W.A., Squires, J.E., Angus, D.E. et al. (2018). Managerial leadership for research use in nursing and allied health care professions: a systematic review. *Implementation Science* 13: 1–23. https://doi.org/10.1186/s13012-018-0817-7.

Gifford, W., Lewis, K.B., Eldh, A.C. et al. (2019). Feasibility and usefulness of a leadership intervention to implement evidence-based falls prevention practices in residential care in Canada. *Pilot and Feasibility Studies* 5: 103. https://doi.org/10.1186/s40814-019-0485-7.

Grol, R. and Grimshaw, J. (2003). From best evidence to best practice: effective implementation of change in patients' care. *Lancet* 362: 1225–1230. https://doi.org/10.1016/S0140-6736(03)14546-1.

Harrison, M.B. and Graham, I.D. (2012). Roadmap for a participatory research-practice partnership to implement evidence. *Worldviews on Evidence-Based Nursing* 9: 210–220. https://doi.org/10.1111/j.1741-6787.2012.00256.x.

Harrison, M.B., van den Hoek, J., and Graham, I.D. (2014). *CAN-IMPLEMENT: Planning for Best-Practice Implementation (Book 20)*. Philadelphia: Lippincott Williams & Wilkins.

Harvey, G. and Kitson, A. (2015). *Implementing Evidence-Based Practice in Healthcare: A Facilitation Guide*. Abingdon: Routledge.

Harvey, G., Loftus-Hills, A., Rycroft-Malone, J. et al. (2002). Getting evidence into practice: the role and function of facilitation. *Journal of Advanced Nursing* 37: 577–588. https://doi.org/10.1046/j.1365-2648.2002.02126.x.

Harvey, G., McCormack, B., Kitson, A. et al. (2018). Designing and implementing two facilitation interventions within the 'Facilitating Implementation of Research Evidence (FIRE)' study: a qualitative analysis from an external facilitators' perspective. *Implementation Science* 13: 141. https://doi.org/10.1186/s13012-018-0812-z.

Hu, J., Gifford, W., Harrison, D. et al. (2019a). 'Leadership for Implementing Evidence-Based Pediatric Pain Management: An International Research Program.' *Sigma Theta Tau International Congress*, Calgary, Alberta: Sigma Theta Tau International Congress.

Hu, J., Gifford, W., Ruan, H. et al. (2019b). Translation and linguistic validation of the implementation leadership scale in Chinese nursing context. *Journal of Nursing Management* 27: 1030–1038. https://doi.org/10.1111/jonm.12768.

Kirchner, J.E., Ritchie, M.J., Pitcock, J.A. et al. (2014). Outcomes of a partnered facilitation strategy to implement primary care-mental health. *Journal of General Internal Medicine* 29 (Suppl 4): 904–912. https://doi.org/10.1007/s11606-014-3027-2.

Kitson, A., Harvey, G., and McCormack, B. (1998). Enabling the implementation of evidence based practice: a conceptual framework. *Quality in Health Care* 7: 149–158. https://doi.org/10.1136/qshc.7.3.149.

Kouzes, J. and Posner, B. (2003). *The Leadership Challenge*. San Francisco, CA: Jossey-Bass.

Lessard, S., Bareil, C., Lalonde, L. et al. (2016). External facilitators and interprofessional facilitation teams: a qualitative study of their roles in supporting practice change. *Implementation Science* 11: 97. https://doi.org/10.1186/s13012-016-0458-7.

Midboe, A.M., Martino, S., Krein, S.L. et al. (2018). Testing implementation facilitation of a primary care-based collaborative care clinical program using a hybrid type III interrupted time series design: a study protocol. *Implementation Science* 13: 145. https://doi.org/10.1186/s13012-018-0838-2.

Ritchie, M.J., Dollar, K.M., Miller, C.J. et al. (2017). *Using Implementation Facilitation to Improve Care in the Veterans Health Administration*: Veterans Health Administration, Quality Enhancement Research Initiative (QUERI) for Team-Based Behavioral Health. Available at: https://www.queri.research.va.gov/tools/implementation/Facilitation-Manual.pdf.

Stetler, C.B., Legro, M.W., Rycroft-Malone, J. et al. (2006). Role of "external facilitation" in implementation of research findings: a qualitative evaluation of facilitation experiences in the Veterans Health Administration. *Implementation Science* 1: 23. https://doi.org/10.1186/1748-5908-1-23.

Tiberg, I., Hansson, K., Holmberg, R., and Hallstrom, I. (2017). An ethnographic observation study of the facilitator role in an implementation process. *BMC Research Notes* 10: 630. https://doi.org/10.1186/s13104-017-2962-5.

Tistad, M., Palmcrantz, S., Wallin, L. et al. (2016). Developing leadership in managers to facilitate the implementation of national guideline recommendations: a process evaluation of feasibility and usefulness. *International Journal of Health Policy and Management* 5: 477–486. https://doi.org/10.15171/ijhpm.2016.35.

Yukl, G. (2013). *Leadership in organizations*, 8e. Upper Saddle River, New Jersey: Prentice Hall.

Part 1

Phase I: Issue Identification and Clarification

5

The Call-to-Action

Introduction

In the last chapter you were introduced to Roadmap as a guide to Evidence-Informed Practice. This chapter begins Phase I of Roadmap and is about understanding the importance and necessity of a group coalescing around the concern with care and converting this into a common desire to do something about it. This generally is the first step in the evidence implementation journey.

Implementing evidence is usually not an aim or an end in itself. Nor does it arise out of the blue. Typically, it is set in motion in one of two ways (Graham et al. 2006). One way is when new evidence emerges and becomes available that should guide care. This could be in the form of a new practice guideline or an evidence-informed protocol. The other way is when an indication arises from local data about a problem, from providers' impressions and concerns, or from red flags related to the use of resources. For example, a potential issue or concern with care may become obvious from unit or program quality reports or when change is observed in risk data reported at regular intervals.

To illustrate this point, let us take the example of pressure injury prevention, a quality of care issue across many sectors of care. In some settings, the release of guideline recommendations from reliable government and professional bodies recommending regular head-to-toe skin assessments (one of the key best practice recommendations) may provide the impetus to organize care differently to implement this recommendation. While in other settings, risk management data showing a rise in pressure injury occurrence rates precipitates establishment of benchmarks and then leads the setting to seek out best practices for pressure injuries spurring the adoption of an available guideline or guideline recommendations. Whether the impetus is the release of new best practice recommendations or wanting to better respond to an existing issue or problem, both fuel a focus for teams to begin looking at available external research and local evidence for planning to improve care.

Turning to best available practice housed in appropriate guidelines is both an approach and a potential solution (or part of a solution) for care improvement. Finding this evidence and appraising it for use is an instrumental step toward evidence implementation (described more in Chapter 6).

Knowledge Translation in Nursing and Healthcare: A Roadmap to Evidence-informed Practice, First Edition. Margaret B. Harrison and Ian D. Graham.

Goal: The intent during the Call-to-Action stage is to galvanize interest and generate widespread support to tackle the issue that has been raised. Pertinent questions at this point are:

- What exactly appears to be the issue or problem of concern from the various perspectives? And how do you know?
- Are all the relevant stakeholders involved?
- Has a working group been struck, and does it represent the stakeholders?
- Has the Call-to-Action stage successfully galvanized interest in the issue or problem?
- Is the planning and process being driven by the stakeholders' concerns?
- Has an Action Map and Implementation Plan been developed?

Form a Working Group

The Call-to-Action is about making the issue or problem explicit and forming a committed group to work on it. To do this as a rule requires establishing and engaging a working group that will clarify the driving force behind a proposed best practice implementation and examination of your organizational context. A key element when starting any best practice implementation journey is developing a strategic alliance with all the relevant stakeholders who have an interest in the issue and a role in improving the quality of care provided. Time needed for the Call-to-Action will vary depending on the complexity of the initiative, number of units, agencies, or jurisdictions that are involved, and the characteristics of your population receiving care. It is at this juncture that you identify who needs to be involved in a working group, the availability of members, and the need to source expertise such as assistance of a library scientist. Having some members of your working group with experience with best practice implementation or guideline implementation initiatives can be a huge asset. If you do not have members with implementation experience it is advisable to find and link with those that do have this background.

When beginning an implementation initiative, it is crucial that the working group includes the right people with the expertise and authority for decision-making. In deciding on the working group, membership consideration for the following can be helpful:

- ✓ *Clinical knowledge of the topic area* (e.g. nurses, inter-professional team members) – to address issues related to application of the evidence-informed practice locally and interpret the clinical research.
- ✓ *Policy and administrative expertise* – to identify the impact of implementing the evidence-informed practice on an organization and to anticipate resource requirements resulting from implementation.
- ✓ *Methodological expertise* (e.g. health services researchers) – to apply knowledge of evaluation designs and critical appraisal and play a role in coaching other panel members on issues related to the systematic and rigorous nature of the process.
- ✓ *Information retrieval expertise* (e.g. librarian) – to access and navigate appropriate databases, conduct, and document thorough literature searches as required.

✓ *Project Management skills* – to manage timelines, meetings and conference calls, and ensure that all documents are circulated.

✓ *Facilitation and leadership skills* – to encourage constructive debate, manage group process and decision-making, maintain motivation and direction, and ensure all group members contribute and achieve panel aims. This role may be assumed by the Chair or shared with a designated facilitator or other panel members.

✓ *Implementation know-how and knowledge of implementation issues* – to develop a plan for putting the evidence into practice and spearhead the implementation.

✓ *Personal experience with the practice issue* (e.g. patients, family, and caregivers) – to ensure that issues related to patient/consumer needs are discussed, and that salient outcomes such as quality of life, pain etc. are considered.

Although it may sound simplistic and obvious, the first, and most important task of the working group is to clarify the issue that is raising concerns. This is vital and may take several weeks. It involves extensive communication, and often requires several meetings. Discussions about the targeted practice issue from relevant perspectives is vital. The manager's view may be different than the practitioner's since they have different sources of data and information and both these perspectives might be different again from the individual's or family perspective as a user of the health service. Continuing with the pressure injury example, for the manager, the issue was managing the increased unit workload with pressure injury occurrences, while at the bedside the lack of knowledge about how to accurately assess an individuals' risk, or stage a pressure injury if found, were concerns. For the patient and family, it was about the mobility and discomfort with the condition.

The working group should also begin considering other factors that may influence the course for change. Is there an organizational mandate such as an upcoming accreditation, or an educational agenda driving evidence uptake? What expectations exist at the institutional level (e.g. explicit philosophy for evidence-informed care) and what is the level of support? Is leadership supportive and committed to providing resources to pursue dealing with the issue? Perhaps most importantly, does everyone share the same definition and understanding of the role and use of evidence at your agency? Are the interests of the relevant stakeholders aligned or are some of the interests competing? These sorts of factors may inhibit or facilitate implementation in the long run. For instance, a new director may be keen to tackle a current issue arising from last month's quality report or be hesitant to as there are too many other initiatives underway and resources such as nursing time, are tight. It will be important to be aware of and sensitive to these forces. The addition of members with organizational savvy on the team can contribute to the thinking about how to get around the challenges of getting the unit or organization on board. These individuals can help figure out how to leverage existing people, initiatives, and activities.

Create the Strategic Alliance

Once you have formed a working group and identified other important key stakeholders and advisors to be involved in the implementation journey the real work begins in earnest.

Nurturing the working group will be an on-going task. We learned (sometimes the hard way), several lessons about creating strategic alliances for change that you might wish to consider in building your strategic alliance to implement evidence.

Leverage Committed Partners

The first lesson is choosing strong committed partners for the working group and understanding what may bring partners to the table. In other words, the working group members need to understand what they will get out of engaging (what you and what they get). Where possible, build on existing relationships to strengthen the partnership focused on this new issue. For example, previous experience of members working together on practice or quality committees, may make developing the working relationships easier.

Get the Mindset Right

Although clinical and practice decisions are appropriately made at the level of the individual provider and the individual with the health care issue, the approach to implementation should be focused on health system change rather than individual change. Remember that even the best-intentioned individual providers are seldom able to implement best practices on their own as they often do not have authority over others in their practice setting. They themselves might be constrained by many factors beyond their control (e.g. staffing assignments and ratios, reimbursement policies, patient/client acuity, etc.). The idea is to move away from "do it yourself thinking" – it is about a collective or team mindset to ultimately make a system change. Independent action happens but it is inter-related and should be coordinated for best results. The working group must seek full agreement on direction with the details in moving forward being worked out collectively. Note – *it is true the devil is in the details!*

Keep the Focus on the Issue

Another lesson we learned is that the focus of the working group should always be on the issue, the population, and improving care – not on singling anyone out or assigning blame. If the implementation effort is perceived to be an attempt to simply identify poor quality of care or performance and/or to be punitive, you will never succeed in getting buy-in.

Know and Share the Local Evidence

We have also learned that the use of local data and information can and should be used to get everyone on the same page and seeing the problem or issue comprehensively from all perspectives. Importantly it keeps the conversations objective and focused on solving the issue. It also reinforces the value and role of local data in evidence-informed practice. Without local data, it is too easy to be influenced by individuals' perceptions reflected by comments such as "we just know there is a problem" or "we know our practice is already evidence-based." Lastly, local data provides the basis for effectively aligning the best practices in your setting.

Build Team Capacity

Sometimes we have found there was a need to help the working group in becoming a well-functioning inter-professional team as all group members may not have acquired the skills to work in teams or had the opportunity to practice them. It may be that to achieve successful implementation, it may be necessary to build team members' capacity for evidence-informed practice and implementation. This builds confidence, trust, and an improved ability to work together.

Respect Boundaries

Finally, we have learned the need to appreciate provider and agency boundaries which includes respecting the range and scopes of practice, practice patterns, understanding boundary spanning roles, exploring the opportunities for in-reach and out-reach with care provision, and respecting financial and administrative authority. In the same way fences make for good neighbors, understanding these professional issues and boundaries makes for good professional working relationships.

Summary

This chapter described, the Call-to-Action stage as a very important early part of the Issues Identification and Clarification phase of Roadmap. To illustrate, one of our initiatives focused on a chronic wound population where there was quite a disconnect in terms of the nature of the issue. The regional managers being concerned with the disproportionately rising costs of supplies. Community nurses and case managers were concerned about their knowledge and experience in conducting a comprehensive assessment as well as the lack of necessary equipment available to them. Realizing the potential impact of wound care issues for the clients, nurses' practice, and costs to homecare provider agencies, all those involved agreed something needed to be done. With the Call-to-Action came the realization that to constructively move forward on the issue, a group with broad representation of all the relevant stakeholders needed to be formed to lead the development of an action plan. The bottom line is that awareness of practice issues and agreement about the evidence and need for change, are essential first steps for the adoption of new practices (Greenhalgh et al. 2004) and the Call-to-Action is intended to begin this process.

You will know that the Call-to-Action has been successful if you are able to conclude that:

- The issue is broadly understood from various perspectives.
- All the relevant stakeholders are involved.
- A working group has been struck and represents the stakeholders.
- The relevant partners and advisory stakeholders are identified and are aware they may be called on to engage (e.g. decision-makers, clinical experts).
- The Call-to-Action has successfully galvanized interest in the issue/problem in your setting.
- The planning is being driven by the stakeholders' issues and concerns.

Box 5.1   Working Practically with a Group

During the implementation of best practice with wound care after radiation, the group worked hard to include all key stakeholders. As the implementation crossed several hospital clinics, the emergency room and homecare, it was evident that the best practice recommendations would be carried out in different environments. After a few initial meetings it was clear that two players were missing: an infection control officer and a representative from the regional homecare authority. The group agreed that these people did not have to attend every planning meeting but could be consulted as needed and that they would be sent email notes, especially around decisions made. This kept these important stakeholders involved in a way that was feasible. Their input informed the group of the issues such as use of various modalities for storing sterile materials and the difference in products used by homecare. Practically speaking it is often helpful to have a core working group and a larger consulting group for certain meetings, if the implementation is broad and boundary crossing.

Getting Organized: Draft an Action Map

We have found that constructing and following a detailed action plan ensures that the evidence implementation journey is transparent, and all critical elements are addressed. In the last chapter we introduced the template called the Action Map. The Action Map can be used to document the major issues and considerations and the group's decisions about how to respond to them in real time. The first element of the Action Map is to compile the perspectives on the issue that emerged during the Call-to-Action. By documenting in the Action Map the types of stakeholders (e.g. patients, managers, point of care clinicians) and their differing (and concordant) perspectives helps to ensure their perspectives are all considered during the rest of the Issues Identification and Clarification phase of Roadmap. Documenting the varying perspectives for all to see serves at least three purposes: (i) when a stakeholder sees their perspective accurately reflected in print it reaffirms to them that their voice is being heard by the group, (ii) when a stakeholder reads the perspectives of other stakeholders, it provides another opportunity to understand and ideally appreciate the other perspectives. This can contribute to greater buy-in for the initiative, and (iii) having all the perspectives described in one place may encourage the group to begin considering the issue from a system's perspective, rather than from the perspective of individual stakeholders, this in turn can start to generate solutions-focused thinking within the group.

Now that you are beginning the process of Roadmap it is the time to track progress using the Action Map. It proves very useful because data and information are uncovered to document and keep up with things. The Action Map is used to build the work outline and serve as a documentation tool as groups move through their evidence implementation (see Table 5.1). It can be used as is or modified to document each step of your plan and the decisions made by your group. Information about the questions from the meetings held and dialogs with stakeholders should be documented. As you read through the Roadmap phases, we provide an example (pressure injury prevention recommendations) of the type of information to track. More columns of information are added to the Action Map as you

Table 5.1 Phase I: ACTION MAP for issue identification and clarification (*with wound example*).

Call-to-Action *Thinking about clinical issue, get various perspectives from working group*	External Recommendations *Discuss & identify clinical issue, get external evidence (broadly)*	Assemble local evidence about setting, care providers, & population	Current practice *(audit, focus group, observation)*	Gaps *Discrepancy between recommendation and current practice*
Key information about issues, potential working group	Insert actual external recommendations	Understand the magnitude of the issue, provider considerations caring for these people	Understand how the issue is currently being managed	Decide whether to address the gap and how
Chief nurse concerned with increase in surgical referrals for flap repairs. Clinical nurses anecdotally reporting ++pressure injuries	1. Head to toe skin assessment every 24 hours			
	2. Conduct pressure injury risk assessment using validated scale			
Nurse managers concerned with use of pressure relieving devices	3. Etc.			
Info about population at risk unknown, # hospital patients with pressure injury not known				
Sustainability thinking starts here. . .	External evidence on best practice provides a benchmark for ongoing quality assessment. Select recommendations that could be sustained			
Chapter 5	Chapter 6	Chapter 7	Chapter 7	Chapter 7

move through the chapters following from Phase I: Issues Identification and Clarification into Phase II: Build Solutions and Field Test them, through to Phase III: Implement, Evaluate, and Sustain. Our experience is that it (or some other type of work tool) provides a helpful work-in-progress check and trail to provide historical notes on tasks and activities completed. Also, this is the time when you can use the Action Map information to update your overall Implementation Plan (e.g. record the involved stakeholders and newly formed working group members).

In the next chapter, we focus on the external evidence for best practices and describe how to find and appraise it. It will be a first and important step to be able to compare your current care with what the best available evidence suggests for the issue at hand.

References

Graham, I.D., Logan, J., Harrison, M.B. et al. (2006). Lost in knowledge translation: time for a map? *The Journal of Continuing Education in the Health Professions* 26: 13–24. https://doi.org/10.1002/chp.47.

Greenhalgh, T., Robert, G., Bate, P. et al. (2004). *How to spread good ideas* – A systematic review of the literature on diffusion, dissemination and sustainability of innovations in health service delivery and organisation. Report for the National Co-ordinating centre for NHS Service Delivery and Organisation R & D (NCCSDO), 1–426.

6

Find the Best Practice Evidence

Introduction

Once the Call-to-Action has brought some clarification and focus to the issue, what comes next is finding the best available external evidence that can address the issue. During the Call-to Action the group starts the Action Map by identifying the stakeholders and their perspectives on the issue, and any available data and information on the issue. Stakeholders include those deciding to implement best practice (i.e. have the authority to implement), and those using the best practice (adopters). Now the task at hand is to continue with this Action Map and find the best available external data relevant to the care issue to serve as a benchmark against which current practice can be assessed. This will determine the extent of the evidence-practice gap.

Thinking back to the Knowledge to Action framework (Chapter 3) and specifically the knowledge creation funnel, evidence comes in different forms. The evidence may be at the level of primary studies, or a body of studies that has been synthesized, or in the form of a knowledge product such as a practice guideline. We will discuss appraisal processes to evaluate the quality of the external evidence. The output from this step will be a list of all relevant best practices that have been assessed for currency and content from which the working group will use for the evidence-practice gap analysis. This list will also be used as the foundation for selecting and customizing which best practices to implement (see Chapter 8).

Goal: In this phase, the intent is to identify, appraise the quality of, and assess the currency and content of the best practices (guideline recommendations) based on external evidence. The pertinent questions to consider include:

- What are the relevant best practices related to the identified issue?
- What is the quality of the best practice evidence and is it adequate?
- What is the evidence supporting each best practice recommendation and is it adequate?
- To what extent are the best practices up to date?
- What indicators can be used to measure adherence to each best practice recommendation?

At this juncture, your strategic alliance members have formed the beginning working group. This is typically a smaller, more hands-on group to move the best practice initiative forward. It is informed about the reasons why the issue surfaced, and the issue has been

Knowledge Translation in Nursing and Healthcare: A Roadmap to Evidence-informed Practice, First Edition.
Margaret B. Harrison and Ian D. Graham.
© 2021 John Wiley & Sons, Inc. Published 2021 by John Wiley & Sons, Inc.

clarified from various perspectives. Finding the best available external evidence is now essential in order to determine the best practices and then assess the magnitude of the evidence-practice gap. If you have not already included someone with literature searching expertise, you may wish to supplement the working group with library science expertise to help find and retrieve the evidence for best practices. You may also want to include more practitioners and others (e.g. methodologists), including students, who can assist with the appraisal process. They do not necessarily need to become members of the working group to participate at this point.

This stage of activity provides opportunity for the working group to come together even more as a team. The work by its very nature informs and educates everyone involved about (i) the general principles of evidence-informed practice (searching for evidence, critically appraising it, etc.), (ii) what the best practices are around the area of interest, as well as (iii) different members' strengths to potentially mentor, guide, and/or lead aspects of the implementation. By understanding the evidence and considering its relationship to your day-to-day practices there is a "meeting of the minds" where practice, management, and systems-related players (e.g. quality department, acquisitions services, etc.) focus and come together, strengthening the initial strategic alliance and working group. Successful implementation is the result of coordinated, focused, collective action.

The External Evidence

Depending on the nature of the care issue, available evidence may be at the level of primary studies (first generation knowledge), or a body of studies that has been synthesized (second generation knowledge), or in the form of a knowledge product (third generation knowledge, e.g. practice guideline) (Graham et al. 2006). If your focus is a well-recognized issue with an abundance of research in place and evidence tools such as guidelines already developed, then you should begin there. If not, you will need to travel up the funnel to evidence syntheses where studies on the topic have been amalgamated and possibly pooled and analyzed into a systematic review or meta-analysis (for quantitative research) or a meta-synthesis (for qualitative enquiries). The last option is to search for primary research in the topic of interest. Given the proliferation of guidelines, the chances are good that you will be able to find evidence in this form which will save having to synthesize primary studies which requires considerable expertise and time.

There is a set of logical steps and processes to accomplish gathering and appraising available evidence. In this chapter, we will focus on the process relative to practice guidelines and syntheses. The task with primary studies is one best left to guideline development panels with the time and resources to review the potentially dozens or even hundreds of available studies.

Sifting the Evidence Wheat from the Chaff

Practice guidelines are systematically developed statements to assist practitioner and patient decisions about appropriate health care for specific clinical circumstances (Field and Lohr 1990). In 2011, the Institute of Medicine in the United States defined clinical practice guidelines (CPGs) as "statements that include recommendations intended to optimize patient care that are informed by a systematic review of evidence and an assessment of the benefits and harms of alternative care options" (Institute of Medicine 2011). They are intended to offer concise instructions on how best to manage health conditions. We prefer the earlier description by Field and Lohr (1990), as it makes explicit that practice guidelines are to be used by practitioners and patients in making (shared) decisions about prevention, diagnosis, treatment, and palliation. The most important benefits of practice guidelines are their potential to improve both the process and quality of care provided by health care professionals and to improve patient health outcomes. However, their beneficial effects are contingent upon how they are developed, and this will be explained more when we describe the attributes of high-quality guidelines.

Health care organizations and professional bodies typically develop guidelines; thus, practitioners, and clinical managers are confronted with numerous, sometimes differing, and occasionally contradictory guidelines from which to choose. This situation may be further complicated by concerns about the poor quality of available guidelines. Adoption of guidelines with questionable validity can lead to harm to patients, inefficient use of scarce resources, and possibly ineffective interventions.

A Note on Guidelines and Standards

The working group will need to distinguish between guidelines and standards. A guideline is a set of recommendations about the most appropriate practice for a particular health condition. It should have been developed with all the relevant stakeholders, contain an interpretive summary of the evidence, recommendations about the most appropriate practice for a health condition supported by evidence, and have a transparent description of the process used to develop the recommendations, including how the evidence was interpreted and summarized. A standard on the other hand defines performance expectations and/or structure and processes that must be in place for an organization to provide safe, high-quality services across the continuum. Standards are usually organization-based documents that address service-provider education and roles, organizational behavior and health system requirements (Bahadur 2014). An example of standards in the health care industry would be accreditation standards which may or may not be grounded in evidence but are required if the organization is to become accredited. With standards, there is no latitude to not follow them.

Many documents are referred to as guidelines but may not contain the essential aspects. Practically speaking there are three defining characteristics of a quality guideline to watch for:

1) A synthesis of the body of scientific/research evidence.
2) An interpretive summary of the evidence.
3) Specific evidence-informed recommendations linked to the evidence.

We will now summarize several logical steps in how to go about appraising a practice guideline for use in your context.

Getting Started – Find Best Practices in Guidelines

By now you will have information about the motivation, purpose, and scope of the proposed initiative that will inform designing your approach. Clarity on what is driving the move to evidence-informed practice will help in defining how narrow or broad your search for appropriate guidelines needs to be. What follows draws heavily on our previous work on the ADAPTE (ADAPTE Collaboration 2009) and CAN-IMPLEMENT processes (Harrison et al. 2014) so for more detailed information please refer to these two sources.

Ideally to start, a search question is formulated by the group. A useful guide in doing this is to document the population, intervention, patients/professionals, outcomes, and health care setting(s) – PIPOH (Fervers et al. 2006). PIPOH (see Table 6.1) is based on the concepts of PICO (Population, Intervention, Control, Outcomes) (Richardson et al. 1995). PICOTS refines this approach further (Patient population, Intervention, Comparator, Outcomes, Timing, Settings) (U.S. Food and Drug Administration; Riva et al. 2012; Echevarria and Walker 2014). The term *intervention* is used broadly in nursing; we may not always be dealing with a medical or clinical intervention but rather a phenomenon of interest such as an assessment of a patient's ability to self-care, or family decisions about treatment, or management options in the home environment.

Typically, a series of search questions will be necessary to find the best available evidence and recommendations. For example: what comprises a comprehensive and feasible assessment for community nurses to carry out in the home for people requiring leg ulcer care? What is the most effective and efficient bandaging system for leg ulcer management in the community? What self-care is required to manage leg ulcers?

Using the PIPOH questions improves the precision of searching and screening for guidelines. There are trustworthy sites where you can find guidelines. See Table 6.2 for a sample of such sites. Your library scientist can also develop a strategy to search the peer-reviewed literature and the gray literature (usually non-peer reviewed documents such professional organizational documents, websites, etc.). For information on how to develop these search strategies see (Ross-White et al. 2014).

It is noteworthy that there are many health relevant databases to search. A caution – they often use different search terms for the same topic. This issue, and effective search methods are dealt with in more detail in a Library Supplement of CAN-IMPLEMENT (Ross-White et al. 2014).

Table 6.1 PIPOH.

The <u>P</u>opulation of concern and characteristics of the disease or condition

The <u>I</u>ntervention(s) or diagnostic test(s), etc. of interest

The <u>P</u>rofessionals/Patients to whom the guideline will be targeted (i.e. users)

The expected <u>O</u>utcomes including patient outcomes (e.g. improved disease-free survival, improved quality of life); system outcomes (e.g. decrease in practice variation); and/or public health outcomes (e.g. a decrease in cervical cancer incidence)

The <u>H</u>ealth care setting and context in which the guideline is to be implemented

---

Reprinted with permission from "Guideline adaptation: an approach to enhance efficiency in guideline development and improve utilisation," B Fervers, JS Burgers, R Voellinger, M Brouwers, GP Browman, ID Graham, MB Harrison, J Latreille, N Mlika-Cabane, L Paquet, L Zitzelsberger, B Burnand, The ADAPTE Collaboration, *BMJ Quality & Safety* 2011;20:228–236, ©2011, Published by the BMJ Publishing Group Limited.

Table 6.2 Selected sources of guidelines; systematic reviews, health technology assessments.

Registered Nurses' Association of Ontario (RNAO)
http://rnao.ca/bpg

Canadian Agency for Drugs and Technologies in Health (CADTH)
http://www.cadth.ca

Canadian Medical Association (CMA) Clinical Practice Guidelines CPG InfoBase
https://joulecma.ca/cpg/homepage

American Medical Association (AMA) Guideline Central
https://www.guidelinecentral.com

Canadian Task Force on Preventive Healthcare (CTFPHC)
http://www.canadiantaskforce.ca/

U.S. Preventative Services Task Force (USPSTF)
https://www.uspreventiveservicestaskforce.org

American Society of Clinical Oncology (ASCO)
http://www.asco.org/quality-guidelines

Institute for Clinical Systems Improvement (ICSI)
https://www.icsi.org/guidelines__more/

Canadian Partnership Against Cancer: Cancer Guidelines Database
https://www.partnershipagainstcancer.ca/tools/cancer-guidelines-database/

Strategy for Patient Oriented Research (SPOR): Asset Map of Canadian Clinical Practice Guideline Developers
https://sporevidencealliance.ca/cpg-asset-map/

The Cochrane library
https://www.cochranelibrary.com

Guidelines International Network (G-I-N): International Guidelines Library
http://www.g-i-n.net/library/international-guidelines-library/

The Joanna Briggs Institute
https://joannabriggs.org/

National Health and Medical Research Council of Australia (NHMRC) Clinical Practice Guidelines Portal www.clinicalguidelines.gov.au

National Institute for Health and Care Excellence (NICE)
http://www.nice.org.uk/about

NHS Evidence
https://www.evidence.nhs.uk/

Scottish Intercollegiate Guidelines Network (SIGN)
http://www.sign.ac.uk/index.html

Range of Guidelines

Guidelines have different purposes and deal with different clinical questions such as intervention, diagnosis, prognosis, etiology, screening, and, increasingly, supportive and palliative aspects of care (issues that are not always studied through traditional experimental designs such as randomized controlled trial (RCT) methods). Different topics require different evidence and different evidence hierarchies. Particularly in nursing and health services, there is a growing interest in the role of non-experimental, quantitative designs (e.g. large scale cohort, observational studies, and program evaluation) and qualitative research in guiding healthcare practices. Systematic review methods are evolving to synthesize this range of evidence. For example:

- The Joanna Briggs Institute (JBI), a publisher of systematic reviews and leading international organization for the translation, transfer, and utilization of evidence, uses the FAME system which focuses on **F**easibility, **A**cceptability/Appropriateness, **M**eaningfulness, and **E**ffectiveness. All quantitative and qualitative evidence may be used depending on the question. The JBI QARI (Qualitative Assessment and Review Instrument) is used to appraise qualitative research. See http://www.joannabriggs.org.
- The Cochrane Collaboration, in cooperation with JBI, has started a Qualitative Research Methods Group and provides a database of tools. Further information is available at https://www.cochrane.org.
- The National Institute for Health and Care Excellence (NICE) also provides a methodological checklist for qualitative studies in their Manual, available online at: https://www.nice.org.uk/article/PMG6/chapter/1%20Introduction.

Assess the Quality of a Guideline

Often you may find many guidelines on the same topic and if a large number of relevant and/or up to date guidelines are discovered, consider reducing the number by limiting full appraisal to only the most recent or by using an appraisal instrument such as the Appraisal of Guidelines for REsearch and Evaluation (AGREE II) instrument (http://www.agreetrust.org/agree-II) (Brouwers et al. 2010a; Brouwers et al. 2010b,c) to do an initial screen for "Rigour" (described more fully below). More on the AGREE II instrument later. It may be more expedient to explore a smaller number of quality guidelines from recognized and reputable sources related to your topic. On the other hand, depending on the nature of your health questions and the practice environment, it may be necessary to extract pertinent recommendations from several related but not specifically targeted guidelines. A good example is assessment and management of pain specific to chronic wounds or cancer which may lead to examination of general pain guidelines as well as condition specific ones.

An experienced health sciences librarian or information specialist should plan and document the search. Involving someone with this expertise early in the question development stage enables understanding of the context for which the question is being developed and focuses the search to best suit the needs of the initiative and your context. Taking advantage of a health science librarian's expertise in searching and citation management saves significant time and effort and ensures a process that is exhaustive, transparent, and reproducible. Extensive and detailed information on this aspect can be found in a resource developed by two expert library scientists we have worked with (Ross-White et al. 2014).

Guideline Appraisal Instruments

A review identified 40 appraisal tools for practice guidelines (Siering et al. 2013). We consider the gold standard instrument for guideline appraisal to be the AGREE II instrument http://www.agreetrust.org/agree-II) because of the testing it has undergone and because we were involved in developing the tool and it is the one we have had the most experience with using. It consists of 23, seven-point Likert-type scale items organized in six domains. Each domain is intended to capture a separate dimension of guideline quality. The quality domains assessed are scope and purpose (three items), stakeholder involvement (four items), rigour of development (seven items), clarity of presentation (four items), applicability (three items), and editorial independence (two items).

For each domain, each guideline you are evaluating is given a standardized dimensional score ranging from 0 to 100. To ensure that all questions are interpreted consistently, the instrument comes with a user guide. Complete information about the instrument and how it is scored can be found at https://www.agreetrust.org. It is important to remember that the AGREE II is not intended to give one overall quality score to a guideline as the relative importance of the six domains is not known.

In the US, another guideline appraisal tool is sometimes mentioned: the US Institute Of Medicine Standards for Developing Trustworthy CPGs (Institute of Medicine 2011). This tool is comprised of eight standards: (i) establishing transparency, (ii) management of conflict of interest, (iii) guideline development group composition, (iv) clinical practice guideline–systematic review intersection, (v) establishing evidence foundations for and rating strength of recommendations, (vi) articulation of recommendations, (vii) external review, and (viii) updating. For each standard, there are multiple criteria. Unfortunately, there is no guidance on how to use this checklist to determine guideline quality which makes it somewhat challenging to use. The lack of testing of this tool is also an issue for some.

Prior to the development of the AGREE-REX (Appraisal of Guidelines REsearch and Evaluation–Recommendation EXcellence) tool, there has been no instrument to use to evaluate the quality of practice recommendations. Similar in format to the AGREE II instrument, AGREE-REX is comprised of three domains and a total of nine items. Domain 1 is Clinical Applicability and is comprised of items: (i) Evidence, (ii) Applicability to Target Users, and (iii) Applicability to Patients/Populations. Domain 2 is Values and Preferences and is comprised of the items: (iv) Values and Preferences of Target Users, (v) Values and Preferences of Patients/Populations, (vi) Values and Preferences of Policy/Decision-Makers, and (vii) Values and Preferences of Guideline Developers. The third domain is Implementability and is comprised of: (viii) Purpose, and (ix) Local Application and Adoption. For each of the nine items, raters are asked to rate both the overall quality of the item using a 7-point Likert scale from 1- lowest quality to 7- highest quality and its suitability for use on a 7-point Likert scale going from 1- strongly agree to 7- strongly disagree. Research demonstrates that AGREE-REX can be useful in identifying guideline recommendations that are clinically credible and implementable (Brouwers et al. 2020). AGREE-REX is freely available on the AGREE Trust website along with instructions on how to use it (including how to score it) and a reporting checklist (AGREE Enterprise website 2019). We have not used AGREE-REX in our work given its recent release, but one of us was involved in developing it (IDG).

Assess the Strength of Evidence: Classification Systems

Practice guidelines have improved in quality by adhering to principles such as systematically reviewing relevant evidence and grading the recommendations and the quality of the underlying evidence. Until recently there was no one widely accepted classification system for assessing the strength of evidence. Moreover, most of the available instruments and scales have been designed to rate evidence specific to questions of intervention effectiveness, and not all have been rigorously developed or tested for validity and reliability. Evidence related to appropriateness, acceptability, or feasibility is rarely dealt with in existing taxonomies.

The methodological quality of randomized controlled trials (RCTs) are commonly evaluated to assess the risk of bias of the estimates of treatment effects. The Scottish Intercollegiate Guidelines Network (SIGN) Guideline Developers' Handbook provides extensive, detailed methodological checklists for systematic reviews and meta-analyses, RCTs, cohort studies, case–control studies, studies of diagnostic accuracy and economic evaluations (SIGN 2011).

A grading system that is gaining acceptance internationally is the GRADE approach (Grading of Recommendations, Assessment, Development, and Evaluation) (Guyatt et al. 2008). GRADE has emerged "as a response to the glut of competing grading systems, their limitations and the confusion resulting from a lack of a 'common rubric'" (Brouwers et al. 2008). GRADE is a two-step approach whereby the quality of evidence is evaluated (high, moderate, low, very low) and then a strength of recommendation is formulated (strong or weak). The quality of the evidence is judged relative to the specific context including benefits and harms, costs, and values and preferences. For detailed guidance about how to apply the GRADE methodology and a comprehensive list of publications, visit the GRADE working Group website http://www.gradeworkinggroup.org.

Guidelines, by definition, should be supported with evidence. However, some developers do not grade the evidence or publish the strength of the evidence supporting each recommendation in their guideline report. It may be necessary to contact the developer and gather the original evidence tables. If the evidence is available but not graded, it might be possible to identify and list the actual type of study data supporting each recommendation.

Determine Guideline Currency, Content, and Consistency

Guideline Currency

It is important to assess whether the guidelines identified are sufficiently current for use. Evidence in rapidly evolving fields may be quickly outdated. Even with current sources, there is an inevitable delay between the final search for the evidence and publication of the guideline. Review the publication date of the guideline as well as the dates and period covered by the supporting literature search to determine if the most current evidence has been included. Some developers publish this information in the guideline itself or on their web sites. If the source guidelines are good quality but the literature is not up to date, the literature, or evidence must be updated. We recommend a top-up search using the same search terms as the source guideline. The ADAPTE Collaboration (2009) makes several recommendations for updating evidence:

- Conduct a quick scan of the literature. Remember to document the search strategy and seek help from an information specialist/health services librarian if necessary. Perform a literature search of web sites most likely to provide up-to-date information and look for systematic reviews, as these provide a rigorous synthesis of primary evidence.

- Contact the guideline developer directly for further information on currency. Determine if there is a more recent version of the guideline, whether the developer intends to update the guideline in the future, or if they are aware of any new evidence that might affect the guideline recommendations.

Assess Guideline Content: Prepare a Recommendations Matrix

As we have noted, by definition, a practice guideline should provide recommendations that are explicitly linked to evidence. A significant advantage in using existing quality guidelines is that the supporting evidence has already been synthesized and graded. In this step of the process, the working group reviews and makes decisions about the strength of the supporting evidence presented in the selected guidelines. A table or matrix which compares similar recommendations across multiple guidelines and displays relative levels of evidence is helpful to effectively guide this discussion. This Recommendations Matrix will be the source document upon which some of the decisions described in Chapter 8 will be made.

The notion behind a Recommendations Matrix is to group recommendations from various guidelines together to compare similarities and differences, identifying all recommendations supported by strong evidence, enabling a comparison of the wording of recommendations to assist working groups in drafting actionable messages, and providing a basis for a discussion about the clinical relevance of each recommendation. To ensure that no recommendation is taken out of context, a practitioner who specializes in the area is in the best position to produce and review the matrix. While the structure and content of the matrix is flexible according to the needs of a specific initiative, a Recommendation Matrix table typically includes a list of recommendations down the left column with the names of the source guidelines across the top. We have found it helpful to order source guidelines across the table by:

- Date (most to least current).
- Best fit or most complete response to specified health questions.
- AGREE II quality scores on specific dimensions (e.g. rigour) plus the overall guideline assessment item.
- The strength of supporting evidence associated with each recommendation.
- The determination of whether the guideline is current.

A matrix may also include recommendations from systematic reviews or health technology assessments. CAN-IMPLEMENT provides a template for building a Recommendations Matrix (Table 6.3).

The quality of the guideline and strength of evidence are important to understand before making changes to care in your local context. If the evidence is weak for a guideline recommendation it may not be worth changing how you currently do things.

You may run into the situation where the guideline(s) does not cover all aspects of the practice issue. You will have to dig deeper into the evidence. In this instance, you return to the literature to seek syntheses specific to the issue. An example from our wound care work relates to our need to better understand the most effective and efficient care models to organize for best wound care practices in the community. This information was not contained in the practice recommendations. Thus, we turned to the health services

Table 6.3 Template for a Recommendations Matrix (to compare details across guidelines).

	Guideline 1	Guideline 2	Guideline 3
Publication Year			
AGREE II Rigour Scores			
Overall Quality Assessment by working group members	Strongly recommend:	Strongly recommend:	Strongly recommend:
	Recommend with proviso:	Recommend with proviso:	Recommend with proviso:
	Would not recommend:	Would not recommend:	Would not recommend:
Guideline Strengths or Limitations	*Strengths:*	*Strengths:*	*Strengths:*
Algorithms or Tools	*describe*	*Describe*	*describe*
Health Question 1:	e.g. What criteria are used to assess the symptom?		
Is question addressed?	Yes ☐ No ☐	Yes ☐ No ☐	Yes ☐ No ☐
Answer to question – the guideline recommendation (plus strength of evidence)			
Is guideline current?	Yes ☐ No ☐	Yes ☐ No ☐	Yes ☐ No ☐
What is an indicator for this recommendation			
Source of recommendation (reference)			

literature for reviews of service delivery models to discuss with the decision-makers and practitioners to support evidence-informed changes.

Assess Guideline Consistency

It is common to find similar recommendations in different guidelines. In building a Recommendations Matrix it is easy to see similar recommendations and how they are worded and their sources. See Table 6.4 for a simplified version of the Recommendations Matrix that facilitates this comparison. For example, if several guidelines have the same recommendation but have different literature sources but they are all current, this adds to the confidence and you might choose the recommendation worded most clearly for your context. If the recommendations are saying different things you may need to investigate more. Is it because they are from different countries, or the currency is older and evidence has evolved, or the population is specific, e.g. meant only for older populations?

Another scenario is that you may find several similar recommendations, but the evidence is not strong in that area. The reality is that practice decisions have to be made, so if you have a similar set of recommendations based on expert opinion then the sum of these recommendations represents an expert consensus. This may be more helpful than individual decision-making.

Table 6.4 Template for a Recommendations Matrix (simplified).

Recommendations Being Considered	Guideline 1	Guideline 2	Guideline 3
Recommendation 1 (with variations in wording) • strength of evidence • AGREE-REX rating			
Recommendation 2 (with variations in wording) • strength of evidence • AGREE-REX rating			
Recommendation 3 (with variations in wording) • strength of evidence • AGREE-REX rating			

Identify Indicators of Best Practice

Once the group has identified what the relevant best practices are from the external evidence, the next step is identify or develop indicators for each recommendation. These indicators are critically important for being able to assess adherence to the recommendations. It is essential to differentiate indicators of uptake (process, e.g. full assessment and plan of care) versus indicators of outcome (clinical improvement, e.g. wound reduction or healing).

The process indicators will be used to conduct the assessment of current practice and in determining the evidence-practice gap. They will also be used in the ongoing monitoring of the implementation of best practice to determine whether the implementation strategies have been successful in bringing about change in practice (adherence with the recommendations).

As an example, with our study of leg ulcer care, one best practice recommendation was the use of compression bandages for venous disease. As none of the guidelines we considered provided any performance indicators, the clinical group created a relevant indicator to signify the proportion of patients appropriately receiving compression therapy. The indicator was operationalized as the number of patients with ulcers of venous disease etiology receiving compression therapy divided by the total number of leg ulcer patients with venous disease multiplied by 100% (a score of 100% indicating all appropriate patients were receiving compression therapy as recommended and 0% indicating no appropriate patients were not receiving the therapy). The indicator was then used in a chart audit to determine the extent to which this recommendation was being adhered to in the local community services.

More recently we are seeing more guidelines provide performance indicators or performance measures for each guideline recommendation. For example, one national guideline on best practices for stroke prevention, treatment, and rehabilitation provides performance measures for each recommendation along with measurement notes on how to measure or what to include. One recommendation under Screening for Post Stroke Depression is that all patients with stroke should be screened for depressive symptoms using a validated tool (Heart and Stroke Foundation of Canada 2018; Lanctot et al. 2019). The related performance measure is the proportion of acute stroke admissions with documentation indicating initial screening for post-stroke depression was performed (either informally or using a formal screening tool). It is calculated by taking the number assessed divided by the number of admissions X 100). This is to be done in the acute care, rehabilitation, long-term care, and community settings (e.g. homecare). This a very clear performance measure with how, when, and where to carry it out.

Unfortunately, many guideline developers have yet to embrace their role in providing indicators to assess adherence to their recommendations making it necessary to often develop your own or finding existing ones in the literature that might be appropriate. The Appendix to Chapter 12 has a more fulsome discussion of how to develop and use indicators of guideline adherence.

A Note on Renewal

In reviewing guidelines and their content, currency, and consistency it is prudent for your group to now consider the timing of an update and renewal. You will have a good sense of how quickly the field is changing and if you need to keep an eye on new research in a year or two or longer. In our work with pressure injury guidelines we could see that little had changed in a five year time span in the evidence supporting various guidelines, thus we set the renewal to happen in three years' time.

Summary

You will know that this stage of finding best practice evidence has been achieved when the working group has identified best practices based on evidence from external research, made decisions about how to operationalize the recommendations so that they can be measured, and can proceed to understanding the gap between their practice and evidence-informed care. The information you should now have at this juncture includes:

- Knowledge of the relevant best practices related to the identified issue.
- An understanding of the quality of the best practice evidence.
- The evidence supporting each best practice.
- The extent to which the best practices are up to date.
- Indicators that might be used to measure adherence to each best practice.
- Consideration of when to do an update of the recommendations to see if new evidence has emerged.

In continuing with the Action Map, the answers to the questions asked at the outset should be used to populate the second column (Table 6.5). This will provide a

Table 6.5 Phase 1: ACTION MAP for Issue Identification and Clarification (*with Wound Example*).

Call-to-Action *Thinking about clinical issue, get various perspectives from working group*	External Recommendations *Discuss & identify clinical issue, get external evidence (broadly)*	Assemble local evidence about setting, care providers, & population	Current Practice *(audit, focus group, observation)*	Gaps *Discrepancy between recommendation and current practice*
Key information about issues, potential working group	**Insert actual external recommendations**	**Understand the magnitude of the issue, provider considerations caring for these people**	**Understand how the issue is currently being managed**	**Decide whether to address the gap and how**
Chief nurse concerned with increase in surgical referrals for flap repairs. Clinical nurses anecdotally reporting ++pressure injuries	1. Head to toe skin assessment every 24 hours 2. Conduct pressure injury risk assessment using validated scale 3. Etc.			
Nurse managers concerned with use of pressure relieving devices				
Info about population at risk unknown, # hospital patients with pressure injury not known				
Sustainability thinking starts here. . .	External evidence on best practice provides a benchmark for ongoing quality assessment. Select recommendations that could be sustained			
Chapter 5	Chapter 6	Chapter 7	Chapter 7	Chapter 7

foundation on which the group's work will continue to better understand what ought to be done and information about how close or not the current practices are to evidence-informed practice. The details about how the best practices were identified, appraised, and assessed can now be added to your Implementation Plan. Given your familiarity with the guidelines and their currency you could add the update and renewal timing to the Implementation Plan.

At this stage the external evidence, in the form of a guideline, is clear to your group. It has been scrutinized for quality and potential performance measures identified. Next major process will be to align the external evidence with your local context. This will first involve gathering "local" evidence. This evidence is needed to be able to compare and understand how closely the local practice and health services is to the external evidence-informed practices.

References

ADAPTE Collaboration (2009). *The ADAPTE Process: Resource Toolkit for Guideline Adaptation. Version 2.0*, (Online), Available: https://www.g-i-n.net/document-store/working-groups-documents/adaptation/adapte-resource-toolkit-guideline-adaptation-2-0.pdf (26 July 2019).

AGREE Enterprise website (2010). *AGREE II*, (Online), Available: http://www.agreetrust.org/agree-II (6 Sept 2019).

AGREE Enterprise website (2019). *AGREE-REX: Recommendation EXcellence*, (Online), Available: https://www.agreetrust.org/resource-centre/agree-rex-recommendation-excellence (9 June 2020).

Bahadur, P. (2014). *Difference between Guideline, Procedure, Standard and Policy*, (Online), Available: http://www.hrsuccessguide.com/2014/01/Guideline-Procedure-Standard-Policy.html (27 Apr 2018).

Brouwers, M.C., Somerfield, M.R., and Browman, G.P. (2008). A for effort: learning from the application of the GRADE approach to cancer guideline development. *Journal of Clinical Oncology* 26: 1025–1026. https://doi.org/10.1200/JCO.2007.14.6373.

Brouwers, M.C., Kho, M.E., Browman, G.P. et al. (2010a). AGREE II: advancing guideline development, reporting, and evaluation in health care. *Preventive Medicine* 51: 421–424.

Brouwers, M.C., Kho, M.E., Browman, G.P. et al. (2010b). Development of the AGREE II, part 1: performance, usefulness and areas for improvement. *Canadian Medical Association Journal* 182: 1045–1052. https://doi.org/10.1503/cmaj.091714.

Brouwers, M.C., Kho, M.E., Browman, G.P. et al. (2010c). Development of the AGREE II, part 2: assessment of validity of items and tools to support application. *Canadian Medical Association Journal* 182: E472–E478. https://doi.org/10.1503/cmaj.091716.

Brouwers, M.C., Spithoff, K., Kerkvliet, K. et al. (2020). Development and validation of a tool to assess the quality of clinical practice guideline recommendations. *JAMA Network Open* 3: e205535. https://doi.org/10.1001/jamanetworkopen.2020.5535.

Echevarria, I.M. and Walker, S. (2014). To make your case, start with a PICOT question. *Nursing* 44: 18–19. https://doi.org/10.1097/01.NURSE.0000442594.00242.f9.

Fervers, B., Burgers, J.S., Haugh, M.C. et al. (2006). Adaptation of clinical guidelines: literature review and proposition for a framework and procedure. *International Journal for Quality in Health Care* 18: 167–176. https://doi.org/10.1093/intqhc/mzi108.

Field, M.J. and Lohr, K.N. (eds.) (1990). *Clinical Practice Guidelines: Directions for a New Program*. Washington, DC: Institute of Medicine, National Academy Press.

Grade Working Group (2020). *GRADE Working Group Organizational Website*, (Online), Available: http://www.gradeworkinggroup.org (6 Sept 2019).

Graham, I.D., Logan, J., Harrison, M.B. et al. (2006). Lost in knowledge translation: time for a map? *The Journal of Continuing Education in the Health Professions* 26: 13–24. https://doi.org/10.1002/chp.47.

Guyatt, G.H., Oxman, A.D., Vist, G.E. et al. (2008). GRADE: an emerging consensus on rating quality of evidence and strength of recommendations. *BMJ* 336: 924–926. https://doi.org/10.1136/bmj.39489.470347.AD, https://www.ncbi.nlm.nih.gov/pmc/articles/PMC2335261/.

Harrison, M.B., van den Hoek, J., and Graham, I.D. (2014). *CAN-IMPLEMENT: Planning for Best-Practice Implementation (Book 20)*. Philadelphia: Lippincott Williams & Wilkins.

Heart and Stroke Foundation of Canada (2018). *Canadian Stroke Best Practices: Mood, Cognition and Fatigue following Stroke*, (Online), Available: https://www.strokebestpractices.ca/recommendations/mood-cognition-and-fatigue-following-stroke (9 June 2020).

Institute of Medicine (2011). *Clinical Practice Guidelines We Can Trust*. Washington, DC: National Academies Press https://www.awmf.org/fileadmin/user_upload/Leitlinien/International/IOM_CPG_lang_2011.pdf.

Lanctot, K.L., Lindsay, M.P., Smith, E.E. et al. (2019). Canadian stroke best practice recommendations: mood, cognition and fatigue following stroke, 6th edition update 2019. *International Journal of Stroke* https://doi.org/10.1177/1747493019847334.

National Institute for Health and Clinical Excellence (2012). *The Guidelines Manual*. London: National Institute for Health and Clinical Excellence www.nice.org.uk.

Scottish Intercollegiate Guidelines Network (2011). *SIGN 50: A guideline Developers Handbook*. Revised Edition. Edinburgh: Scottish Intercollegiate Guidelines Network https://www.sign.ac.uk/assets/sign50_2011.pdf.

Richardson, W.S., Wilson, M.C., Nishikawa, J., and Hayward, R.S. (1995). The well-built clinical question: a key to evidence-based decisions. *ACP Journal Club* 123: A12–A13.

Riva, J.J., Malik, K.M., Burnie, S.J. et al. (2012). What is your research question? An introduction to the PICOT format for clinicians. *The Journal of the Canadian Chiropractic Association* 56: 167–171. https://www.ncbi.nlm.nih.gov/pmc/articles/PMC3430448/.

Ross-White, A., Oakley, P., and Lockwood, C. (2014). *Guideline Adaptation: Conducting Systematic, Exhaustive, and Reproducible Searches (Book 19)*. Philadelphia: Lippincott Williams & Wilkins.

Siering, U., Eikermann, M., Hausner, E. et al. (2013). Appraisal tools for clinical practice guidelines: a systematic review. *PLoS One* 8: e82915. https://doi.org/10.1371/journal.pone.0082915.

The Cochrane Collaboration (2020). (Online), Available: http://www.cochrane.org
(27 Apr 2018).

The Joanna Briggs Institute (2019). (Online), Available: http://joannabriggs.org
(27 Apr 2018).

U.S. Food and Drug Administration. Using the PICOTS Framework to Strengthen Evidence
Gathered in Clinical Trials—Guidance from the AHRQ's Evidence-based Practice
Centers Program, (Online), Available: https://www.fda.gov/media/109448/download
(9 June 2020).

7

Assemble Local Evidence on Context and Current Practices

Introduction

In the Call-to-Action there was initially a focus on the issue and understanding it from various perspectives and gathering an interested group to work on the practice concern. Then the effort turned to finding the best available evidence to deal with the problem. At this point in the Issue Identification and Clarification Phase, action turns to marshaling local evidence to get as complete as possible a picture of the magnitude of the issue, documenting current practice, and determining the evidence–practice gap from patient, provider, and health system perspectives so as to fully understand context of care.

Goals: To understand: (i) the magnitude of the issue/problem within the local context, (ii) to determine how it is being addressed in day-to-day practice, and (iii) what is the evidence-practice gap.

To begin work on this aspect of Roadmap, there are several pertinent questions that drive the enquiry into local evidence:

- What is the context for the practice issue?
  - How many (and what proportion of) individuals have the condition of interest?
  - What is the demographic and clinical profile of these individuals?
- What is known about current practice (the care these individuals receive) and the outcomes produced by current practice?
- What healthcare providers are addressing the concern?
  - What types of healthcare providers are providing care?
  - What are the providers' scopes of practice?
- What are the resource implications of providing care for these individuals currently (what does it cost)?
- What is the extent of the evidence-practice gap?

The answers to these questions can be used to determine how similar your patients are compared to those in the studies used to generate best practice evidence. It will also be used in determining the size of the population with the condition and may also permit an assessment of the "economy of scale" for how to deal with the condition, e.g. a few suffer greatly from the condition versus many suffer a little from the condition. The findings that

Knowledge Translation in Nursing and Healthcare: A Roadmap to Evidence-informed Practice, First Edition.
Margaret B. Harrison and Ian D. Graham.
© 2021 John Wiley & Sons, Inc. Published 2021 by John Wiley & Sons, Inc.

emerge from goals one and two provide critical information needed to determine the evidence-practice gap. In other words, it will provide an indication of the true extent of how different current practice is from what is considered best practice. Importantly this activity also provides crucial information the working group will need when it begins to consider how the issue/problem might be addressed by best practices.

At this phase, the working group will want to ensure that the perspectives of managers, clinicians, patients, and any other key stakeholders are included. It is essential that the views of those making the decision to implement or fund the best practice as well as those who will be using the best practice are considered. This can be done through membership on the working group but also by collecting information directly from the stakeholders.

Where previously it was about finding best practices as determined by external evidence, some of the stakeholders may not have felt empowered to be fully engaged particularly if they lacked skills in assessing or using evidence in their practice. At this juncture however, almost all the stakeholders can contribute with providing or collecting local evidence. Everyone has a perspective on the local context so take advantage of this to keep working group members involved. Accept all perspectives respectfully.

Determine the Magnitude of the Issue Within the Local Context

To sort out the potential magnitude of the population affected, some questions may be answered by the organization through their available internal administrative databases such as the health record, patient rosters or registries to determine the number of people with the condition on service. Other questions may necessitate gathering new data not readily available and require time and expertise absent within the setting itself. Partnering with researchers may provide the expertise required if there is a need to gather primary data through a local study. These sorts of questions make good thesis topics so keep graduate students and students needing to do practicums in mind if assistance is needed to conduct such enquiries. Methods may include prevalence, incidence and population profiling studies, environmental scans, and qualitative inquiries. Mixed methods are often best suited for producing *local evidence* about the issue and the affected population.

Population Prevalence and Profile Studies

It is important to understand your population of interest and ensure cases are appropriately classified and counted. Questions guiding these inquiries include:

- How many individuals (on service or on and off service combined) have the condition at this moment in time (prevalence rate)?
- How many new cases are there in a given time period (3-month incidence rate)?
- What is the profile (clinical, socio-demographic, circumstance of living) of the affected individuals?

Box 7.1   Making Sure the Problem is Clear

In a wound care implementation that we assisted with, it was next to impossible to separate out the different types of chronic wounds in the community administrative database. Thus, we undertook a primary survey to determine the number and general characteristics of the community-based population. This information was highly valuable in planning the resources for care in both the nurse clinics and in individuals' homes, e.g. numbers as well as age and mobility characteristics. Circumstance-of-living data was useful to understand if there was anyone in the same home able to assist with bandaging.

Keep in mind that you may be unable to determine the size and profile of the population from administrative databases alone, or at all. For example, with one project we were involved with, for planning purposes, the regional health care authority was interested in the magnitude of the issue in the region and managers suspected that documentation of the condition may not have consistently been recorded in either the health record or other agency administrative databases. The only way to get a handle on how many individuals had the condition was to undertake a regional prevalence and profile study to assess if the local population was similar to those reported in the literature and whether the prevalence of the condition was the same, higher or lower in our region compared to what was reported in the literature.

Box 7.2   Big or Little Problem?

With the community leg ulcer initiative, the supply expenditure database was used to identify all possible cases receiving wound care supplies. Then nurses followed up with each individual and conducted a clinical assessment and determined if they actually had a wound of interest (Friedberg et al. 2002). This process let us identify known cases in care but did not help us identify those with the condition not in care but who should or might be referred to care. Therefore, to identify all individuals in the region with the condition, we surveyed all family physicians, podiatrists, and long-term care facilities in the catchment area to identify cases in addition to those receiving home care. For good measure, we also placed advertisements in 15 local and community papers asking for individuals with the condition to self-identify. Combining the results of these inquiries provided us with a satisfactory estimate of all the cases within the jurisdiction of interest. We recognized however, that this approach was probably providing the highest estimate as we could not be assured whether some individuals were counted more than once.

Acquiring information on the entire population can be very helpful when planning potential changes in health services delivery. Keep in mind that surveys can be quite simple and easy to administer. In the example in call out box 7.2, it consisted of only two questions (Do you currently have any patients with the condition not receiving home-care? If yes, how many?). Or they can be more complex and epidemiological in nature (see Graham et al. (2003) for examples). The key is always to choose the method that is most appropriate for meeting your objectives, i.e. pragmatic, feasible, and providing reliable data.

Profiling Studies

Profiling studies typically involve collecting detailed information on individuals with the condition (often the ones identified or a representative portion of those in the prevalence and incidence studies). The profile information may be found in the health record or other administrative databases or you may need to collect this information directly from individuals or families. Chart audit is a common method for extracting data from the health record (electronic and/or hard copy) to examine some component of performance, to determine what has been done, and see if can be done better. It is a practical and relatively straightforward way to collect information (Agency for Healthcare Research and Quality 2013; Bissonnette 2016).

Making use of existing data sources is usually very efficient but only if the data are comprehensive enough. It must provide the information you are seeking and be reliable and accurate. If the group determines that primary data collection is required (either because the information they are wanting has not previously been collected or if it has, is not as complete as required or there are concerns about its quality), you should carefully consider what information is needed and weigh it against the effort and resources needed to collect it. It can be a temptation to want to collect more information than is essential to profile the population. You often hear comments such as, *"Wouldn't it be interesting if we collected data on . . .."* The group should resist this as the more information to be collected the greater the response burden for patients and others and the more it costs in terms of time and money to collect it. If the data are not necessary for planning and/or not going to be used for additional purposes other than to satisfy someone's curiosity – do not collect it.

The most useful types of information for profiling the population of concern include information on individuals' socio-demographic characteristics (e.g. age, sex, gender, geographic location, education, health literacy, race and ethnicity, etc.), circumstance-of-living (e.g. marital status, social support network, income, health insurance, etc.), general health history (co-morbidities, medications, disabilities, mobility, health related quality of life, etc.), and health history specific to the condition of interest (e.g. wound – number and types of ulcers, recurrences, healing rates, etc.). All this information becomes invaluable when the group considers how best practice recommendations may apply to their population, the practice context, and when the group begins to think about potential strategies to implement best practices.

Box 7.3 Important Planning Details

With one project where a potential solution was to set up a community clinic, it was important to know in advance that the average age of potential clients would be over 65 years but that 80% were mobile and could drive or had access to transportation to attend a community clinic to receive their care.

Determine Current Practice – What Are We Doing Now?

The last chapter described how to identify best practice for addressing the condition based on best available external evidence and the indicators that could be used to measure best practice. Now the group must figure out and describe the current practice related to the issue and compare with the available evidence recommendations.

There are several ways to determine current practice. Routinely collected patient data from the health record, or registries of individuals with specific conditions can provide information on diagnosis, type, frequency, and intensity of care provided and by whom. Clinical datasets can be used to identify patterns in service utilization, and local audit data can be used to monitor activity. The use of quality and safety datasets is useful to show trends in patient events (e.g. infections, falls, various adverse events). If the behaviors or outcomes you are interested in are not routinely collected, you can also do primary data collection, observe practice, and interview individuals about their experiences.

It is important to balance the reliability and validity of the data with the effort and expense needed to acquire it. Ideally relying on routinely collected data is more efficient and less time consuming. However, you must consider and assess the reliability and validity of the data. For example, practitioners may be using some, or all the best practice recommendations but not documenting them. This will lead to under-reporting of the best practice, if you rely solely on health record data. For example, we know that while the health record may commonly report information on diagnostic tests, they often omit details on other interventions such as counseling (Rethans et al. 1994). Relying on self-report also has limitations as practitioners may not accurately recall how often they have performed a specific clinical behavior.

Another crucial consideration is the sample that will be used for your analysis.

- What is the most appropriate sample?
  - a sample of the population of interest (only those with the condition) or
  - the entire population (everyone regardless of whether they have the condition)? (Celentano and Szklo 2019)
- How will patients/healthcare providers be identified?
- How large should the sample be? How representative is it (age, sex, gender, etc.)?

In addition to determining current practice, it is also useful to investigate the role of healthcare providers in delivering current practice, the perspectives of recipients of care, and the expenditures related to current practice.

Health Care Provider Review

To be able to really understand the role that health care providers play in managing the condition it is essential to be able to answer questions such as:

- What healthcare providers are involved in care delivery for individuals with this condition (e.g. range of providers – nurse practitioners, acute care nurses, homecare nurses, registered practical nurses, rehabilitation professionals, personal support workers, primary care physicians, specialist physicians, etc.)?

- What are their scopes of practice related to care provided (e.g. Who is permitted [legally] and expected to do which aspects)?
- How often do they see these people (e.g. What is the frequency of visits/consultations/ hospitalizations, etc.)?

Box 7.4   Really understand current practice

In the wound care example, the profiling study revealed 40% of people were receiving daily or twice daily nursing visits (i.e. a high demand on nursing time which was a scarce resource) and that the average patient was seen by 19 different nurses (registered nurses (RNs), licensed practical nurses (LPNs)) for their condition during a 1 month period (i.e. the lack of continuity of provider being suggestive of the potential for lack of continuity of care).

Appreciating that current practice is highly relevant, especially if the required change in practice will have an impact on a provider's scope of practice (e.g. certain level of provider required to deliver).

Box 7.5   Where are changes required?

Continuing with our wound care example, best practices indicate that aspects of the assessment should only be conducted by registered nurses. However, we found that care was also delivered by unregulated care providers, highlighting a fundamental area for changes in team assignment.

Perspectives of the Recipients of Care

To be able to incorporate the viewpoint of individuals and their families it is important to answer questions such as: What is their experience receiving care? What are their preferences?

Qualitative approaches are useful to document care recipients' experience and how they might like to see things improved. This can be done through several straightforward methods such as setting up a focus group or town hall meetings especially if there is a regular clinic or other meeting opportunity for your population of interest. Brief surveys can also be used to elicit the views of patients and their carers.

Expenditure Review

This involves understanding the economic context of caring for individuals with the condition. Guiding questions to uncover relevant costs include, what are the costs related to:

- Provider fees/time (e.g. costs of nursing time, physician consultation fees, travel time in the case of home visits by providers, etc.),
- Health care supplies (e.g. expenditures on medical devices, dressings, bandages, etc.), as well as

• Any out-of-pocket expenses patients may cover (travel for appointments, parking, over the counter medications, medications not covered by health insurance, etc.).

Administrative databases are a good place to start to find some of these expenditures. It may be practical for the group to sample a proportion of individuals to fully determine what services they receive and estimate the associated costs. Undertaking the expenditure review concurrently with the assessment of current practice is often an efficient way to proceed.

It will be important to understand and document the results of current care – clinically, resource use, and economically to develop a sound assessment for a change to best practice. Available administrative and quality data often provide this information. For example, the current healing rates, resource use (nursing time) and cost of materials (e.g. dressings, ointments, stockings, bandages). When there is not sufficient information, then primary data collection may be necessary, e.g. interview or survey a sample of individuals from the service.

You may want more information on how to go about collecting some of the various types of data described above using qualitative methods. An excellent resource is Leeman and Sandelowski's (2012) paper about using qualitative inquiry to obtain practice-based evidence derived from the experiences and practices of healthcare providers and the contexts of healthcare provision.

Measure the Evidence-Practice Gap

After determining and documenting current practice, the third goal of this stage is to determine the extent to which current practice aligns (or not) with best practice that has been determined by external (research) evidence, in this case the guideline.

To assess current practice, it is usually easiest to start with a best practice guideline. As noted in Chapter 6, check practice guidelines for suggested best practice indicators. As already noted, essentially practice indicators are measures of process – they indicate the extent to which care activities are undertaken (i.e. the proportion of patients with venous leg ulcers with a determination of the etiology of the leg ulcer or the proportion who receive compression therapy).

In much of our work, best practice guideline recommendations have been relatively straightforward and so developing best practice indicators has not been difficult. For example, in the project on community leg ulcer care (Chapter 2, case 1), the recommendations for best practice were easy to turn into indicators. As an example, Table 7.1 presents the best practices reported in practice guidelines and the best practice indicators we developed to measure current practice. Measuring the ulcer was an obvious one but all the stakeholders had to confer and agree upon how to safely, and effectively, conduct that assessment in the home setting with acetate tracings, or ruler measures. We have also found it very helpful to engage practitioners with extensive experience and expertise in the topic area, to assist in thinking through how to convert recommendations into viable indicators. They not only understand the nuances of the recommendations but also understand the charting system and potential administrative databases and all their limitations.

Table 7.1 Examples of best practice recommendations for leg ulcer care along with their indicators. *Note the specificity of the numerators and denominators.*

Best practice recommendation	Best practice indicator
Identification of ulcer etiology	Proportion of clients with venous leg ulcers recorded *# clients with venous leg ulcers recorded/total # clients with leg ulcers X 100*
ABPI prior to initiating compression	Proportion of Venous Leg Ulcer (VLU) clients with ankle-brachial pressure index (ABPI) recorded *# VLU clients with ABPI identified/total # VLU clients*100*
Serial ulcer measurement	Proportion of clients with serial ulcer measurement recorded *#VLU clients with serial ulcer measurement recorded/total # VLU clients*100*
Compression bandage initiated for venous ulcers	Proportion of clients with venous leg ulcers receiving compression (appropriate care) *# VLU clients receiving compression/total # VLU clients*100* Proportion of clients with arterial leg ulcers receiving compression (inappropriate care) *# clients with arterial leg ulcers receiving compression/total # clients with arterial leg ulcers*100*
Pain assessment	Proportion of VLU clients with pain assessment recorded *# VLU clients with pain assessment recorded/total # VLU clients*100*

For more advice on how to measure the gap at the population, organizational and care provider level and the different data sources that may be used for each level see "Identifying Knowledge to Action Gaps" by Kitson and Straus (2013, pp. 97–109).

When determining current practice and the extent to which it adheres to best practice, the working group will need to decide on what the appropriate population is (numerator and denominator), consider what an adequate sample size for the analysis needs to be (so the findings will be credible to stakeholders), and assess the reliability of data sources (health records, primary data collection, etc.). We have found it helpful to enter the current practice indicators into a table that includes actual numbers as well as percentages (%) (n=50/100, 50%) to document evidence-practice gaps. See Table 7.2 for an example of an evidence-practice gap table from the community leg ulcer project.

Finally, when assembling local data (e.g. prevalence data, clinical profiling data, health services utilization and expenditure reviews, or monitoring current practice to be able to measure knowledge to action/evidence-practice gaps), always consider the privacy and security of the health information collected according to policy and privacy laws in your region. Privacy regulations vary between jurisdictions and a chart audit or patient/provider survey may require prior ethics approval in some institutions while in others it is considered part of standard care or considered quality improvement and not subject to institutional review requirements. Figure out whether you need ethics approval for any audit/data collection and if you do, seek necessary approvals before you start your project (Baily et al. 2006; DHA Human Research

Table 7.2 Example of adherence rates to evidence-based recommendations for leg ulcer care.

	Pre guideline adoption (n = 66)	Post Guideline adoption (n = 238)
	n (%)	n (%)
Identification of ulcer etiology	35 (53)	238 (100)
ABPI prior to initiating compression (n = 44)	21 (47)	227 (95)
Serial ulcer measurement recorded (n = 64)	7 (11)	208 (88)
Compression bandage initiated for venous ulcers	44 (66)	206 (86)
Pain assessment documented	10 (15)	215 (90)

Protection Program 2013). Keep in mind that if the group is thinking it might like to publish the data collected, some journals will only publish studies involving humans if there was an a priori ethics approval (even if the project was deemed quality improvement and not requiring ethics approval in your jurisdiction). If the intent is to publish your experience it may be useful to seek ethics approval or at a minimum have the ethics committee confirm in writing that the group does not require ethics approval for the type of data collection proposed.

By the end of this stage, the working group should more fully appreciate the following:

- The context for the practice issue
  - Number of patients/clients/residents that have the condition of interest
  - The demographic and clinical profile of these individuals
- Provision of care
  - The current practice (the care these individuals receive) and the outcomes produced by current practice
  - Which healthcare providers are addressing the concern
  - The providers' scopes of practice relative to the issue
  - The perspectives from the recipients of care on current practice
  - The economic implications of providing care for these individuals (resources used, what it costs)
- Extent of the evidence-practice gap
  - Entirely different than recommended practice and needing a major overhaul
  - Or somewhat different but needing changes to align with best practice

Documenting and Synthesizing the Local Evidence

This is a good point to begin populating your Action Map (introduced at the end of Chapter 5, see Table 7.3). Questions contained in the grid serve to guide information gathering. The information on your context can be summarized into key points for consideration with planning the best practice implementation. Do not forget to also add details about this stage to your Implementation Plan.

Table 7.3 Phase 1: ACTION MAP for issue identification and clarification *(with Wound Example)*.

Call-to-Action *Thinking about clinical issue, get various perspectives from working group*	External Recommendations *Discuss and identify clinical issue, get external evidence (broadly)*	Assemble local evidence about setting, care providers, and population	Current practice *(audit, focus group, observation)*	Gaps *Discrepancy between recommendation and current practice*
Key information about issues, potential working group	Insert with actual external recommendations	Understand the magnitude of the issue, provider considerations caring for these people	Understand how the issue is currently being managed	Need to decide whether to address the gap and how
Chief nurse concerned with increase in surgical referrals for flap repairs. Clinical nurses anecdotally reporting ++pressure injuries	1) Head to toe skin assessment every 24 hours	High risk population for pressure injuries on orthopedics (25%)	Variable, often depends on assigned nurse, floor workload	Conducted assessment of hospital population for risk and occurrence
		Assessment not in the Care Assistants scope of practice	Usual routine is an assessment few times week	Inconsistent timing of assessments in practice
			<30–50% patients assessed based on chart audit of 10 units	30–50% considered too low
Nurse managers concerned with use of pressure relieving devices	2) Conduct pressure injury risk assessment using validated scale	Nurses very busy on day shift, lifting help limited	Risk assessment not routinely conducted using validated scale or documented as done if not using a scale	Managers & nurses decide 30-50% is inadequate, action required to use a validated scale and created a documentation scheme
		No tool currently in use, no place to document risk in health record		
Info about population at risk unknown, # hospital patients with pressure injury not known	3) Etc.	Most nurses unfamiliar with risk scales		
Sustainability thinking continues here. . .	External evidence on best practice provides a benchmark for ongoing quality assessment. Select recommendations that could be sustained	Strategies used for collecting data chosen because they can be sustained.	Information on current practice to acknowledge what is being done well -build on it as move forward with change. Indicators and their collection are sustainable	Gap analysis designed to be used again in future When issue is widespread this provides leverage to continue and sustain best practice.
Chapter 5	Chapter 6	Chapter 7	Chapter 7	Chapter 7

Summary

Now you have covered topics on how to increase your understanding of the population with the relevant condition and those providing care to them. This chapter has also described the need to determine the current care received by this population. This context and population information is "local" evidence that will need to be aligned with the "external" best practice recommendations. Importantly it has highlighted the need for stakeholder engagement in this process to ensure a good understanding of the perspectives of all those involved. While presented here as temporally discrete activities, in reality data collection for the prevalence/incidence studies, profiling studies, current practice, etc. may occur simultaneously. For example, a comprehensive chart audit can be used to provide data for several of the enquiry questions described in this chapter.

At this juncture you should have a good deal of information about the context and the issue. On the Action Map you can fill in the third column with what has been gathered to help synthesize the information to assess the gap with best practices.

All these data serve to determine the nature and extent of the local evidence-practice gap. Now the next major task is to use this information to assist in aligning the best practice recommendations to your context. Understanding the "fit" is vital to a successful implementation and in the next chapter this alignment and customizing recommendations will be described.

References

Agency for Healthcare Research and Quality (2013). *Module 8. Collecting Data With Chart Audits. Content last reviewed May 2013*, [Online], Available: https://www.ahrq.gov/ncepcr/tools/pf-handbook/mod8.html (6 Sept 2019).

Baily, M.A., Bottrell, M.M., Lynn, J., and Jennings, B. (2006). The ethics of using QI methods to improve health care quality and safety. *Hastings Center Report* 36: S1–S40. https://www.thehastingscenter.org/wp-content/uploads/The-Ethics-of-Using-QI-Methods.pdf.

Bissonnette, J. (2016). *Chart Audits: Pros and Cons as a Research/QI & Data Collection Methodology*, [Online], Available: http://www.ohri.ca/clinicalresearchtraining/documents/0820 Chart Audits.pdf (6 Sept 2019).

Celentano, D.D. and Szklo, M. (2019). *Gordis Epidemiology*, 6e. Philidelphia, PA: Elsevier.

DHA Human Research Protection Program (2013). *Human Subject Research versus Quality Improvement Activity*, Falls Church, VA. Report number DHA-HRPP-001.

Friedberg, E.H., Harrison, M.B., and Graham, I.D. (2002). Current home care expenditures for persons with leg ulcers. *Journal of Wound, Ostomy, and Continence Nursing* 29 (4): 186–192. https://doi.org/10.1067/mjw.2002.125137.

Graham, I.D., Harrison, M.B., Nelson, E.A. et al. (2003). Prevalence of lower-limb ulceration: a systematic review of prevalence studies. *Advances in Skin & Wound Care* 16: 305–316. https://doi.org/10.1097/00129334-200311000-00013.

Kitson, A. and Straus, S.E. (2013). Identifying knowledge to action gaps. In: *Knowledge Translation in Health Care: Moving from Evidence to Practice* (eds. S. Straus, J. Tetroe and I.D. Graham), 97–109. Oxford, UK: Wiley Blackwell BMJ Books.

Leeman, J. and Sandelowski, M. (2012). Practice-based evidence and qualitative inquiry. *Journal of Nursing Scholarship* 44: 171–179. https://doi.org/10.1111/ j.1547-5069.2012.01449.x.

Rethans, J.J., Martin, E., and Metsemakers, J. (1994). To what extent do clinical notes by general practitioners reflect actual medical performance? A study using simulated patients. *The British Journal of General Practice* 44: 153–156. https://www.ncbi.nlm.nih.gov/pmc/ articles/PMC1238838/.

Part 2

Phase II: Build Solutions

8

Customize Best Practices to the Local Context

Introduction

Now that the group has determined that there is an evidence-practice gap and that it is sufficiently wide to justify addressing it (Chapter 7), this chapter describes a process by which best practice recommendations can be reviewed and prioritized, selected and customized for implementation in your setting.

Goal: The intent at this stage is to develop a local guideline or protocol that is aligned to your context and population of interest and endorsed by policy makers in the setting. There are a number of pertinent questions for this stage including:

- Are all relevant stakeholders represented on the interdisciplinary working group?
- Are the guideline recommendations of sufficient quality to be considered for implementation?
- Are the guideline recommendations current or out-of-date?
- Are the guideline recommendations adequately addressing the issue of concern?
- Are the guideline recommendations clinically useful?
- Is the strength of the evidence for each guideline recommendation adequate?
- Are the guideline recommendations acceptable, implementable, and sustainable?
- Having assessed the above what are the selected guideline recommendations for local use?
- How should the best practice be customized for local use?
- What indicators will be used to measure uptake of the best practice and its impact?
- Have the stakeholders endorsed the best practice?

Who Should Be Involved in Selecting Best Practices?

This phase starts by convening an interdisciplinary working group. This usually involves someone assuming leadership and convening the group (who may or may not assume the role of group leader). The ultimate success of this, and every phase of Roadmap is in part attributable to the group lead. This may be the members who worked on finding the best practice evidence (Chapter 6) or additional members depending on the expertise you feel is

Knowledge Translation in Nursing and Healthcare: A Roadmap to Evidence-informed Practice, First Edition.
Margaret B. Harrison and Ian D. Graham.
© 2021 John Wiley & Sons, Inc. Published 2021 by John Wiley & Sons, Inc.

needed. For instance, this working group may include people with decision-making responsibility for the implementation area, especially if there are resource implications. Practitioners will be especially helpful as they understand how best to customize the recommendations for their practice.

Now that the focus is on reviewing and selecting best practices that will be implemented, there are a few things to consider. It is important that the group include all relevant interprofessional health care provider groups that may be implicated with the delivery of any of the best practice recommendations. The group must include clinical experts who have content expertise in the area of focus. Depending on the skills and experiences of group members, it may be helpful to include a library scientist or information specialist to assist with finding more recent evidence since the publication of best practices. Individuals with expertise in research methods and critical appraisal can be very useful additions as well. Individuals from the quality portfolio would bring the institutional quality improvement perspective and possibly resources from their department. Clinical educators provide valuable input as they will certainly be an important component of the implementation strategy. Students and trainees could be included as they provide extra hands and could benefit from the learning experience in evidence-informed practice and critical appraisal. In some cases, we have also included researchers who bring evaluation knowledge and expertise as well as implementation scientists. Both groups bring their unique perspectives to the work at hand and including them provides an opportunity to develop a relationship should your group want or need to conduct some research in future to inform decisions. Researchers from a local or affiliate university or college might engage in such activity.

Do not forget to include those who have organizational decision-making authority (e.g. managers, clinical leaders, directors) as these are the people who can approve all the plans and provide access to needed resources and possibly remove barriers to implementation. Last but certainly not least, care recipients and their carers must always be included. It may even be appropriate to have members of the public and other relevant stakeholders, e.g. local health charity or support network included. The rational for including patients and their carers as part of the group is that the recommendations directly impact them. They bring their experiences living with the condition, their experiences navigating, interacting with and negotiating the health system, as well as identifying possible patient preferences (DiCenso et al. 2005) related to recommendations. All these factors can have implementation implications and should be considered during best practice customization.

Depending on who may be involved in delivering the best practices in your particular context, the following questions can help frame thinking about who should be included on your working group:

- Who will lead or co-lead the working group? What are important attributes this person should have?
- Who will be affected by the new best practices? (e.g. patients, nurses, allied health, physicians, etc.)
- Who are all the stakeholders that need to be on board? (e.g. recipients of care, carers, case managers, homecare and rehabilitation, etc. if the practice has implications across health sectors, etc.)

- What are the key departments that should be involved? (e.g. quality, professional development, housekeeping, etc.)
- Who has authority to approve or endorse the best practices and who has resources that could help with implementing them?

It may not always be possible to include everyone on the working group because it might make the group too large to function effectively. When this is the case, find other ways to keep all relevant stakeholder groups that may not be represented on the working group informed of the group's processes and activities as well as seek their input on decisions. Finally, remember that how the working group functions (inclusive, transparent, respectful of different disciplinary perspectives, promoting a team ethos, etc.) can influence the ultimate acceptance of the selected best practice and the cohesiveness of collective action.

Determine the Best Practice

Once the group is assembled or reassembled, the first activity is to revisit the Recommendations Matrix that was developed in preparation for undertaking the analysis of the evidence-practice gap (refer to Chapter 6). This involves going through all the potentially relevant best practices that address your identified issue of interest. The goal is to rule out ones the group will no longer consider, leaving in contention recommendations that could be selected for adoption. At this point it is not about determining whether the best practice(s) is right for the organization but rather, which ones will NOT work for the organization based on predetermined criteria. Figure 8.1 visually presents the decisions that need to be made at this stage of Roadmap.

Determining what and how best practice could be implemented locally is the objective of the customization step. If it was not already done as part of identifying best practice, the group must first appraise the candidate guidelines and recommendations (Chapter 6).

Consider Guideline Quality

Carefully examining the quality of the candidate guideline(s) is essential as this information can be used to prioritize which guideline(s) the group should consider using. Some (Semlitsch et al. 2015) have suggested a "rapid and rough" assessment as a first assessment or to use in conjunction with AGREE II. In their 2015 review of tools to evaluate guidelines, these authors noted that recently developed instruments for a rapid review of guidelines mainly consisted of four key questions: (i) Was the evidence analyzed systematically? (ii) Does the evidence support the recommendations? (iii) Is the goal of the guidelines formulated, and are the authors named? Is the organization of the guideline easy to follow, and (iv) Are the recommendations clearly signposted? (Semlitsch et al. 2015). These questions may provide a quick and simple way to focus the working group on guideline selection.

As described earlier in Chapter 6, the AGREE II instrument is the gold standard for appraising the quality of practice guidelines (PGs) (Brouwers et al. 2010) and AGREE-REX to assess the quality of recommendations (https://jamanetwork.com/journals/jamanetworkopen/fullarticle/2766238). For additional support including links to online training tools see

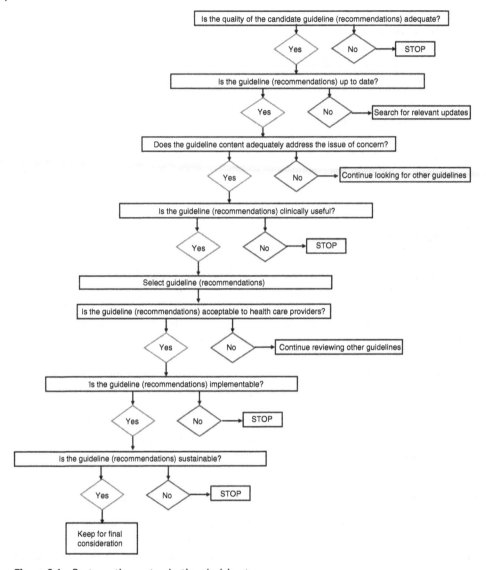

Figure 8.1 Best practice customization decision tree.

Appendix 8.A. We have often used the AGREE II rigour domain score to weed out the guidelines that have not used sufficiently rigorous guideline development methods. Depending on the views of the group, the rigour domain cut off score below which a guideline will no longer be considered can be customized (e.g. 50, 60, 70% or higher or lower). The actual cut off threshold is less important than the group's rationale for selecting it and arriving at a consensus on what it should be. We often require the rigour domain score to be above 60% for a guideline to be retained for consideration. The group may also decide to consider other domain scores when getting a sense of which guidelines should be retained or removed from consideration. This worksheet can then be reviewed by the group as they deliberate about which guidelines (or specific recommendations) to keep or drop from consideration. Remember that the AGREE II domain scores are about how the guideline was developed. It does not assess the clinical usefulness of individual recommendations, nor the quality of specific recommendations. AGREE-REX is for that purpose. Keep in mind that the AGREE II process takes time and effort as people must learn the process to conduct the AGREE II assessment. On the other hand, we have found healthcare providers who have learned to use the AGREE II instrument, are able to discuss the guidelines they appraise in greater depth because they have typically read the guideline document and reflected on it as they were completing the AGREE II instrument.

The U.S. Institute of Medicine's (IOM) (2011) Clinical Practice Guidelines We Can Trust tool can also be used to decide which candidate guidelines are of sufficient quality to keep for consideration. Unlike the AGREE II instrument, however, the IOM tool does not come with a validated scoring system (Hayawi et al. 2018).

We also have experience working with groups where the decision was to select one guideline because it was developed by a known credible developer recognized for producing high quality guidelines and widely accepted by local practitioners. In these cases, the group did not undertake guideline quality appraisal using the AGREE II instrument. This approach can be quite efficient when the guideline developer and its products are well known, evidence-informed, and respected by members of the group.

Consider Guideline Currency (Is the Guideline up-to-Date?)

At the same time as guideline quality is being considered the currency of the guideline should also be considered. What we mean by current or currency is essentially that the guideline is not past its "sell by date." This means the recommendations are still valid (or more precisely, the evidence supporting the recommendations is still valid). Information on when each candidate guideline was released and the dates when the underlying evidence were published should also be collected and considered by the group. These dates give a sense of the currency of the guidelines under consideration. However, it is also dependent on how quickly new research is coming out on a topic area. For example, after using an initial guideline in pressure ulcer risk assessment, a five-year review did not produce any new evidence to change recommendations. When thinking about the currency of

---

Box 8.1   Building Capacity

Encouraging group members to complete the AGREE II instrument with guidelines can be challenging as it requires reading a guideline, learning about the AGREE II instrument and then answering the 23 items of the instrument. The AGREE website (https://www.agreetrust.org) has online training materials that are very helpful. Getting busy clinicians to find time to do this can be difficult. On the other hand, our experience is that when clinicians participate in appraising guidelines, it can build their critical appraisal skills, reveal guidelines that they thought were high quality may be lacking in different ways, and can result in more in depth group discussion during the customization phase because of the greater knowledge of the recommendations that group members may have acquired through the appraisal process (i.e. reading the guideline document more carefully to answer the appraisal questions).

the candidate guidelines you are considering, it might be wise to contact the guideline developers to ask if, and when they are updating (or planning to update their documents). We always encourage conducting a quick search for systematic reviews on the topic of interest that may have been published after the guidelines were released. Refer to the CAN-IMPLEMENT Library Supplement (Ross-White et al. 2014) for advice on how to search for guidelines and systematic reviews.

The group will need to discuss their comfort level related to whether an out-of-date guideline should be retained for consideration for implementation. In some cases, research in an area may be slow to change and recommendations in a guideline that is several years old may still be relevant and appropriate to use. In other cases, there may be new research that makes a relatively recent guideline obsolete. This is where your clinical experts need to weigh in and offer insight about whether there are concerns about the currency of the guidelines under consideration.

Consider Adequacy of the Guideline Content (Does the Content of the Guideline Adequately Address the Issue of Concern?)

Having determined that the guideline is of sufficient quality and up to date, the working group now needs to consider if the content of the guideline adequately addresses the issue of concern. This can be done by going back the PIPOH question that was created at the beginning of the initiative and reviewing the guideline to ensure that all the issues of interest are dealt with in the guideline (see Chapter 6 for discussion of PIPOH and PICOTS).

Consider Clinical Usefulness (Is Each Recommendation Clinically Sound?)

Once the group has agreed upon the guidelines or best practices that should be retained because it/they meet adequate quality levels, are considered sufficiently up to date, and address the issue of concern, the group now needs to turn to the recommendations found within these guidelines. This stage is about reviewing the specific recommendations from the candidate guidelines in anticipation of making decisions about which guideline (or guidelines) and which recommendations the group will want to accept and implement. Keep in mind that in some cases, a bundle of recommendations may be recommended by a guideline. It is usually unwise to break up bundled recommendations, especially if the supporting evidence relates to the bundle versus the individual recommendations.

We have found it helpful to take the Recommendations Matrix and now reorder the recommendations (rows) by clustering similar recommendations to make it easier to see the differences in wording and intent related to similar recommendations contained in different guidelines (see Chapter 6 Tables 6.3 and 4). Keep in mind that this is critical as organizations and health care providers typically implement specific recommendations which may not represent the entirety of one guideline.

As already suggested, this stage involves first and foremost assessing the substance of the recommendations from a practical perspective to identify what the group considers would be clinically useful recommendations. We encourage the group to discuss each row of the Recommendations Matrix (i.e. each similar recommendation) and reflect on the clinical utility of each. When reviewing the substance of the recommendations listed in the Recommendations Matrix, the group will want to ask:

- Are different guidelines making the same recommendations? or Are there recommendations that substantively differ by guideline?
- Are these differences clinically meaningful or important?
- Are delivering the recommendations possible in our setting (e.g. within our scope of practice)?
- Is each recommendation clinically useful and addresses the issue of concern?

Select Guideline and Recommendations for Local Use as Best Practice

Having assessed each potential guideline and recommendation based on quality, currency, content, and clinical usefulness the group has now ruled out the guidelines and recommendations that did not meet these criteria. The Recommendations Matrix should be revised accordingly to reflect these deletions and should now only include guidelines and recommendations that in theory, would be worthy to implement. When thinking of recommendations to implement, the challenge is often that there is more than one relevant guideline to choose from and many more recommendations than any organization would be able to implement at once. The goal at this point is to cull the guidelines and recommendations into a workable number. In some cases, essentially the same recommendation with slightly different wording is being made by different guidelines so the decision is about choosing which wording to go with. In other cases, it may involve choosing between different recommendations from different guidelines (which may not agree with each other). There are also context specific considerations that can influence a decision to accept a recommendation as well. There can be very good reasons not to implement a potentially clinically useful, up-to-date recommendation from a quality guideline. Not every recommendation meeting these criteria needs to or necessarily should be implemented. For example, there may be more recommendations available than groups are able to implement at a given time. Or the ability to implement is hindered by current resources or staffing in the local context. For example, working in more rural or remote communities, guideline recommendations often must be modified due to the limited availability of specialists.

As before, what is critical to successful decision making at this step is ensuring that the group remains inclusive and interdisciplinary with all relevant stakeholders involved. This contributes to the legitimacy of the process and improves the quality of the process because those affected by the decisions are the ones making the decisions.

The Recommendations Matrix becomes a major source of the evidence upon which discussion and decisions are made. Seeking and listening to all group members' perspectives on the recommendations, respecting everyone's opinions, and remaining focused on the decisions that need to be made is how the process should unfold. The group also needs to set rules for this discussion (e.g. agree upon criteria). This will contribute to the group making systematic and transparent decisions about selecting recommendations to accept from all the ones still left in contention. Document the decisions in the Action Map. Remember that at this point, the goal switches from ruling out recommendations to deciding on which ones to accept as is or accept in principle. Criteria we have used with groups at this step include: starting with recommendations with the strongest level of supporting evidence and then working through to recommendations to the weakest levels of evidence or, starting with recommendations believed to have the greatest potential for improving health outcomes. Another approach is to work through the nursing process, e.g. in one of our projects we began with assessment recommendations for pressure ulcer injury risk and then tackled the pressure ulcer injury risk reduction recommendations.

Criteria such as the strength of the evidence for the recommendation, acceptability of the recommendation to the organization, implementability, and sustainability of the recommendation can all be useful in helping to decide which recommendations to adopt.

Consider Strength of the Evidence

The strength of the evidence for a recommendation is an important discussion point and whether the group considers it adequate to change practice. This is an essential criterion if the desire is for care to be evidence informed. As noted in Chapter 6, there are several systems that guideline developers use to grade the strength of the evidence for specific recommendations. In recent years the GRADE approach (Grade Working Group 2019) has become more common and allows for comparison of the strength of the evidence across different guidelines using this system. Keep in mind that a recommendation may make great clinical sense but have little supporting evidence for it and the opposite may also be true. A win-win situation is when a recommendation makes good clinical sense and is supported by strong evidence. Depending on when the guidelines were released and when the supporting evidence in those guidelines was published, it may be prudent to search for recent systematic reviews that could provide more recent evidence summaries related to the recommendations. Your clinical experts on the group may also be aware of more recent relevant evidence that should be considered.

It is through open dialogue that the group can weigh the clinical utility and strength of the evidence of each recommendation. Discussion questions can be:

- Is the strength of the evidence supporting the recommendation adequate for our local context?
- To what extent is our patient population like those upon which the primary studies were conducted? (e.g. is our frail population too different from the younger sample in the studies?)
- Is the recommendation stated in a manner that will be clearly understood?
- Do we have the resources and clinical capacity to deliver the recommendation?
- Are there any equity or diversity aspects to the recommendation that may make it unacceptable in our context? (for example would using the recommendation provide greater benefit for men or women?)
- Are there components of different recommendations that are critical for guideline effectiveness?

Box 8.2   Careful Consideration with Local Factors

In one implementation we found it necessary to include a guideline that did not score well on the Rigour domain. However, the guideline was already implemented in many settings and favored as it came from the national wound care association. Thus, we included it in the Recommendations Matrix and after analyzing the content found it was similar to all the other highly rated guidelines on the topic. The reasons for this were the developing panel's process was not well documented and some recent research papers were not included. Given the recommendations were similar and the group felt were better worded, it was decided to use this guideline and provide further support for recommendation by referencing the higher scoring ones.

Additional Considerations

In addition to recommendations being clinically useful and based on evidence, the group should simultaneously consider whether the potential recommendations are acceptable, implementable and sustainable and essential to guideline effectiveness. These are considerations that can affect the potential implementation and ongoing use of the recommendations. Excellent clinical recommendations may not be implemented or not completely implemented because: 1) they are not acceptable to health care providers or patients (e.g. are not aligned with patient preferences); 2) are impossible to implement (e.g. the required equipment needed to adhere to the recommendation is not available); 3) or cannot be sustained over time, and will not have their desired impact (i.e. which denies patients effective care and results in inefficient use of existing resources, etc.). Furthermore, failed implementation efforts waste scarce healthcare resources. The rationale for beginning to consider implementation issues when selecting best practices to implement should be strategic and can improve future implementation success.

Is the Recommendation Acceptable?

The group needs to reflect on whether each recommendation will be acceptable in their clinical setting. When the group is contemplating the implementation of a recommendation, we have found it is common to deliberate on whether the recommendation will be acceptable to different provider groups as well as patients and carers. For example, a recommendation encouraging specialist clinics to be set up in the community to manage wounds may be favored by the nurses but not be acceptable to older patients, who are concerned about going out in harsh winter conditions or those who do not have reasonable access to transportation. By considering how acceptable the recommendations may be in their setting, the group can plan how to overcome potential acceptability challenges. Following through with the example above, providing transportation options to the clinics might make it more acceptable but this will only partially deal with the concern about snow and ice and treacherous walking conditions in winter.

Many factors may influence the perceived acceptability of recommendations. For example, managers may be concerned that recommendations are too costly to implement, clinicians may think following the recommendations will be too time consuming, and patients may have preferences for other options. If the overall feeling is that the recommendations are not going to be acceptable, then the group may want to exclude them from future consideration. On the other hand, the group may be convinced of the value of the recommendations and decide on the need to find ways to increase their acceptability to stakeholders. For example, when the acceptability of a recommendation is anticipated to be low, the group can begin exploring the reasons it is not seen to be acceptable.

We have found a common concern affecting the perceived acceptability of a new practice is the belief by providers that the practice will take too much time to carry out. This can be addressed by establishing how much time it will actually take to do the practice and share this with the potential adopters. When the recommendation is being implemented, we have also encouraged groups facing potential resistance related to time, to have discussions with point-of-care providers about the time issue. This discussion should include how current practice processes might be reorganized to free up time. This could include practices that are not supported by evidence or have been shown to be ineffective being discontinued. Other approaches to dealing with the time issue might be to consider whether a recommendation could be carried out during a quieter time or whether an alternate provider could deliver it.

The point here is about the group thinking through each candidate recommendation and considering how acceptable it will be to the potential adopters and deciding whether those recommendations that may not seem acceptable on the surface could become acceptable if the underlying concern can be adequately addressed. Sometimes this is about changing people's misunderstanding about a candidate recommendation. In other cases, it is about finding ways to convince them their negative views may not be accurate. While a somewhat rare occurrence, we have worked with some groups that have taken the decision that a specific recommendation was simply not acceptable. When this happens, it was often because the recommendation was based on expert opinion and adhering to the recommendation would require deployment of considerable resources or major changes to the way things were done. In this instance the group felt it would be unjustified because of the lack of empirical evidence for the recommendation. We have also had groups decide recommendations based on expert opinion were acceptable because the recommendations were aligned with their current practice. When recommendations in a guideline are arrived at through a consensus of expert opinion when there is poor or no empirical evidence, this may still be better guidance than "just the way we have been doing it." Chapter 9 describes how to systematically assess barriers and drivers to implementing best practice once the best practices have been selected, as this information is used to help select implementation strategies. Questions that can be used to stimulate discussion about recommendation acceptability include:

- Will this recommendation be acceptable to our health care providers (think specifically about which providers: nurses, physicians, allied health, managers, etc.)? If not, why not?
- Will this recommendation be acceptable to our patients and carers? If not, why not?
- If not acceptable, what would it take to make it acceptable?

Is the Recommendation Implementable?

Even when a recommendation may be considered clinically useful and acceptable it does not mean that it will always be possible or feasible to implement it. For example, the concern may be that the implementability of a practice may be low because the organization does not have the required equipment to follow the recommendations (e.g. insufficient number of pressure relieving devices for all the patients requiring them) but identifying this when selecting the best practices to implement means that the group can take proactive action to overcome the identified implementation barriers. Chapters 10 and 11 focus on implementation strategies and how to select them. Asking the group to contemplate the implementability of each recommendation lets them begin to think about implementation issues. It is far better to begin thinking about implementation while making decisions about which recommendations to adopt than to assume implementation considerations will be dealt with later – as it may be too late then. Of course, if the group concludes that the recommendations are not implementable in their setting, then they will not select them. This is a reasonable decision but should only be taken when the group has convinced itself that the implementation issues are truly insurmountable (e.g. the site is not physically capable of delivering the best practice because it lacks specific infrastructure to do so and there are no resources available to build the needed infrastructure). Specific questions that may help the group think about the implementability of recommendations include:

- How difficult or feasible will it be to implement this recommendation? Why?
- What factors or issues could hinder or facilitate implementing this recommendation?
- How modifiable are these factors/issues?

Is the Recommendation Sustainable?

The final consideration during this phase of selecting recommendations for adoption is their sustainability. Implementing a recommendation that cannot be sustained over the long run wastes the initial resources used to implement the recommendation since the impacts of adhering to the recommendation will not be achieved. Things that can affect sustainability can include: changes within the organization (e.g. reorganization of departments or divisions, changes in executive leadership, change fatigue, etc.), staff changes (e.g. turnover of a large proportion of staff, best practice champions changing positions, staff burnout, changes in scopes of practice of health care professionals, etc.), and external changes that affects the organization (e.g. mergers of healthcare facilities, etc.). Specific questions that may help the group think about the sustainability of recommendations include:

- After initial implementation of the best practice, how likely is it that the best practice will be continued?
- What would be the main reasons it might not be continued?
- What might be the resource implications or costs of sustaining use of the best practices?
- Are there organizational changes planned that would affect the continuation of the best practices? (e.g. change in the provider team reducing [or increasing] the number of registered nurses needed to carry out the recommended assessment)
- Are there broader changes at the municipal, state or province, or national level that will affect the organization's ability to implement best practice? (e.g. regional health services move the care to a different sector such as from hospital clinic to homecare).

While these criteria are the ones, we and the CAN-IMPLEMENT process suggest using to help with the group's decision making about which recommendations to adopt, the group may also decide to use other criteria. If this happens, documenting these criteria and providing a rationale for their selection will be important. Add more rows to the Recommendations Matrix for these criteria.

What Might the Discussion Sound Like?

With the Recommendation Matrix in front of the members of the group, they start going through the rows of the Matrix which represent unique recommendations. Consider all like recommendations at the same time. The Chair or lead of the group should guide the discussion of each recommendation and seek the group's agreement that it is clinically useful, supported by strong (adequate) evidence, would be generally thought to be acceptable (or not), would/would not have major implementation issues, and whether there are any concerns about sustainability. These points can be used to prompt discussion. Finally, the group needs to reach agreement on whether the recommendation should be kept or dismissed. Agreement can be reached through open discussion and consensus (everyone agrees; a majority agrees and a minority dissents) or voting if a more formal process is preferred.

When there are several recommendations along the same lines, the group needs to decide whether to accept the general intent of these recommendations. If the decision is to accept, then it needs to consider if the wording of one of the recommendations is preferable to the others and adopt that one. It is best not to spend a lot of time wordsmithing at this time as the group will have another opportunity to look at the wording of all kept recommendations and make wording modifications at that time.

Someone should take notes on the decision to keep or reject a recommendation and the rationale for the decision. Dissenting opinions should be captured and documented. Documenting this process ensures the reasons for all the decisions cannot be forgotten as membership of the group may change (See Appendix 8.B for a best practice protocol/guideline report template). Importantly, it supports the transparency of the group's work. This information can be useful during the implementation phase to demonstrate how carefully the group deliberated during its decision-making process and the reasons for its decisions.

Once the group has rejected some of the recommendations in the Recommendations Matrix (or kept all the recommendation in the Matrix), the group must decide about whether one of the candidate guidelines (columns in the matrix) covers all the recommendations the group is interested in implementing. If one guideline meets the group's need, then it can simply endorse the "winning" guideline. If one guideline does not contain all the recommendations of interest, then the group will need to create its own local "guideline" or best practice protocol by assembling recommendations originating from multiple guidelines.

Before finishing this step, the group should go through each selected recommendation and review its wording and make minor editorial changes to make the recommendations easier to interpret or to make the behavior change required more explicit. This step is about wordsmithing the recommendations, **not** about changing the substance or essence of recommendations that are based on evidence. For example, a guideline from a different country might use terminology or language that is unfamiliar to your context, so the wording should be modified accordingly.

The decisions to be made at this step are:

- Is there one guideline that the group wants to endorse?
- Whether one guideline or considering multiple ones, is there a need to modify recommendations?

Figure 8.2 presents a decision tree listing the various decisions at this point in the process.

Customize Selected Best Practice (What Will Work Here and How?)

Once the final recommendations to be implemented have been selected and assembled into the local protocol, the final step of this phase is about contextualizing or aligning the recommendations to the local context, as necessary. This involves reviewing each recommendation one last time and considering how the prescribed behavior could be undertaken in the local context. It involves thinking about who needs to do what, how, under what conditions and when. For example, a recommendation might state that nurses should conduct a specific type of assessment on patients. When the group thinks about how this would work in their context, they realize that nurses may not have the time or capacity to do the assessment, but the social worker does, so they modify the recommendation to state the social worker will perform the assessment as prescribed. A different example might be that the recommendation requires a 30–60 minute thorough assessment on admission to a complex care facility, but the group feels that patients are already overwhelmed with the number of admission assessments they are exposed to on admission day. Additionally, the nurses voice the concern that there currently is not time to add another long assessment. They decide to customize the recommendation by stating the assessment must be done within 48 hours of admission rather than on admission after having determined that delaying the assessment by a couple of days would not pose a health risk to patients.

The group may have thought about customizing issues during the recommendation selection process, but at that stage, the final set of recommendations had not been chosen and so they could not have foreseen exactly how all the recommendations would fit together. Hence the need to review the final package of recommendations from both an operational and logistical perspective and make modifications to the recommendations about who will need to do what exactly. This customization discussion is also a good opportunity to again consider implementation issues such as: opportunities to link with quality improvement, risk reduction and safety initiatives within the organization, identify resource requirements, and consider the impact of the best practices on interdependent relationships between health care provider groups. Documentation is a critical issue that should enter the discussion here and requires careful consideration and planning as it often takes months to change documentation processes. Now the best practice should be in a ready state to begin aligning it to your local context.

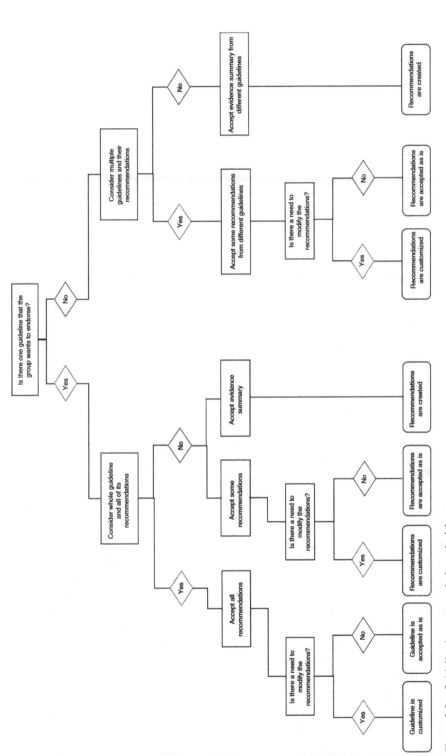

Figure 8.2 Guideline/recommendations decision tree.

All that is left is to do at this stage is for the group to draft the local best practice protocol/ guideline report. This ideally should detail the package of selected recommendations, the decision-making process, and reasons for its decisions. Appendix 8.B provides a template for the best practice report. It is this draft document that will now need to go out for consultation and feedback from healthcare providers, patients, managers, etc. This consultation/feedback can take the form of a meeting and/or a survey. It is important for successful implementation that issues raised are addressed and revision done accordingly. Once the feedback issues are addressed, the final version of the report will then be ready to go for formal endorsement by the organization. Describing the feedback received and how it was or was not incorporated into the best practice report contributes to transparency. Our experience has been that when individuals see that their concerns have been heard and considered, they realize the consulta-tion process is authentic and meaningful and this contributes to their trusting the guideline customization process and wanting to provide feedback in future.

Decide on Indicators of Best Practice Use and Impact

There is one more detail to attend to before completing the local best practice document. The working group needs to identify all the specific best practice recommendations and identify or develop indicators for them. If the source guidelines do not provide indicators that can be used to measure adherence to them, the group will need to develop their own indicators. In line with the concept of conceptual and instrumental knowledge use (see Chapter 12 and Chapter 12 Appendix), the process indicators need to measure the extent to which each recommendation is being used. We have found that sometimes guideline devel-opers do not provide indicators and when the working group is trying to develop them, it becomes clear that the actual recommendations are not worded in a way that allows them to be measured. For example, a recommendation states that, all patients should be assessed using a given measure, and those scoring high should be referred to specialist care. To meas-ure adherence to this recommendation, one wants to know what proportion of presenting patients are being assessed (# assessed/total # of appropriate patients *100) and what pro-portion are being appropriately referred (number being referred/ number scoring high on the assessment *100). The first indicator is fairly easy to operationalize but the second is problematic if it is not clear what a high score on the assessment is (it is also problematic as healthcare providers will be left to their own discretion to decide what the cutoff point for referral is). By thinking through what the adherence indicators should be, the working group may need some further customization of the recommendations by refining the word-ing of recommendations to make sure that each one is measurable.

Similarly, the working group should identify indicators of impact that may be of interest to the group. That is, if a best practice recommendation is followed, what impact does it have on health outcomes or health system outcomes. For example, if the patient received the appropriate treatment for a wound, what is the effect on healing rates or patients' quality of life, or what are the resource implications of receiving best practice.

There are also a number of data collection issues that the group must consider when making decisions about what indicators to adopt, these include: what data are already available, what data may need to be collected, how it will be collected, and the resources required to collect it. Decisions about indicators must consider these feasibility issues. Given the ongoing measuring of the indicators will inform how well the organization is adhering to the best practice over time, it is important to be able to continue this data collection after the initial implementation of the best practice. Ongoing monitoring of best practice and impact is an important strategy for sustaining the use of best practice. It can be used to reveal when adherence to the best practice is declining and the need for more or different implementation strategies to reverse the decline (for more on this see Chapter 14).

Establish a Renewal Plan

The working group should also devote some time to thinking through the process by which the customized best practice will be kept up to date. The best practice renewal process will require scanning for new guidelines and literature which may change the existing recommendations. There needs to be a process for continuously monitoring the source guidelines to identify when they are updated or retired. The approach to the searching needs to be systematic and ongoing, and ideally guided by a library scientist. The group's clinical experts can be used to flag new evidence but should not be solely relied on for this. The group will need to decide on rules for updating their customized best practice. What criteria will be used to decide if the entire customized best practice should be retired, whether specific recommendations should be retired, or new recommendations added? The group needs to decide who will be responsible for this task and where any needed resources will come from. Not keeping a customized best practice up to date can have serious implications if users of the best practice realize it is no longer evidence informed. This can pose a major threat to the credibility of the best practice and to the working group. Keeping the best practice current is a critical strategy for sustaining use of the best practice after its initial implementation and warrants regular attention of the working group.

Seek Endorsement of the Proposed Best Practice

Once the best practice has been carefully customized and is now more-or-less complete, there is one last step which is ensuring that all the key stakeholders approve of the best practice. This is done by sending the proposed best practice report out to all relevant stakeholders and seeking their feedback. This can be done by sending the best practice report out with a brief survey that asks if the respondent agrees with the best practice and if not, asks for the reason why not. The survey can also ask participants if they have intentions to adhere to the best practices. The responses to the best practice should be discussed by the working group and decisions made about whether the best practice document requires modification to address identified concerns. Any changes made should be documented in the local best practice report as well as reasons for not making suggested changes. Being explicit and transparent about the process will increase the credibility of the process among potential users of the best practice.

Once finalized, official endorsement of the best practice report should be sought from policy makers who have responsibility for clinical practice where the best practice will be implemented. This step involves leaders (committees) within the organization reviewing the proposed best practice (which may have been modified based on feedback) and making the

Table 8.1 Phase 2: ACTION MAP for solution building (*with Wound Example*).

Adopted external recommendations *Operationalization of recommendation*	Customize best practice recommendations by aligning them with context to become local best practice intervention (who, what/how, when/timing)	Barriers and facilitating factors (drivers)
Guideline/recommendations selected for local use	Guideline/recommendations customized for local use	Factors related to each recommendation, potential adopters, or context. *What would aid or prevent implementation?*
1. Q 24 hr skin and risk assessment, document on flow chart	Who: attending evening RN What/how: skin and risk assessment during HS care, document on flow chart When: daily, evening shift when units are generally less busy 1. Evening RN to daily conduct a head to toe assessment during HS care and document in flow chart	Most nurses familiar with head-to-toe skin assessment Currently not in orientation for new staff HS routine happens with every patient so will be an incremental extra
2. Risk Assessment with Braden Scale	Who: evening RN What/how: Braden Risk assessment, (6 sub-scales); each subscale document in flow chart When: during head to toe skin assessment, on evening shift 2. Braden Risk assessment conducted with head to toe skin assessment by attending RN on evening shift daily and documented in nursing notes	Staff on several units not familiar with risk assessment scale (6 sub-scales), questioning total score, perceived as a lot of work Currently not in orientation for new staff
3. etc.		
Sustainability thinking continues here. . .	Consider and reconsider the "fit" to ensure customized best practice is achievable to encourage ongoing uptake	Barriers assessment conducted such that it can be redone in future, if necessary. Target implementation strategies to known barriers and drivers to improve the uptake and ongoing maintenance
Chapter 8	Chapter 8 and 9	Chapter 8 and 9

decision to formally sanction or adopt it, thereby giving it official status. This is done, for example, when an organization endorses a guideline as policy. This administrative step provides the organization with a final opportunity to consider the effects of the proposed best practice on its functioning. The formal decision making, and procedural process required to endorse a best practice needs to be explicit and documented by the organization. Once the organization provides its "seal of approval," the guideline is ready for dissemination and implementation. Obtaining formal endorsement of the best practice is an important milestone that signals that the best practice has been adopted within the organization. Now the work turns to how to ensure that all the relevant stakeholders change their practice to align with the best practice.

Summary

This chapter has described the process by which the working group can systematically review, prioritize, select, and customize best practices for their local context. At the completion of this phase, the group has:

- Selected the best practices to implement and considered their quality, currency, clinical usefulness, strength of the evidence, acceptability, implementability and sustainability.
- Customized the chosen best practice(s) for the local context and drafted the local best practice report.
- Chosen the indicators or measures that will be used to determine whether the best practice is being adhered to and the impact of its use.
- Draft best practice report sent to healthcare providers, patients, managers, and other relevant stakeholders for consultation/feedback and revised accordingly before it has been officially adopted by the organization.

Again, it is imperative to update the Action Map (Table 8.1) to document all these activities and any decisions made. If the group is drafting an Implementation Plan, that should also be updated at this juncture.

The next chapter describes how to undertake a barriers assessment of the factors that might interfere with or drive implementing the best practice. This information will enable the group to better plan its implementation strategy.

Appendix 8.A

The AGREE II Instrument – Online Access and Support

The AGREE II Instrument

The AGREE II Instrument (Appraisal of Guidelines for REsearch and Evaluation) provides a framework for assessing the *methodological quality* of clinical practice guidelines; it *does not assess the clinical content* of the recommendations. The 23 items in the AGREE II Instrument examine the methods used for developing the guideline and the quality of the reporting. A final Overall Assessment item allows appraisers to make a judgment on the quality of the guideline as a whole. The AGREE II Instrument is available at http://www.agreetrust.org.

AGREE II Instrument Training Tools

Two training tools have been developed to assist AGREE II users to effectively apply the tool. The tools were evaluated in a randomized research study. The training tools are available at https://www.agreetrust.org/resource-centre/agree-ii/agree-ii-training-tools.

The AGREE II Overview Tutorial provides an Avatar-guided overview of the AGREE II tool. This tool takes approximately 10 minutes to complete: http://agree2.machealth.ca/players/open/index.html.

The AGREE II Tutorial + Practice Exercise expands upon the Avatar-guided tutorial. The "Practice Exercise" tool provides trainees with the opportunity to appraise a test practice guideline with the AGREE II; upon submitting their ratings, the training tool system provides immediate feedback on how the trainees' responses compare with those of expert ratings. On average, completion of this tool takes approximately one hour:

http://agree2.machealth.ca/openinstrumentfeedback.aspx?id=918e38c1-a84d-45aa-8343-145c06eea243.

AGREE-REX

The AGREE-REX is a newly developed tool designed to evaluate the clinical credibility and implementability of practice guidelines (PGs) recommendations.

https://www.agreetrust.org/resource-centre/agree-rex-recommendation-excellence.

My AGREE Plus

By registering for the AGREE website, volunteer raters can create their own personal account allowing them to conduct practice guideline appraisals online and save them for future reference, create a personal library of practice guideline appraisals, and share appraisals with colleagues.

My AGREE PLUS is available at https://www.agreetrust.org/resource-centre/agree-plus.

Additional AGREE II Resources

Additional resources for the AGREE II Instrument are available on the AGREE website:
https://www.agreetrust.org/resource-centre.

Appendix 8.B

Best Practice Protocol/Guideline Report Template

Source: Adapted with permission from: Harrison et al. (2014).

[Insert Facility/Health Authority responsible for Guideline]
[Insert Logo]
[Insert the Guideline Title]
[Insert the Guideline Sub-title]

[Insert the name(s) of the author(s)]
[Insert date]

	Revision History		
Revision #	**Date of Release**	**Owner**	**Summary of Changes**

[To maintain the integrity of this document, include a revision history in the working file]

Overview

Abstract

(The abstract is typically a short summary of the contents of the document. A traditional three to four part structure may be used to highlight key points. Include the release date plus print and electronic sources.)

Introduction: (A brief context of the work. Include the purpose of the guideline initiative and the questions to be answered.)

Methods: (A description of the methodology/procedures followed to answer the health questions.)

Results and Discussion *(may be combined):* [Key results in answer to your health questions, along with comments re: importance, relevance, application].

Institutional Affiliation of Adaptation Panel

(Name and institutional or health authority/regional affiliation(s) of the adaptation panel.)

Introduction and Background

(The Introduction and Background typically clarify the subject matter [definitions, historical background] and provide the necessary contextual information to outline the practice problem [e.g. current practices and outcomes, burden associated with a disease]. This section should end with a brief statement of what is being reported in the guideline. The following sections describe the objective[s], target users, target population, and health questions covered by the guideline.)

Scope and Purpose

(The Scope and Purpose typically describe the rationale or need for the guideline and overall objective[s]. Potential health intent[s] [i.e. prevention, screening, diagnosis, etc.], health impact[s] [expected benefits or outcomes], and target populations of patients or individuals should be communicated. The anticipated health benefits from the guideline should be specific to the clinical problem or health issue.); *Consider adding links to supporting tools or documents/outputs here.*

Target Users

(Target users of the guideline are identified in this section. A precise description will immediately inform readers as to the relevancy of the guideline to their issue. Include a well-defined description of the intended audience [i.e. health care professionals, administrators, patients/families] and an explanation of how the guideline is intended to be used.); *Consider adding links to supporting tools or documents/outputs here.*

Target (Patient) Population

(The Target Population [patients, individuals] is described in this section. All parameters for inclusion [i.e. gender, age, clinical circumstances, disease site/severity, psychosocial, cultural] and exclusion criteria should be specifically stated.); *Consider adding links to supporting tools or documents/outputs here.*

Health Questions

(The Health/Clinical Questions addressed by the guideline are clearly defined in this section. The following criteria are important to include when stating the health questions: target population, intervention[s], professionals, comparisons, outcomes, and health care setting/context.); *Consider adding links to supporting tools or documents/outputs here.*

Documentation Checklist[1]: Introduction and Background

✓ The overall objective(s) of the guideline is (are) specifically described.
✓ The target users of the guideline are clearly defined.
✓ The population (patients, public, etc.) to whom the guideline is meant to apply is specifically described.
✓ The health question(s) covered by the guideline is (are) specifically described.

[1] Documentation Checklist items have been adapted from the AGREE II Instrument, available at http://www.agreetrust.org.

Recommendations

(The adapted recommendations, their associated health risks and benefits, and circumstances in which they apply are stated in the following sections.)

Recommendations

(The Recommendations, which include different options for management of the condition/health issue, are clearly stated in this section. Under what circumstance [when/for whom] each option is appropriate in addition to the intent or purpose of the recommendation should be described. The strength of each recommendation based on stated recommendation grading criteria and links to the supporting evidence [summaries/tables/references] on which the recommendation was formulated must be clearly specified. Presenting the recommendations as a group, in boldface, underlined, or in a flowchart or algorithm format will help to make them easily identifiable to the target audience.); *Consider adding links to supporting tools or documents/outputs here.*

Health Risks and Benefits

(The health benefits, side effects, and risks associated with the recommendations are clearly stated in this section. Topics such as potential adverse effects, impact on survival and quality of life, symptom management and alternative treatment options should be addressed. Include supporting data of benefits and harms and discuss balance/trade-off between benefits and harms/side effects/risks.); *Consider adding links to supporting tools or documents/outputs here.*

Supporting Evidence and Information

(The supporting evidence and panel rational for formulating the recommendations is clearly described in this section. Criteria for selecting the evidence [i.e. target population, study design, outcomes, language, and context] and the methods for formulating the recommendations should be explained in this section *or in an Appendix*. Present additional evidence/and or the results of the updating process. If existing recommendations were modified, an explanation is warranted.); *Consider adding links to supporting tools or documents/outputs here.*

External Review and Consultation Process

(The purpose of the external review [i.e. gather feedback, seek patient input, improve quality, obtain endorsement] is described in this section. A description of the reviewers, methods, and collection of feedback from external reviewers of the guideline are outlined in the following sections); *Consider adding links to supporting tools or documents/ outputs here.*

Documentation Checklist[1]: Recommendations

✓ The different options for management of the condition or health issue are clearly presented.
✓ The recommendations are specific and unambiguous.
✓ Key recommendations are easily identifiable.
✓ There is an explicit link between the recommendations and the supporting evidence.
✓ The health benefits, side effects, and risks have been considered in formulating the recommendations.
✓ The criteria for selecting the evidence are clearly described.

External Review Panel

(Reviewers of the guideline [who were not involved in the development of the guideline] are described in this section. In addition to providing a list of reviewers and their affiliation, include a description of their clinical or methodological expertise, or whether they are part of the target population [patients, public].); *Consider adding links to supporting tools or documents/outputs here.*

External Review Process and Methods

(The methods used to conduct the external review and how the information was gathered is clearly described in this section. It is important to document how the feedback was gathered [i.e. surveys, hard copy edits to a draft] and the type of survey methods used if applicable [i.e. rating scale, open-ended questionnaire].); *Consider adding links to supporting tools or documents/outputs here.*

Discussion of Feedback

(Discussion of feedback that was incorporated into the final document is addressed in this section. A summary of the key findings from the external review and reasons for not including reviewer's feedback [if applicable] should be discussed.); *Consider adding links to supporting tools or documents/outputs here.*

Documentation Checklist[1]: External Review and Consultation Process

✓ The guideline has been externally reviewed by experts prior to its publication.
✓ The views and preferences of the target population (patients, public, etc.) have been sought.

Plan for Scheduled Review and Update

(The plan for a scheduled review and update of the guideline is clearly described in this section. Explicitly state the planned scheduled date [or time interval] of review of the guideline. Report the plan and methodology that will be used to update and review the guideline.); *Consider adding links to supporting tools or documents/outputs here.*

Documentation Checklist[1]: Plan for Scheduled Review and Update

✓ A procedure for updating the guideline is provided.

Algorithm or Summary Document

(Additional materials such as algorithms, summary tables, quick reference guides, educational tools, patient information pamphlets, and links to online resources, should be provided in this section to aid users in implementation of the recommendations into practice. A description of how users can access tools and resources should also be included.); *Consider adding links to supporting tools or documents/outputs here.*

Documentation Checklist[1]: Algorithm or Summary Document

✓ The guideline provides advice and/or tools on how the recommendations can be put into practice.

Implementation Considerations

(Implementation considerations including facilitators and barriers, resource implications, and criteria for monitoring/auditing usage of the guideline are described in the following sections.)

Facilitators and Barriers

Facilitators and barriers which may impact the uptake of the guideline into practice are discussed in this section. It is important to describe the procedures that were used to gather information regarding the facilitators and barriers to implementing the recommendations [e.g. feedback from key stakeholders, usability testing]. Include a description of how the information influenced the guideline development process and/or formation of the recommendations.); *Consider adding links to supporting tools or documents/outputs here.*

Resource Implications

(The potential resource implications of applying the recommendations are described in this section [i.e. types of cost information, methods used to gather the data, how the information was used to inform the recommendations].); *Consider adding links to supporting tools or documents/outputs here.*

Monitoring Guideline Adherence

(The strategies that will be used to monitor the uptake and adherence to the guideline are described in this section. The criteria that will be used to measure if the guideline has been successfully implemented into practice [using key recommendations as indicators] should be clearly stated.); *Consider adding links to supporting tools or documents/outputs here*

 Documentation Checklist[1]: Implementation Considerations

✓ The guideline describes facilitators and barriers to its application.
✓ The potential resource implications of applying the recommendations have been considered.
✓ The guideline presents monitoring and/or auditing criteria.

Glossary of Unfamiliar Terms

(An alphabetized list of terms which are newly introduced, uncommon or specialized are included in this section of the report. [Tip: using a tabular format will allow for quick alphabetical sorting of terms. With cursor placed anywhere on the table access the Table Tools Layout tab, then choose "Sort" from the menu])

Term	Definition

References

(All reference material used in creating the guideline is documented in this section of the guideline report.)

Acknowledgement of Source Guidelines

(The acknowledgement of source guideline developers and permissions granted [where necessary] are included in this section of the report.); *Consider adding links to supporting tools or documents/outputs here.*

Guideline Adaptation Panel

(The guideline adaptation panel, conflicts of interest, and sources of funding are described in the following sections.)

Membership and Role

(List the names of all panel members, and include their credentials, area of expertise, institution, geographical location, and role on the panel.); *Consider adding links to supporting tools or documents/outputs here.*

Conflicts of Interest

(An explicit statement as to whether members declared whether or not they had any conflicts of interest is included in this section.); *Consider adding links to supporting tools or documents/ outputs here.*

Funding Sources

(List all funding sources for the development of the guideline. It is equally important to document in the case that there was no external funding source. If the views or interests of the funding body have not influenced the final recommendations, it is important to include a statement to that effect.); *Consider adding links to supporting tools or documents/outputs here.*

Documentation Checklist[1]: Guideline Adaptation Panel

- ✓ The guideline development group includes individuals from all relevant professional groups.
- ✓ Competing interests of guideline development group members have been recorded and addressed.
- ✓ The views of the funding body have not influenced the content of the guideline.

Appendix

Guideline Search and Retrieval

([Details regarding the systematic search and retrieval of guidelines are described in this section. A detailed description of the search strategy should include the search terms used, database sources consulted (e.g. MEDLINE, EMBASE, PsychINFO, CINAHL)], and time periods included. Hand searching methods should also be documented. A list of guidelines identified in the search, and whether or not they were considered for use in the guideline adaptation and why, should be provided.]; *Consider adding links to supporting tools or documents/outputs here.*

Guideline Assessments

[Guideline assessments conducted on the retrieved guidelines are described in this section. Which assessments were conducted, in what order, and a summary of results for each assessment (including AGREE scores) should be provided. The strengths and limitations of the evidence should be discussed in detail (e.g. risk of bias, consistency, applicability, etc.).]; *Consider adding links to supporting tools or documents/outputs here.*

Decision Processes

[The decision processes used by the panel to formulate the recommendations are described in this section. A description of the methods the panel used to come to consensus (e.g. Delphi method, Nominal group technique) and resolve disagreements should be explicitly stated.]; *Consider adding links to supporting tools or documents/outputs here.*

Evaluation Results and Decisions

[The results and decisions of each evaluation are described in this section.]; *Consider adding links to supporting tools or documents/outputs here.*

Documentation Checklist[1]: Appendix

✓ Systematic methods were used to search for evidence.
✓ The strengths and limitations of the body of evidence are clearly described.
✓ The methods for formulating the recommendations are clearly described.

References

Brouwers, M.C., Kho, M.E., Browman, G.P. et al. (2010). AGREE II: advancing guideline development, reporting, and evaluation in health care. *Preventive Medicine* 51: 421–424. https://doi.org/10.1016/j.ypmed.2010.08.005.

DiCenso, A., Guyatt, G., and Ciliska, D. (2005). *Evidence-Based Nursing: A Guide to Clinical Practice*. St. Louis, MO: Elsevier Health Sciences.

Grade Working Group (2020). *GRADE Working Group Organizational Website*, [Online], Available: http://www.gradeworkinggroup.org (6 Sept 2019).

Harrison, M.B., van den Hoek, J., and Graham, I.D. (2014). *CAN-IMPLEMENT: Planning for Best-Practice Implementation (Book 20, Appendix 13)*. Philadelphia: Lippincott Williams & Wilkins.

Hayawi, L.M., Graham, I.D., Tugwell, P., and Yousef Abdelrazeq, S. (2018). Screening for osteoporosis: a systematic assessment of the quality and content of clinical practice guidelines, using the AGREE II instrument and the IOM Standards for Trustworthy Guidelines. *PLoS One* 13: e0208251. https://doi.org/10.1371/journal.pone.0208251.

Institute of Medicine (2011). *Clinical Practice Guidelines We Can Trust*. Washington, DC: National Academies Press.

Ross-White, A., Oakley, P., and Lockwood, C. (2014). *Guideline Adaptation: Conducting Systematic, Exhaustive, and Reproducible Searches (Book 19)*. Philadelphia: Lippincott Williams & Wilkins.

Semlitsch, T., Blank, W.A., Kopp, I.B. et al. (2015). Evaluating guidelines: a review of key quality criteria. *Deutsches Ärzteblatt International* 112: 471–478. https://doi.org/10.3238/arztebl.2015.0471.

9

Discover Barriers and Drivers to Best Practice Implementation

Introduction

Now that the group has established and worked through a process by which best practice recommendations were reviewed, prioritized, selected and finally customized for implementation in your setting, this chapter focuses on how to determine the barriers and drivers to implementation that may need to be addressed if successful implementation is to occur.

The purpose of this chapter is to: (i) review the different types of barriers and drivers of implementation of proposed best practices, (ii) describe strategies for assessing these determinants of practice, and (iii) provide guidance on how to assess for barriers and drivers.

Goal: The intent of this stage of Roadmap is to identify and understand the determinants of implementation, both positive and negative so as to be able to effectively select implementation strategies to overcome the barriers and leverage the drivers of change.

Pertinent questions that can be used to guide action and discussion at this stage are:

- Who are the key stakeholders and what are their levels of support for implementation and their ability to influence uptake?
- What are the barriers/drivers to implementation related to perceptions of the best practice, potential adopters, and stakeholders (e.g. point-of-care providers, management), and the context or practice setting?
- What are the barriers at the individual, team, organization, and system (e.g. health ministry) levels?

Why Is it Important to Assess What Might Be Barriers and Drivers to Implementing Best Practice?

Within the field of implementation science, knowledge about determinants of change has been evolving over time. Rogers' theory of diffusion of innovations was very influential in initially shaping thinking about the importance of understanding how people perceive

Knowledge Translation in Nursing and Healthcare: A Roadmap to Evidence-informed Practice, First Edition. Margaret B. Harrison and Ian D. Graham.
© 2021 John Wiley & Sons, Inc. Published 2021 by John Wiley & Sons, Inc.

innovations as these perceptions affect their intentions and decisions to adopt, adapt or abandon their use (Rogers 1995). By understanding the barriers and drivers that might affect implementation, it then becomes possible to select and tailor implementation strategies to overcome the barriers and build on the drivers. Chapter 11 discusses how to map implementation strategies to identified barriers and drivers to support successful implementation.

Frameworks for Thinking About Determinants of Implementation

The Ottawa Model of Research Use (OMRU) identifies three categories of factors that can hinder or promote uptake of best practice (Logan and Graham 1998, 2010; Graham and Logan 2004). They are factors related to the best practice or innovation, factors related to the potential adopter and factors related to the practice setting or context in which the implementation is to take place. The *innovation* comprises perceived attributes related to how the innovation was developed and the innovation itself. Factors related to the *potential adopter* relate to knowledge of the best practice, attitudes toward the best practice and professional role and skills related to using or doing the best practice. The *practice setting or context* includes: structural factors such as decision making structures, policies and rules, physical structures within the setting, workload, professional standards, leadership; cultural and social factors such as local customs, politics and personalities, opinion leaders; patient and consumer factors such as patient needs and preferences, patient acuity; and economic factors such as available resources, remuneration, and incentives.

Several frameworks or taxonomies of factors that can positively or negatively influence implementation have been published over the years. One of the earliest is the Clinical Practice Guidelines Framework for Improvement by Cabana et al. (1999) that identified potential barriers to guideline adherence as: awareness of the guideline, familiarity with the recommendations, agreement with the recommendations, self-efficacy (feeling one can carry out the recommendations), outcome expectancy (perception that adhering to the recommendations will improve patient outcomes), ability to overcome inertia of previous practice, and absence of external factors that impede use of the recommendations. Espeland and Baerheim (2003) and Légaré et al. (2008) subsequently expanded the taxonomy of barriers and facilitators to knowledge use classifying the major categories as knowledge, attitudes, and behavior and including numerous subcategories. The Model of Evidence-Based Clinical Decision Making (EBCDM) identifies four main factors influencing decision making: research evidence, patients' preferences, clinical expertise and resources (DiCenso et al. 1998).

There are also more recent frameworks that can be used to categorize barriers and drivers to implementation. For example, the Consolidated Framework for Implementation Research (CFIR) identifies the key implementation factors as: the intervention (evidence, strength, quality), individual characteristics, inner setting (culture, leadership engagement), outer setting (patient needs and resources), process (plan, evaluate, reflect) (Damschroder et al. 2009). The Integrated framework for Promoting Action on Research Implementation in Health Services (I-PARIHS) identifies implementation factors as: the innovation/evidence, the recipients, characteristics of the setting or context and the way in which the evidence is introduced or facilitated into practice (Harvey and Kitson 2016).

The Theoretical Domains Framework-2 (TDF) is both a taxonomy of determinants of behavior and an instrument for assessing barriers and drivers (Cane et al. 2012). It has become one of the most common approaches for assessing barriers and drivers of behavior change (Tabak et al. 2012; Skolarus et al. 2017). The TDF is based on 33 theories with 128 constructs distilled into 14 domains that may explain health-related behavior change. These domains are: knowledge; skills; social professional role and identity; beliefs about capabilities; optimism; beliefs about consequences; reinforcement; intention; goals; memory, attention and decision processes; environmental context and resources; social influences; emotion and behavioral regulation. Atkins et al. (2017) have published a guide to using the TDF. For an example of a TDF interview guide see Appendix 9.A. The interview guide was used in a study to identify barriers and facilitators of physician hand hygiene compliance (Squires et al. 2014).

One other framework that can be used to classify determinants of behavior change as well as design behavior change interventions is the Behavior Change Wheel (Michie et al. 2011). This framework was developed from 19 behavior change frameworks and identifies Capacity, Motivation, Opportunity (COM) as the three major determinants of behavior change.

As we have just revealed, there is no shortage of frameworks and taxonomies of barriers and drivers of change. While each presents a different way to think about determinants of implementation, in many cases the frameworks about implementation factors can be boiled down to the three factors included in the OMRU: the innovation (evidence or best practice), the potential adopters (individuals doing or receiving the best practice), and the context in which the best practice and implementation is to occur. The key is for the working group to select a taxonomy or framework of barriers and drivers to guide the assessment of implementation determinants that best fit with your context. The next section will provide more information on the three factors common in many of the frameworks.

Attributes of Innovations

Decades ago Rogers (1995) described five attributes of innovations that influence decisions about their use. These attributes are: relative advantage (the degree to which an innovation is perceived as better than the idea it supersedes); compatibility (the degree to which an innovation is perceived as being consistent with existing values, past experiences, and needs of potential adopters); complexity (the degree to which an innovation is perceived as difficult to understand and use); trialability (the degree to which an innovation may be experimented with on a limited basis before deciding to permanently adopt it); and observability (the extent to which the results of an innovation are visible to others (or the implementers). The theory posits that innovations that are considered by potential adopters to be more useful than the current approach (relative advantage), fit with existing practice and norms (compatible), are easy to understand and use (low complexity), can be tried without having to permanently commit to the change (trialability), and permits the adopter and others to see the outcomes/benefits of using the innovation (observability) are more likely to be taken up. Of course, having all these positive attributes does not guarantee uptake of an innovation as factors unrelated to the innovation may also discourage adoption (e.g. adopter knowledge, attitudes, skills or aspects of the context such as availability of resources, supportive leadership, etc.).

Others have identified the same and other attributes of innovations that can influence adoption. Tornatzky and Klein (1982) included 75 studies in a meta-analysis of the literature that identified the 10 most common attributes of innovations to be: compatibility, relative advantage, complexity, cost, communicability, divisibility, profitability, social approval, trialability, and observability. Specifically in the field of health, Grilli and Lomas (1994) were the first to confirm that clinical practice guidelines that are low in complexity, high in trialability, and high in observability were more likely to be adhered to by physicians. Grol et al. (1998) studied 47 recommendations, 12 attributes of the recommendations and 12880 decisions about using the recommendations by 61 general practitioners in the Netherlands. They found the factors influencing physicians' adherence to the recommendations to be recommendations that were not controversial (compatible), not vague or non-specific (i.e. were clear), not requiring change (compatible), and were evidence-based.

Much more recently, Kastner et al. (2015) undertook a review of 278 articles and identified over 1700 guideline attributes which they synthesized into 16 categories (credibility of guideline development group, disclosure of conflict of interest, reporting of what is needed, execution of what is needed, updating of guidelines, clinical applicability, values, local applicability, resource constraints, novelty, simple, clear, persuasive, multiple versions, components and presentation). These were organized over six domains of guideline implementability (stakeholder involvement, evidence synthesis, considered judgment, feasibility, message and format). Table 9.1 summarizes the findings from this realist review. They found that the six domains affected the uptake of guideline recommendations within two broad categories: the "creation" of guideline content (including stakeholder involvement in guidelines, evidence synthesis, considered judgment, and implementation feasibility) and the "communication" of this content by fine-tuning the guideline's message and format. They concluded that how guidelines are developed and written influences how often they are used (Kastner et al. 2015). This is a very important aspect as the group customizes and develops the guideline for local use (Table 9.1).

The purpose of this brief historical review about attributes of innovations is to highlight the notion that how people perceive a best practice can affect their intentions to adopt it. When thinking about how to go about implementing best practice, we have found it useful to distinguish between potential adopters' perceptions of the attributes of how the best practice was developed and their perceptions of attributes of the best practice. If the process used to develop the best practice is not seen to be credible, then the likelihood of it being adopted is reduced. But even if the best practice was developed in a rigorous, transparent, and evidence-informed way, this does not guarantee that it will be adopted if perceptions of the best practice are not positive. For example, a guideline maybe considered credible by a group but judged totally impractical to implement. For this reason, it may be necessary to get a sense of both your group's perception of the

Table 9.1 Final list of attribute categories across six domains of guideline implementability.

Category (N = 16)	Major attributes	Domain (N = 6)
Credibility of guideline development group	Credibility	Stakeholder involvement
Disclosure of conflict of interest	Conflict of interest; Transparency; Funding sources; Editorial independence	
Reporting of what is needed	Scope; Patient preferences; Cost and resource requirements; Outcomes data; Harms and benefits	Evidence synthesis
Execution of what is needed	Evidence-based; Valid and reliable; Transparent	
Updating of guidelines	Updating; Currency	
Clinical applicability	Clinical relevance; Appropriateness of patient population; Considered implementation	Considered judgment
Values	Professional/provider values (clinical judgment, clinical freedom); Patient values (acceptability, patient preferences); Guideline developer values	
Local applicability	Adaptation; Application tools	Feasibility
Resource constraints	Availability of resources; Economic outcomes	
Novelty	Compatibility; Requires new knowledge and skills	
Simple	Information overload; Complexity	Message
Clear	Actionability (specificity, ambiguity); Effective writing	
Persuasive	Framing; Relative advantage	
Multiple versions	End-users; Versions (flat, dynamic); Document type	Format
Components	Components to include in guidelines (e.g. purpose, target audience, methods)	
Presentation	Layout of full document (placement, length); Structure within sections (match the system to the real world, sequential bundling); Information visualization (information display [e.g. algorithms, pictures], information context [e.g. framing, vividness])	

Source: Reproduced with permission from: Kastner et al. (2015), © 2015 The Authors. Published by Elsevier Inc.

development process as well as their perceptions of the actual guideline and its recommendations.

Conduct a Stakeholder Analysis

As a first step toward understanding the barriers and drivers of implementation, we recommend conducting a stakeholder analysis. A stakeholder is an individual, group, or organization with a vested interest or concern in the proposed implementation and may be directly or indirectly affected by the implementation of best practice or more importantly affect the implementation of best practice (Baker et al. 1999; Registered Nurses' Association of Ontario 2012). These are the people who are critical to the success (or failure) of implementation efforts. We also find it useful to distinguish three types of stakeholders: (i) those having to adopt the best evidence (e.g. patients or nurses at the point of care enacting an evidence informed recommendation), (ii) those affected by the implementation but who are not themselves implementing the best practice (e.g. managers may support the best practice but do not adhere to the recommendations as they do not provide direct care for patients, or a physician or other health care provider who may be affected by a change in nursing practice), and (iii) those who may be generally interested in the best practice implementation while not directly affected by it (e.g. an allied health professional for whom the best practice is not relevant and the change in nursing practice has no effect on them). We often refer to the first category of stakeholder as a knowledge user to distinguish them from the other categories given their critical role in the implementation process.

Classifying stakeholders in this way helps one think about how the barriers and drivers of best practice may differ by category of stakeholder. We also encourage thinking about implementation at the individual healthcare provider and patient levels, team or unit level, organizational level, and system level (Gifford et al. 2013) as determinants of change may be quite unique at these different levels. Others have suggested considering barriers and drivers that are internal, external, and at the interface (Registered Nurses' Association of Ontario 2012).

The aims of a stakeholder analysis are to: (i) maximize congruence between stakeholder interests and the goals of implementation, and (ii) manage and/or minimize risks associated with stakeholder non-support (Registered Nurses' Association of Ontario 2012). A stakeholder analysis involves assessing (Registered Nurses' Association of Ontario 2012):

- Stakeholder characteristics (e.g. knowledge, perspectives, vested interests, experience with teams, decision making abilities).
- Potential stakeholder influence based on their position.
- Considering ways to engage stakeholder interests to ensure as much support as possible.

These data can be collected qualitatively or quantitatively as described above. Creating a grid showing stakeholders influence and support facilitates analysis (see Figure 9.1).

STAKEHOLDER INFLUENCE & SUPPORT GRID		
Low	**← INFLUENCE →**	**High**
• Least able to influence dissemination and adoption • Could have negative impact on plans • Some attention to obtain support &/or maintain neutrality • Work towards project buy-in	• Can negatively affect dissemination and adoption in a big way • Need great amount of attention to obtain support &/or neutrality • Work towards buy-in	
Low Support Low Influence	High Support Low Influence	
High Support Low Influence	High Support High Influence	
• Can positively affect dissemination and adoption if given attention • Need attention to maintain buy-in and prevent development of neutrality	• Will positively affect dissemination and adoption • Need a great deal of attention and information to maintain their buy-in	

(left axis label: **SUPPORT** with Low ↑ and High ↓)

Figure 9.1   Stakeholder influence and support grid. (*Source:* Adapted from RNAO Toolkit. Reprinted with permission from Registered Nurses' Association of Ontario (2012).)

Barriers Assessment

By this point in the Roadmap journey, the working group will have already started to think about some of these questions, but it is good to ask them again and document the responses.
   Pertinent questions that can be used to guide action and discussion at this stage are:

• What exactly is the best practice? (who needs to do what, how, under what circumstances, with whom, when)
• What is the message(s) that needs to be transferred or the behavior to be adopted?
• What will be the barriers (and drivers) related to implementing the best practice (innovation) in our setting?
   – What are adopters' perceptions of how the best practice recommendations were developed?
   – What are adopters' perceptions of the attributes or characteristics of the best practice?
   – Are there other barriers or drivers specific to the best practice that should be considered?

Assess Factors Related to the Best Practice

As has been described above, it is important for the working group to assess potential adopters' perceptions of the best practice. How people perceive the best practice can determine their willingness to adopt it. We have often used Rogers' attributes of innovations as a starting point to guide data collection on perceptions of the attributes of the best practice.

Questions to consider related to potential adopters' perceptions of the best practice include:

- What do they think about how it was developed?
- What do they think about the recommendations?
- What factors related to their perception of the recommendations will discourage or encourage their use of the recommendations?
- Which factors are amenable to being altered?

Assess Factors Related to Potential Adopters

Factors related to potential adopters that can influence the uptake of best practices also need to be considered. To use a best practice, a potential adopter needs to know about and understand the best practice, but also have the relevant skills to perform it. In healthcare, there is often a strong reliance on education and training which can deal with these issues. However, knowing how to do something often does not translate into doing it because of the nature and complexity of human behavior. Other things to be aware of related to the potential adopters that can influence best practice uptake include having generally positive attitudes toward best practice (i.e. believing the provision of best practice is an expectation of professional practice). While positive attitudes may encourage uptake, that alone is seldom enough to change practice. Conversely, negative attitudes toward a best practice do not preclude adoption of it, especially when incentives to do so, or sanctions for not using it, trump the negative attitudes one may have. For example, a clinician may not view a best practice positively and if left to their own devices would not adopt it but do adopt the practice because it is an expectation in their performance plan and pay raises are related to achieving outcomes set in the performance plan. Individuals' motivation to adopt a best practice can also serve to promote or discourage uptake and having a sense of what might influence intentions to change can offer insight into how to motivate and support uptake. Keep in mind that motivation can be intrinsic (for example, the desire for one's practice to be evidence-informed), or extrinsic (for example remuneration for performing the best practice or sanctions that may be imposed for not performing it). Finally, there may also be other concerns or issues relevant to the potential adopters that should be considered so as not to scuttle attempts to implement the best practice. For example, in healthcare, professional college requirements and/or fear of medico-legal consequences can be a significant inhibitor of practice change.

Questions that are important for the working group to consider are:

- Do the potential adopters know about and understand the best practice?
- Do the potential adopters have the skills necessary to perform the best practice?
- Do the potential adopters have positive attitudes toward the best practice?
- What could motivate (or discourage) potential adopters' use of the best practice?
- Are there other issues or concerns the potential adopters have about adopting the best practice?
- What are the potential adopters' intentions to use (or not use) the best practice?

Assess Characteristics of the Context

Even though healthcare providers usually have autonomy to use best practice in their clinical encounters, the practice setting, or context can exert considerable influence on what they should and can do and the nature of the practice setting can also affect the ease of implementing best practice. For example, despite knowing what to do and having good intentions to use best practice, the chaotic clinical setting may cause a practitioner to forget to use the best practice. The setting may also not be organized to make it easy to do the best practice (e.g. the equipment needed to perform the best practice is located at the other end of the unit requiring extra trips to retrieve it when the nurse is already short on time). The leadership in the setting might be very supportive and encouraging of the best practice or be ambivalent toward it or even explicitly not support it. The setting may or may not have the necessary resources to appropriately implement the best practice or there may not be sufficient staffing to make it feasible. Recent studies by Squires et al. (2015) have examined the concept of context and they suggest that there are six overarching domains (users of context, providers/workers within context, internal arrangements of context, internal infrastructure/networks, responsiveness to change, and broader system related to change) that consist of 20 attributes and 136 feature of context.

While the nature and effect of context on implementation will continue to be studied for years to come, when implementing best practice, the key is to develop an understanding of the critical aspects of the context that may need to be addressed, keeping in mind some aspects of the context may be modifiable while other may not.

Questions to consider about the influence of context on best practice implementation include:

- Is leadership (executive and managerial levels) supportive (or not) of the proposed implementation of best practice?
- Are there patient considerations that could influence implementation? (e.g. patient acuity, preferences, etc.)
- Are there aspects about how the health care providers or the setting are organized that could influence best practice uptake? (e.g. scopes of practice, staff-patient ratios, etc.)
- Are there adequate resources to support implementation? (e.g. people, equipment, supplies, etc.)
- Are there infrastructure considerations that could influence implementation? (e.g. reorganization of outpatient and inpatient areas)
- Is there organizational readiness for change?
- Are there factors or pressures external to the organization that could influence implementation? (e.g. accreditation requirements, changes in funding models, health ministry restructuring, etc.)

Measures and Means of Assessing Barriers and Drivers

Barriers and drivers of implementation can be identified qualitatively, quantitatively, and by using mixed methods. *Qualitative* approaches can range from having conversations with key informants in the practice setting to conducting one-on-one interviews, to holding focus groups, or conducting workshops with potential adopters and stakeholders. The guiding questions can be made up by the working group or be more structured such as questions based on the Theoretical Domains Framework (Cane et al. 2012). A common question is, from whom should we collect data about perceived barriers and drivers? There is no one answer and usually a purposeful sample works well. It can help to consider who might be key informants (e.g. individuals because of their positions or views would be considered essential to interview), typical informants (e.g. health care providers expected to adopt the best practice), or extreme informants (e.g. individuals with strong views either in favor of, or opposed to, implementing the best practice). When using a qualitative approach to barriers assessment, we have used the following questions to guide who we approach:

- Who are the key opinion leaders in the setting?
- Who are the formal leaders?
- Who are the individuals known to be typically enthusiastic about change, or resistant?
- Who are the individuals who may be particularly affected by implementing the best practices?
- Who is willing to speak with us?

Quantitative approaches typically involve administering paper or internet surveys to potential adopters and stakeholders. The surveys can be validated questionnaires or scales such as those discussed later in the chapter and listed in Table 9.2 or they can be developed for the purpose at hand or a combination of both. As it was with using a qualitative approach, there are no set rules for whose opinions and views to elicit about perceived barriers and drivers. In some cases, it may be reasonable and practical to survey all who will be affected and involved (a census approach). If the group is large, then a random or a convenience sample of participants may be more feasible.

We often use a mixed-methods approach which involves combining approaches. Sometimes during guideline reviewing, members of the group begin discussing barriers and drivers. Reflect on notes you have from that stage. More formally, to identify barriers we first interview a few people (and in some cases just have a quick chat) to get a sense of the potential barriers and drivers, and then develop a questionnaire to survey a more representative sample. See Appendix 9.B for an example of a baseline barriers survey.

Légaré and Zhang (2013) provide a useful review of other approaches for identifying barriers and drivers. While not framed in terms of barriers or drivers, Chaudoir et al. (2013) have undertaken a systematic review of structural, organizational, provider, patient, and innovation level measures. They identified 62 measures which have potential relevance for barriers assessment. Unfortunately, there is no one measure for assessing barriers and drivers of practice change. Table 9.2 provides a list of some quantitative measures to assess barriers and drivers we have come across over the years.

This list is not exhaustive and is only intended to identify possible resources. Note that the measures are divided into clinician barriers to carrying out evidence-informed practice and context measures. These measures can be used to survey potential adopters/knowledge users and stakeholders about their perceptions of best practice and context. While it is advisable to use measures or scales in their entirety, sometimes tailoring a survey using elements from different measures as well as adding new questions specifically related to the best practice of interest can also be defended. Dillman's Total Design Method for surveys is an excellent reference on best practices for conducting surveys (Dillman et al. 2014). Our advice is to keep it short and simple to maximize response rates.

Table 9.2 Examples of instruments and measures to assess determinants of research use.

Authors (Year)	Measure name	Description of the measure
Perceived attributes of practice guidelines		
Brouwers et al. (2004)	Clinicians Assessment of Practice Guidelines in Oncology (CAPGO)	18 items, 5-point Likert scale. 4 factors predict guideline endorsement and intention to use: guideline quality; acceptance of recommendations; application of recommendations; comparative value
Clinician barriers		
Evidence Based Practice		
Aarons (2004)	Evidence Based Practice Attitude Scale (EBPAS)	18 items, 5-point Likert scale. 4 domains: attitudes toward appeal of EBP; requirements to adopt EBP; openness to innovation in general; perceived divergence between current work processes and requirements of EBP
Rye et al. (2017)	Evidence-based Practice Attitude Scale-36 (EBPAS-36)	36 items, 5-point Likert scale 12 subscales: requirements; appeal; openness; divergence; limitations; fit; monitoring; balance; burden; job security; organizational support; feedback
Jette et al. (2003)	Evidence Based Practice Knowledge, Attitudes, and Belief Scale	51 items, 31 items with 5-point Likert Scale divided into four domains: attitudes and beliefs about EBP; behaviors regarding reading literature and using guidelines; – access to resources and personal skills; barrier (indicate top 3)
McEvoy et al. (2010)	Evidence Based Practice Profile	58 items. 5-point Likert scale. 5 factors: relevance; technology; confidence; practice; sympathy
Melnyk et al. (2008)	Evidence Based Practice Belief Scale (EBPBS)	EBPBS- 16 items, 5-point Likert scale. • Measures beliefs about the value of EBP and ability to implement it
	Evidence Based Practice Implementation Scale (EBPIS)	EBPIS- 18 items, 5-point Likert scale • Measures the extent to which EBP is implemented
Salbach et al. (2007)	Evidence Based Practice Belief, Attitude and Skills Scale	11 items. 5-point Likert scale Practitioner barriers: education; attitudes and beliefs; interest, perceived role; engage in EBP; self-efficacy Barriers: perceived organizational barriers (perceived support and resources)
Salbach and Jaglal (2011) Clyde et al. (2016)	Evidence-Based Practice Confidence (EPIC) Scale	11 items, scored 0–100

(Continued)

Table 9.2 (Continued)

Authors (Year)	Measure name	Description of the measure
Shi et al. (2014)	Evidence Based Practice Knowledge Attitudes, Behavior Questionnaire (EBP-KABQ)	33 items, 7-point Likert scale. 4 domains: knowledge; attitudes; behavior; outcomes/decisions
Ritchie et al. (2019)	Evidence Based Practice-Knowledge Attitudes and Practices	23 items across three domains: knowledge, attitudes, practice
Menon et al. (2010)	PERFECT (Professional Evaluation and Reflection on Change Tool)	Clinicians asked to recall behaviors 6 months ago and 1 year ago; cues for each question. 33 questions, 4 domains: Problem Identifications (integrating information); – Assessment Practices; Treatment Practices; Referral Practices
Funk et al. (1991)	BARRIERS scale	29 items. 4-point Likert scale. 4 key dimensions: nurse, setting, research, presentation
Huijg et al. (2014)	Determinants of Implementation Behavior Questionnaire (DIBQ) – Theoretical Domains Framework Questionnaire	93 items. 7-point Likert Scale 18 domains: knowledge; skill; social/professional role and identity; belief about capabilities; optimism; beliefs about consequences; intentions; goals; innovation; socio political context; organization; patient; innovation strategy; social influences; positive emotions; negative emotions; behavior regulation; nature of behavior
Context		
Hoben et al. (2016)	Alberta Context Tool (ACT)	56 items, 5-point Likert scale. 8 core context dimensions: leadership; culture; evaluation; social capital; structural and electronic resources; formal interactions; – informal interactions; organizational slack; Permission for use is needed (Knowledge Utilization Studies Program-KUSP-UALberta)
Aarons et al. (2014)	Implementation Leadership Scale (ILS)	12 items. 5- point Likert scale. 4 domains: proactive, knowable, supportive, perseverant 2 scales: One for supervisor to rate themselves; One for staff to rate the supervisor
Helfrich et al. (2009)	Organizational Readiness to Change Assessment (ORCA)	77 items, 5-point Likert scale. 3 domains: Evidence (4 subscales), organizational context (6 subscales), facilitation (9 subscales)
Shea et al. (2014)	Organizational Readiness for Implementing Change (ORIC)	12 items, 5-point scale on change commitment and change valence

Table 9.2 (Continued)

Authors (Year)	Measure name	Description of the measure
McCormack et al. (2009)	Context Assessment Instrument (CAI)	37 items, 4-point Likert scale. Five domains: collaborative practice, evidence-informed practice, respect for persons, practice boundaries, evaluation
Gagnon et al. (2011) Gagnon et al. (2014) Gagnon et al. (2018)	Organizational readiness for knowledge translation (OR4KT)	59 items, 5-point Likert scale. Six domains: organizational climate for change, organizational contextual factors, change content, leadership, organizational support, motivation
Keith et al. (2017); Fernandez et al. (2018)	Consolidated Framework for Implementation Research (CFIR)	5 major domains, each of which may affect an intervention's implementation: Intervention characteristics; Inner setting; Outer setting; Characteristics of individuals involved in implementation that might influence implementation; Implementation process
Timmings et al. (2016)	Ready, Set, Change! online decision support tool	The purpose of the tool is to guide users through the process of selecting a valid and reliable readiness assessment measure that is appropriate for your organizational setting

There are also several measures of organizational readiness for change that can be used to get a sense of potential barriers and drivers to implementation. There is a useful online decision support tool called Ready, Set, Change! that can be used by the working group to help select the organizational readiness measure that is most appropriate for the group's needs (Ready, Set, Change! online decision support tool 2014; Timmings et al. 2016). This tool categorizes the determinants of readiness for change into individual psychological, individual structural, organizational psychology and organization structural factors.

On an experiential note, we have had good results conducting Knowledge, Attitude, Practice (KAP) surveys to assess barriers and drivers of best practice implementation. We tailor these surveys to the specific project. These surveys include questions to get at the potential adopters' knowledge of the best practice to be implemented and sometimes also ask about their knowledge of the evidence supporting the best practice. We ask attitude questions to determine whether potential adopters think the best practice was well developed, credible, and their perceptions of the attributes of the best practice. Both these sets of questions help us determine the extent to which education might be required to reduce knowledge deficits and improve attitudes about the best practices. The "practice" part of the survey usually gets at respondents' views on scopes of practice, their usual practice, perceptions of others' practices. We also include questions about perceptions of barriers and drivers to the proposed change. The surveys are typically easy to complete and designed so as not to not take too much time to complete. We have distributed surveys to staff on paper and have also administered them as e-surveys. We have surveyed nurses and physicians about their perceptions sometimes using the same question or mirror questions for both groups to show differences in perspectives. For an example of a KAP survey, see Appendix 9.C.

Box 9.1   Some surprises uncovered!

In the community leg ulcer project, our survey revealed important barriers and drivers of change. In the survey, the family physicians revealed they lacked confidence in managing the condition while the nurses suggested a need for continuing education in assessment. Both the physicians and nurses' knowledge of effective management of wounds was suboptimal but the nurses were more likely to know what best practice actually was.

We have developed and validated a brief survey with questions to specifically assess the health care providers' intentions to use a best practice and their perceptions of it and factors potentially related to their use of it (Brouwers et al. 2004, 2009). We have used these questions in some of our barriers assessment surveys. The survey items are listed in Appendix 9.D.

Most of the time we simply use the local data we collected for internal implementation planning purposes. However, if the barriers assessment is conducted in a sufficiently rigorous way, they may be of interest beyond the local group (Graham et al. 2001, 2003). Publishing the barriers assessment can add credibility to the working group's efforts and generate greater interest in the implementation project. For some members of the group, authorship on a peer reviewed publication may be highly valued and desired. Members of our teams have always been keen on publishing their work with us. If the working group decides to publish, it is important that all members of the group understand and meet journal authorship guidelines (International Committee of Medical Journal Editors 2020) and that data collection received research ethics board approval, if that was required.

What is critical, regardless of how the barriers assessment is conducted, is to find ways to minimize the burden on individuals (e.g. nurses and patients) to participate in these assessments. This usually means balancing what is essential to learn about the potential implementation determinants and how much time and effort a participant can be expected to contribute to elicit them. In our experience, there is usually a temptation to want to collect much more information than is needed at this stage, often because members of the group are interested to find out what their patients and colleagues think. Resist the temptation by thinking about the respondents and how to minimize the burden on them. Pilot your assessment process with a few individuals to make sure the questions make sense and the data collection process works efficiently. Revise the data collection methods if necessary; it is better to get it right than frustrate respondents which can affect the quality of the information they provide.

It is also important for the working group to remember that it may be desirable to conduct sequential or longitudinal monitoring of barriers and drivers to change. Perceived barriers elicited prior to implementing a best practice may turn out not to be a barrier after all once adopters have an opportunity to use the best practice. Also, things that were never contemplated as a potential barrier may emerge once the best practice is being used and adopters have experience using it. Ongoing monitoring of the implementation determinants will permit better tailoring of implementation strategies (more about this to come in Chapter 12).

Summary

This chapter has described the importance of assessing the barriers and drivers to best practice implementation and reviewed frameworks that classify types of determinants of change. In general, factors typically relate to the best practice, potential adopters, and the context. The chapter described how to do a stakeholder analysis and how to assess for barriers and drivers to using best practice. By identifying and understanding the potential determinants of implementation, it is possible to better select and tailor implementation strategies to these factors thereby improving the likelihood of successful implementation.

The key message from this chapter is that the working group must understand as many of the possible factors that could promote or inhibit best practice uptake as possible. This information is needed to effectively plan strategies to overcome barriers. The group should also keep in mind that the same factor can be perceived by some as a barrier and a driver by others. Collecting these data should be done in a systematic fashion that produces reliable information. It is also important to ensure that the data collection process (whether this be interviews or surveys) is not onerous or burdens the respondents especially if health care providers are busy or patients unwell, for example.

The working group will know it has successfully completed this stage of Roadmap if it has:

- Identified the key stakeholders and determined their level of support for implementation and their ability to influence uptake.
- Identified the barriers/drivers to implementation related to perceptions of best practices, potential adopters (e.g. point of care, management), and the context or practice setting.
- Recognized what are the barriers/drivers to implementation related to the potential adopters? (e.g. point-of-care, management).
- What are the barriers/drivers to implementation related to the context generally or the practice setting?
- What are the barriers/drivers at the individual, team, organization, and system (e.g. health ministry) levels?

Returning to the Action Map (Table 9.3) and our implementation example, we are now able to complete the barriers and drivers' column based on the barriers assessment that was undertaken. The group assessed barriers and drivers by having discussions with nurses on the units, nurse managers, and the executive team and the Chief Nursing Officer (who had raised the concern early on because of the referrals for surgery). In this case, we assessed Knowledge Attitudes and Practice more informally. Keep in mind that it is always critical to determine as part of the barriers assessment where providers are at "knowledge wise" as this information will be instrumental in organizing the appropriate educational sessions.

When the analysis of the barriers assessment is complete, it is a good time to add to the draft Implementation Plan how the barriers assessment was conducted and what were the results.

In the next chapter we discuss what we know about the effectiveness of implementation strategies to increase the uptake of best practice. Following that (in Chapter 11) we focus on how to tailor those implementation strategies to the barriers and drivers that have been identified. Your solutions are building!

Table 9.3   Phase 2: ACTION MAP for Solution Building (*with Wound Example*).

Adopted external recommendations *Operationalization of recommendation*	Customize best practice recommendations by aligning them with context to become local best practice intervention *(who, what/how, when/timing)*	Barriers and facilitating factors (drivers)
Guideline/recommendations selected for local use	Guideline/recommendations customized for local use	Factors related to each recommendation, potential adopters, or context. *What would aid or prevent implementation?*
1. Q 24 hr. skin and risk assessment, document on flow chart	Who: attending evening RN What/how: skin and risk assessment during HS care, document on flow chart When: daily, evening shift when units are generally less busy 1. Evening RN to daily conduct a head to toe assessment during HS care and document in flow chart	Most nurses familiar with head-to-toe skin assessment Currently not in orientation for new staff HS routine happens with every patient so will be an incremental extra
2. Risk Assessment with Braden Scale	Who: evening RN What/how: Braden Risk assessment, (6 sub-scales); each subscale document in flow chart When: during head to toe skin assessment, on evening shift 2. Braden Risk assessment conducted with head to toe skin assessment by attending RN on evening shift daily and documented in nursing notes	Staff on several units not familiar with risk assessment scale (6 sub-scales), questioning total score, perceived as a lot of work Currently not in orientation for new staff
3. etc.		
Sustainability thinking continues here. . .	Consider and reconsider the "fit" to ensure customized best practice is achievable to encourage ongoing uptake	Barriers assessment conducted such that it can be redone in future, if necessary. Target implementation strategies to known barriers and drivers to improve the uptake and ongoing maintenance
Chapter 8	Chapters 8 and 9	Chapters 8 and 9

Appendix 9.A: Improving Physician Hand Hygiene Compliance Using Behavioural Theories

Interview Schedule

Explanation

Thank you for agreeing to speak with me today about hand hygiene practice. There may appear to be overlap between questions but each question is worded to obtain specific information and therefore you may find that answers are repeated. It is important to note that there are no right or wrong answers to the questions and that no one will know what your specific answers were.

The interview should take approximately 15 to 20 minutes and will be audio-recorded to ensure that all key points are accurately documented. Any identifying information (for example the names of other individuals) that you use in the course of our discussion will be removed from the interview transcripts. If you wish to end the interview before I have asked all of the questions or if you wish to withdraw from the study you are free to do so.

Background
- Male or Female (to keep track of, will not be asked)
- Confirm if right campus documented (for staff physicians)
- Age range- <30, 31–40, 41–50, 51–60, 61+
- How long have you been a physician?
- What year of residency? (if applies)
- How long have you been at TOH?
- Have you done any of your training at TOH in the past 10 years (medical school, residency, fellowship)?

1) Knowledge
   - Are you aware of any guidelines about hand hygiene?
     - i) If yes, what are they?
     - ii) Are you familiar with the 4 moments of hand hygiene?
   - Are you aware of any evidence that links hand hygiene to healthcare associated infections?
     - i) If yes, what are your thoughts about this evidence? (prompt: do you agree? etc.)
   - Do you feel as though you have a sufficiently strong background in infection control training?
     - i) If yes, what is the training?
     - ii) If no, what would you like to know more about?
   - When do you think that you need to practice hand hygiene?
2) Skills
   - Were you ever trained in the proper technique for hand hygiene?
   - Do you think proper hand hygiene is a skill?

3) Social/Professional Role and Identity
   - Is hand hygiene a standard part of your patient consultations?
   - Is hand hygiene something specific to [residents] [staff physicians] [surgeons] [general medicine]?
   - What is your impression of the compliance of others in your profession with hand hygiene guidelines? Do you feel as though your hand hygiene practice is in line with your peers?
4) Beliefs about Capabilities
   - How easy or difficult is it for you to practice hand hygiene? What made it easy what made it difficult?
   - Do you believe that what you consider to be good hand hygiene fits with the current guidelines?
   - Are you confident that you are following the guidelines when practicing hand hygiene?
5) Beliefs about consequences
   - What are the benefits when good hand hygiene is practiced? (prompts: patients, yourself)
   - What are the negative aspects when good hand hygiene is practiced? (prompts: patients, yourself)
   - In what situations do you think hand hygiene is necessary/unnecessary?
6) Optimism
   - What do you think will happen if you are not able to practice hand hygiene (prompt: the 4 moments)?
   - In your opinion, how likely is it that improper hand hygiene will lead to a healthcare associated infection?
7) Intentions
   - Do you intend to practice hand hygiene (prompt: the 4 moments)?
     i) If no, why?
     ii) If yes, do you anticipate any problems?

   - What will make the process of hand hygiene easier?
8) Memory, Attention, and Decision Processes
   - Is hand hygiene automatic or do you need to remember or be reminded to do it?
   - Is practicing or not practicing hand hygiene ever a conscious decision?
   - Do you have any triggers for remembering to practice hand hygiene? What would make it easier to remember hand hygiene?
   - Are there certain situations where you find yourself forgetting to practice hand hygiene more often than others?
   - In what situations might you find it difficult to follow the hand hygiene guidelines?
9) Environmental context and resources
   - Have you found hand hygiene audits to be successful at promoting compliance? If yes, what aspects of this intervention encourage hand hygiene? If no, what could be done to improve this intervention?

- What resources would make it easier for you to practice hand hygiene?
- What aspects of your work environment influence whether you practice hand hygiene? (PROMPT: any trigger or prompts in clinic?)
- Are there any competing tasks or time constraints that might influence whether or not you practice hand hygiene? What would help you overcome these problems/difficulties?

10) Social influences
- Do other team members influence your decision to practice hand hygiene?
  i) If yes, how?
  ii) If no, prompt (co-workers / team lead / department / overall workplace)
- Do the expectations of your patients and their families influence you to practice hand hygiene?
  i) If yes, how?

11) Emotion
- Do you have any strong feelings about current hand hygiene guidelines (prompt: 4 moments)?
- Do your emotions or mood ever influence whether you practice hand hygiene?
- Does not practicing hand hygiene evoke worry or concern in you?

12) Goals
- Do you want to practice hand hygiene (prompt: the 4 moments)?
- In what situations do you want to practice hand hygiene?
- Considering your other priorities, on a scale of 1 to 10 with 10 being very important, how important do you think it is for you to practice hand hygiene (prompt: the 4 moments)?
  i) (If not 10), what is a higher priority?

13) Behavioural regulation
- What could you personally do to increase your hand hygiene practice? (prompt: within your everyday practice)
- What do you think is needed to ensure that you consistently practice hand hygiene?
- Within your healthcare team Are there procedures or ways of working that encourage hand hygiene?

14) Reinforcement
- In the past, are there any personal or external incentives that you have experienced to be effective to improve hand hygiene? (prompt: yourself, or others)
- Have your views toward hand hygiene evolved from your time in medical school up until now?
  i) If so, how?

Appendix 9.B: Factors Influencing Nurses Using Symptom Practice Guides for Remote Support of Patients Undergoing Cancer Treatments

Factors Influencing Nurses Using Symptom Practice Guides for Remote Support of Patients Undergoing Cancer Treatments ©2015 Stacey for the COSTaRS Team. Ottawa Hospital Research Institute & University of Ottawa, Canada.

The Baseline Barriers Survey is freely available on the COSTaRS Website https://ktcan-ada.ohri.ca/costars/Research/. The adapted survey was reprinted with permission under the terms of the Creative Commons Attribution 4.0 International License (http://crea-tivecommons.org/licenses/by/2.0) from Graham, I.D., Logan, J., Bennett, C.L., Presseau, J., O'Connor, A.M., Mitchell, S.l., et al., 2007. Physicians' intentions and use of three patient decision aids. BMC Medical Informatics and Decision Making 7, 1e10.

Baseline Survey

1) Have you reviewed the evidence-informed symptom practice guides by COSTaRS?
   ☐ Yes   ☐ No

2) Do you currently provide remote support (e.g. telephone, email) to oncology patients undergoing cancer treatment?
   ☐ Yes   ☐ No
   If yes, go to Section 3   *If no, go to Section 4.*

Section 3.0: To be completed by participants that provide remote support

3.1 During what hours are patients able to contact you or a colleague for remote support (e.g. telephone, email)?
   ☐ During regular hours only (Monday to Friday daytime)
   ☐ Weekend/evening coverage (mostly outside of regular hours)
   ☐ 24 hours a day, 7 days a week
   ☐ Other *(please specify):*

3.2 Do you document calls in the health record?
   ☐ No; *go to question 3.4*
   ☐ Yes, routinely
   ☐ Yes, as necessary

3.3 If yes, what format is used:
   ☐ Computer-based documentation
   ☐ Documented on paper-based forms that are placed in the health record

3.4 Do you use practice guides or guidelines for triaging symptom calls?
   ☐ Yes   ☐ No   *If no, go to 3.7*

3.5 If yes, which practice guides/guidelines are used?
   Please specify:

3.6 If yes, how are practice guides/guidelines used?
   ☐ Used primarily for orientation of nurses to their role in providing remote support
   ☐ Used by nurses as a reference (as needed) on their desk

- ☐ Used by nurses as an app on their smartphone
- ☐ Integrated into the computer-based documentation system
- ☐ Used as a paper-based documentation form
- ☐ Other *(please specify):*

3.7 What are three barriers interfering with you using symptom practice guides to provide remote support to patients undergoing cancer treatments (please list them from first priority to third highest priority)?

1st priority _____

2nd highest priority _____

3rd highest priority_____

Section 4.0: To be completed by all participants

Please tell us how much to you agree or disagree with the following statements.

	Strongly disagree	Disagree	Neutral	Agree	Strongly Agree
Issues related to the development of the symptom practice guides					
4.1 The developers of the symptom practice guides are credible	☐	☐	☐	☐	☐
4.2 The information provided within the symptom practice guides is supported by evidence	☐	☐	☐	☐	☐
4.3 The symptom practice guides are well developed	☐	☐	☐	☐	☐
4.4 The development of the symptom practice guides was not influenced by vested interests	☐	☐	☐	☐	☐
4.5 Other:	☐	☐	☐	☐	☐
Issues related to the content and format					
The symptom practice guides contains essential information to					
4.6 Assess the symptom	☐	☐	☐	☐	☐
4.7 Triage based on symptom severity	☐	☐	☐	☐	☐
4.8 Review medications used for symptom	☐	☐	☐	☐	☐
4.9 Guide the patients to manage their symptoms	☐	☐	☐	☐	☐
4.10 The symptom practice guides are well-organized	☐	☐	☐	☐	☐
4.11 Summarize and document plan agreed upon	☐	☐	☐	☐	☐
4.12 The evidence described in the symptom practice guides reflects my understanding of symptom management	☐	☐	☐	☐	☐
4.13 The evidence is presented in an unbiased manner	☐	☐	☐	☐	☐
4.14 The evidence is up-to-date	☐	☐	☐	☐	☐

	Strongly disagree	Disagree	Neutral	Agree	Strongly Agree
4.15 The practice guides are compatible with how I think patients undergoing cancer treatment should be supported when experiencing symptoms	☐	☐	☐	☐	☐
4.16 Other:	☐	☐	☐	☐	☐
For nurses using the symptom practice guides, these practice guides will					
4.17 Be acceptable	☐	☐	☐	☐	☐
4.18 Be simple to use	☐	☐	☐	☐	☐
4.19 Be too complex to use	☐	☐	☐	☐	☐
4.20 Guide nurses through the process of assessing, triaging and helping patients manage their symptoms in a logical fashion	☐	☐	☐	☐	☐
4.21 Improve the quality of symptom management	☐	☐	☐	☐	☐
4.22 Apply to a sizeable proportion of patients	☐	☐	☐	☐	☐
4.23 Other:	☐	☐	☐	☐	☐
Issues related to my current knowledge, skills and confidence in providing remote support to patients					
4.24 I need to enhance my knowledge about using symptom practice guides when providing remote support to patients undergoing cancer treatment	☐	☐	☐	☐	☐
4.25 I feel confident in my ability to use symptom practice guides when providing remote support to patients undergoing cancer treatment	☐	☐	☐	☐	☐
4.26 I need to enhance my skills in using symptom practice guides to provide remote support to patients undergoing cancer treatment	☐	☐	☐	☐	☐
4.27 Other:	☐	☐	☐	☐	☐
Issues about implementation; from my perspective					
4.28 The symptom practice guides will be easy to use in our oncology program	☐	☐	☐	☐	☐
4.29 The symptom practice guides will save time	☐	☐	☐	☐	☐
4.30 There is clear direction within our oncology program that we need to provide remote support using practice guides	☐	☐	☐	☐	☐
4.31 There is adequate time to provide remote support using these practice guides	☐	☐	☐	☐	☐

	Strongly disagree	Disagree	Neutral	Agree	Strongly Agree
4.32 Using these practice guides will require reorganization in the way we provide remote support within our oncology program	☐	☐	☐	☐	☐
4.33 Using these symptom practice guides will not require major changes to the way we currently providing remote support	☐	☐	☐	☐	☐
4.34 Using these symptom practice guides will help me tailor my support to patients' needs	☐	☐	☐	☐	☐
4.35 Using these symptom practice guides will affect my relationship with patients in a positive way	☐	☐	☐	☐	☐
4.36 Using these symptom practice guides will provide easily observable benefits to the patients.	☐	☐	☐	☐	☐
4.37 The symptom practice guides will be easy to experiment with before deciding to adopt them in our oncology program	☐	☐	☐	☐	☐
4.38 The symptom practice guides are likely to be used by most of my colleagues.	☐	☐	☐	☐	☐
4.39 Other	☐	☐	☐	☐	☐

5) How comfortable would you be using the symptom practice guides when providing remote support to patients in your oncology program?

☐	☐	☐	☐	☐
Very uncomfortable	Uncomfortable	Neutral	Comfortable	Very Comfortable

6) How likely are you to tell someone about these symptom practice guides as a resource for providing remote support to patients undergoing cancer treatment?

☐	☐	☐	☐	☐
Not at all	Very Unlikely	Somewhat likely	Likely	Very likely

7) What changes need to be made to the symptom practice guides to make them more relevant to your oncology program?

8) What are two to three factors that would make it easier for nurses to use these evidence-based symptom practice guides for providing remote support to patients undergoing cancer treatment (please list them in order of importance, starting with the most important)?

Most important _____

2nd highest _____

3rd highest_____

9) Do you have any further comments, questions or suggestions?

10) *Please tell us a little about yourself . . .*

10.1 What is your position within the cancer program?

○ Staff nurse

○ Supervisor / manager

○ Advanced practice nurse

○ Educator

○ Other: _____

10.2 How long have you been working within this position?

○ 6 or fewer months	○ 3 to 5 years
○ 7 to 12 months	○ 6 to 10 years
○ 1 to 2 years	○ more than 10 years

10.3 Are you currently working:

○ Full-time   ○ Regular part-time   ○ Causal

10.4 Your age range?

○ Under 29	○ 40 to 49	○ 60 and older
○ 30 to 39	○ 50 to 59	

10.5 Your sex

○ Female   ○ Male

10.6 What education programs have you completed (check all that apply)?

○ College diploma in nursing

○ Undergraduate university degree in nursing

○ Specialty certification in oncology nursing

○ Graduate university degree in nursing

○ Other _____

10.7 How long have you been working within your profession?

○ Less than 2 years	○ 11 to 15 years	○ 26 to 30 years
○ 2 to 5 years	○ 16 to 20 years	○ more than 30 years
○ 6 to 10 years	○ 20 to 25 years	

10.8 Which province do you work in?

Thank you for completing the survey.

Appendix 9.C: Example of a KAP Survey

 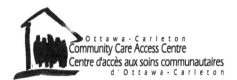

Ottawa-Carleton
Community Care Access Centre
Centre d'accès aux soins communautaires
d ' O t t a w a - C a r l e t o n

**Ottawa-Carleton
Regional Leg
Ulcer Project**

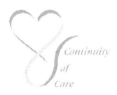 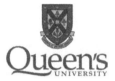 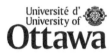

Leg Ulcer Diagnosis

In your experience, what proportion of clients with leg ulcers that are referred by family physicians/GP's have:

	A Few <10%	Some 10–25%	Many 26–50%	Most 51–75%	Almost All >75%	Don't Know
Doppler assessment (ankle/brachial index)	☐	☐	☐	☐	☐	☐
Vascular Studies/Clinical Laboratory WorkUp	☐	☐	☐	☐	☐	☐

In what proportion of your leg ulcer clients is the disease etiology known (ie. it is known that the disease etiology is venous, arterial or mixed)?

	A Few <10%	Some 10–25%	Many 26–50%	Most 51–75%	Almost All >75%	Donot Know
Etiology is known.	☐	☐	☐	☐	☐	☐
Etiology is unknown.	☐	☐	☐	☐	☐	☐

Leg Ulcer Care

Who usually determines the initial treatment for leg ulcers (e.g. type of dressings, bandages, frequency of dressing changes, choice of pharmaceutical products)? *Check more than one if the decision is made collaboratively.*

☐ GP/Family Physician
☐ MD Specialist
☐ Podiatrist/Chiropodist/Foot Specialist
☐ ET
☐ RN

Does your agency have policy and procedures regarding dressing and bandage protocols for leg ulcer care?

☐ Yes   ☐ No   ☐ Don't Know

Does your agency accept physician's standing orders regarding dressing and bandage protocols for leg ulcer care?

☐ Yes   ☐ No   ☐ Don't Know

In your experience, how long does a typical leg ulcer usually take to heal?

☐ < 1 mos ☐ 1–2 mos ☐ 2–3 mos ☐ 3–6 mos ☐ 6–12 mos ☐ 1–3 years
☐ > 3 years ☐ Don't Know

How long do you usually wait with a non-healing ulcer before referring the client for additional care?

☐ < 2 mos   ☐ 2–3 mos   ☐ 3–6 mos   ☐ 6–12 mos   ☐ Don't Know

To whom do you typically refer non-healing ulcer clients?

☐ Other   ☐ RN   ☐ ET   ☐ Vascular Surgeon   ☐ Dermatologist   ☐ Podiatrist

In your experience, how effective is each of the following in healing venous leg ulcers?

Please circle one choice for each.	Never Use	Not Effective	Somewhat Effective	Very Effective	Don't Know
Compression Stockings (e.g. Jobst)	1	2	3	4	5
Tensors	1	2	3	4	5
Zinc oxide boot (e.g. Ichthopaste)	1	2	3	4	5
Zinc oxide boot (e.g. Unnaboot)	1	2	3	4	5
Two layer bandage (e.g. Surepress)	1	2	3	4	5
Four Layer Compression (Profore)	1	2	3	4	5
Other: Specify _____	1	2	3	4	5

Please comment on other treatments you've found useful for venous leg ulcers.

_____

_____

_____

Please indicate how strongly you agree with each of the following statements:

Please circle one choice for each.	Strongly Agree		Neutral		Strongly Disagree
Within my scope of nursing practice, I feel confident in my ability to treat leg ulcers.	1	2	3	4	5
Since being in practice, I could have benefited from ongoing education about leg ulcer care.	1	2	3	4	5
I can rely on the physicians responsible for my clients to have up to date information on how to treat leg ulcers effectively.	1	2	3	4	5
I have learned most of what I know about leg ulcer treatment strategies from other nurses.	1	2	3	4	5
In my experience, a barrier to leg ulcer healing is client compliance with their treatment plan.	1	2	3	4	5
When needed, I have easy access to physician specialist consultation for leg ulcer clients.	1	2	3	4	5
I do not feel I have adequate knowledge of wound care products to use them effectively.	1	2	3	4	5
Evidence-based practice guidelines for leg ulcer care are needed for nurses to give appropriate care.	1	2	3	4	5
Greater access to wound care products is necessary.	1	2	3	4	5
A barrier to leg ulcer healing is inappropriate treatments ordered by physicians.	1	2	3	4	5
Most physician specialists seem disinterested in the care of leg ulcers.	1	2	3	4	5
Nurses need greater input into the products CCAC (Home Care) purchase.	1	2	3	4	5
Caring for clients with leg ulcers is not rewarding.	1	2	3	4	5
The use of evidence-based guidelines for leg ulcer care would improve wound healing.	1	2	3	4	5
Better communication between community nurses and physician specialists is needed to promote continuity of leg ulcer care.	1	2	3	4	5
Clients would benefit from an interdisciplinary wound care centre in this region.	1	2	3	4	5
If I had the option, I would prefer not to care for leg ulcer clients.	1	2	3	4	5

To what extent are each of the following, important sources of information on caring for individuals with leg ulcers?

Please circle one choice for each.	Not at all important	Important	Very important
ET	1	2	3
RN	1	2	3
GP/Family Physician	1	2	3
Podiatrist/Chiropodist/Foot Specialist	1	2	3
Vascular Surgeon	1	2	3
Dermatologist	1	2	3
Representatives of wound care products	1	2	3
Nursing literature/Scientific literature	1	2	3
Internet	1	2	3

Description of Practice

In the past month, approximately how many clients have you cared for? _____

How many of these clients had leg ulcers? _____

Check all that applies to you.

☐ RN   ☐ BSN/BN   ☐ ET   ☐ MSN/MN   ☐ RPN   ☐ Other, specify _____

Are you,

☐ Full-time   ☐ Part-time   ☐ Other _____

THANK YOU

Appendix 9.D: The Clinicians' Assessments of Practice Guidelines in Oncology (CAPGO) Survey

Source: Brouwers, M., Hanna, S., Abdel-Motagally, M. & Yee, J. (2009) Clinicians' evaluations of, endorsements of, and intentions to use practice guidelines change over time: a retrospective analysis from an organized guideline program. Implementation Science 4, 34. https://implementationscience.biomedcentral.com/articles/10.1186/1748-5908-4-34. Licensed under CC BY 2.0.

Item	Domain or Outcome
1. Are you responsible for the care of patients for whom this draft report is relevant? This may include the referral, diagnosis, treatment, or follow-up of patients. ('Yes', 'No' or 'Unsure'. If 'Yes', please answer the questions below.	NA
2. The rationale for developing a guideline, as stated in the 'Introduction' section of this draft report, is clear.	Quality
3. There is a need for a guideline on this topic.	Quality
4. The literature search is relevant and complete (*e.g.,* no key trials were missed nor any included that should not have been).	Quality
5. I agree with the methodology used to summarize the evidence.	Quality
6. The results of the trials described in this draft report are interpreted according to my understanding of the data.	Quality
7. The draft recommendations in this report are clear.	Quality
8. I agree with the draft recommendations as stated.	Acceptability
9. The draft recommendations are suitable for the patients for whom they are intended.	Acceptability
10. The draft recommendations are too rigid to apply to individual patients.	Applicability
11. When applied, the draft recommendations will produce more benefits for patients than harms.	Acceptability
12. The draft report presents options that will be acceptable to patients.	Acceptability
13. To apply the draft recommendations will require reorganization of services/care in my practice setting.	Applicability
14. To apply the draft recommendations will be technically challenging.	Applicability
15. The draft recommendations are too expensive to apply.	Applicability
16. The draft recommendations are likely to be supported by a majority of my colleagues.	Acceptability
17. If I follow the draft recommendations, the expected effects on patient outcomes will be obvious.	Acceptability
18. The draft recommendations reflect a more effective approach for improving patient outcomes than is current usual practice. (if they are the same as current practice, please tick NA).	Comparative

(Continued)

Item	Domain or Outcome
value	
19. When applied, the draft recommendations will result in better use of resources than current usual practice (if they are the same as current practice, please tick NA).	Comparative
value	
20. I would feel comfortable if my patients received the care recommended in the draft report.*	Endorsement
21. This draft report should be approved as a practice guideline.	Endorsement
22. If this draft report were to be approved as a practice guideline, how likely would you be to make use of it in your own practice?	Intentions to use in practice
23. If this draft report were to be approved as a practice guideline, how likely would you be to apply the recommendations to your patients?	Intentions to use with patients

*Items 1, 20, and 23 were not considered in this study.

References

Aarons, G.A. (2004). Mental health provider attitudes toward adoption of evidence-based practice: the Evidence-Based Practice Attitude Scale (EBPAS). *Mental Health Services Research* 6: 61–74. https://doi.org/10.1023/b:mhsr.0000024351.12294.65.

Aarons, G.A., Ehrhart, M.G., and Farahnak, L.R. (2014). The Implementation Leadership Scale (ILS): development of a brief measure of unit level implementation leadership. *Implementation Science* 9: 45. https://doi.org/10.1186/1748-5908-9-45.

Atkins, L., Francis, J., Islam, R. et al. (2017). A guide to using the Theoretical Domains Framework of behaviour change to investigate implementation problems. *Implementation Science* 12: 77. https://doi.org/10.1186/s13012-017-0605-9.

Baker, C.M., Ogden, S.J., Prapaipanich, W. et al. (1999). Hospital consolidation. Applying stakeholder analysis to merger life-cycle. *The Journal of Nursing Administration* 29: 11–20. https://doi.org/10.1097/00005110-199903000-00004.

Brouwers, M.C., Graham, I.D., Hanna, S.E. et al. (2004). Clinicians' assessments of practice guidelines in oncology: the CAPGO survey. *International Journal of Technology Assessment in Health Care* 20: 421–426. https://doi.org/10.1017/s0266462304001308.

Brouwers, M., Hanna, S., Abdel-Motagally, M., and Yee, J. (2009). Clinicians' evaluations of, endorsements of, and intentions to use practice guidelines change over time: a retrospective analysis from an organized guideline program. *Implementation Science* 4: 34. https://doi.org/10.1186/1748-5908-4-34.

Cabana, M.D., Rand, C.S., Powe, N.R. et al. (1999). Why don't physicians follow clinical practice guidelines? A framework for improvement. *Journal of the American Medical Association* 282: 1458–1465. https://doi.org/10.1001/jama.282.15.1458.

Cane, J., O'Connor, D., and Michie, S. (2012). Validation of the theoretical domains framework for use in behaviour change and implementation research. *Implementation Science* 7: 37. https://doi.org/10.1186/1748-5908-7-37.

Chaudoir, S.R., Dugan, A.G., and Barr, C.H. (2013). Measuring factors affecting implementation of health innovations: a systematic review of structural, organizational, provider, patient, and innovation level measures. *Implementation Science* 8: 22. https://doi.org/10.1186/1748-5908-8-22.

Clyde, J.H., Brooks, D., Cameron, J.I., and Salbach, N.M. (2016). Validation of the Evidence-Based Practice Confidence (EPIC) scale with occupational therapists. *The American Journal of Occupational Therapy* 70: 7002280010p1–7002280010p9. https://doi.org/10.5014/ajot.2016.017061.

Damschroder, L.J., Aron, D.C., Keith, R.E. et al. (2009). Fostering implementation of health services research findings into practice: a consolidated framework for advancing implementation science. *Implementation Science* 4: 50. https://doi.org/10.1186/1748-5908-4-50.

DiCenso, A., Cullum, N., and Ciliska, D. (1998). Implementing evidence-based nursing: some misconceptions. *Evidence-Based Nursing* 1: 38–40.

Dillman, D.A., Smyth, J.D., and Christian, L.M. (2014). *Internet, Phone, Mail, and Mixed-Mode Surveys: The Tailored Design Method*. Wiley.

Espeland, A. and Baerheim, A. (2003). Factors affecting general practitioners' decisions about plain radiography for back pain: implications for classification of guideline barriers--a qualitative study. *BMC Health Services Research* 3: 8. https://doi.org/10.1186/1472-6963-3-8.

Fernandez, M.E., Walker, T.J., Weiner, B.J. et al. (2018). Developing measures to assess constructs from the inner setting domain of the consolidated framework for implementation research. *Implementation Science* 13: 52. https://doi.org/10.1186/s13012-018-0736-7.

Funk, S.G., Champagne, M.T., Wiese, R.A., and Tornquist, E.M. (1991). BARRIERS: the barriers to research utilization scale. *Applied Nursing Research* 4: 39–45. https://doi.org/10.1016/s0897-1897(05)80052-7.

Gagnon, M.P., Labarthe, J., Légaré, F. et al. (2011). Measuring organizational readiness for knowledge translation in chronic care. *Implementation Science* 6: 72. https://doi.org/10.1186/1748-5908-6-72.

Gagnon, M.P., Attieh, R., Ghandour el, K. et al. (2014). A systematic review of instruments to assess organizational readiness for knowledge translation in health care. *PLoS One* 9: e114338. https://doi.org/10.1371/journal.pone.0114338.

Gagnon, M.P., Attieh, R., Dunn, S. et al. (2018). Development and content validation of a transcultural instrument to assess organizational readiness for knowledge translation in healthcare organizations: the OR4KT. *International Journal of Health Policy and Management* 7: 791–797. https://doi.org/10.15171/ijhpm.2018.17, https://www.ncbi.nlm.nih.gov/pmc/articles/PMC6186488/.

Gifford, W.A., Graham, I.D., and Davies, B.L. (2013). Multi-level barriers analysis to promote guideline based nursing care: a leadership strategy from home health care. *Journal of Nursing Management* 21: 762–770. https://doi.org/10.1111/jonm.12129.

Graham, I.D. and Logan, J. (2004). Innovations in knowledge transfer and continuity of care. *The Canadian Journal of Nursing Research* 36: 89–103.

Graham, I.D., Harrison, M.B., Moffat, C., and Franks, P. (2001). Leg ulcer care: nursing attitudes and knowledge. *The Canadian Nurse* 97: 19–24.

Graham, I.D., Harrison, M.B., Shafey, M., and Keast, D. (2003). Knowledge and attitudes regarding care of leg ulcers. Survey of family physicians. *Canadian Family Physician* 49: 896–902. https://www.cfp.ca/content/cfp/49/7/896.full.pdf.

Grilli, R. and Lomas, J. (1994). Evaluating the message: the relationship between compliance rate and the subject of a practice guideline. *Medical Care* 32: 202–213. https://doi.org/10.1097/00005650-199403000-00002.

Grol, R., Dalhuijsen, J., Thomas, S. et al. (1998). Attributes of clinical guidelines that influence use of guidelines in general practice: observational study. *British Medical Journal* 317: 858–861. https://doi.org/10.1136/bmj.317.7162.858.

Harvey, G. and Kitson, A. (2016). PARIHS revisited: from heuristic to integrated framework for the successful implementation of knowledge into practice. *Implementation Science* 11: 33. https://doi.org/10.1186/s13012-016-0398-2.

Helfrich, C.D., Li, Y.F., Sharp, N.D., and Sales, A.E. (2009). Organizational readiness to change assessment (ORCA): development of an instrument based on the Promoting Action on Research in Health Services (PARIHS) framework. *Implementation Science* 4: 38. https://doi.org/10.1186/1748-5908-4-38.

Hoben, M., Estabrooks, C.A., Squires, J.E., and Behrens, J. (2016). Factor structure, reliability and measurement invariance of the Alberta context tool and the conceptual research utilization scale, for German residential long term care. *Frontiers in Psychology* 7: 1339. https://doi.org/10.3389/fpsyg.2016.01339.

Huijg, J.M., Gebhardt, W.A., Dusseldorp, E. et al. (2014). Measuring determinants of implementation behavior: psychometric properties of a questionnaire based on the theoretical domains framework. *Implementation Science* 9: 33. https://doi.org/10.1186/1748-5908-9-33.

International Committee of Medical Journal Editors (2020). *Defining the Role of Authors and Contributors*, [Online], Available: http://www.icmje.org/recommendations/browse/roles-and-responsibilities/defining-the-role-of-authors-and-contributors.html.

Jette, D.U., Bacon, K., Batty, C. et al. (2003). Evidence-based practice: beliefs, attitudes, knowledge, and behaviors of physical therapists. *Physical Therapy* 83: 786–805.

Kastner, M., Bhattacharyya, O., Hayden, L. et al. (2015). Guideline uptake is influenced by six implementability domains for creating and communicating guidelines: a realist review. *Journal of Clinical Epidemiology* 68: 498–509. https://doi.org/10.1016/j.jclinepi.2014.12.013.

Keith, R.E., Crosson, J.C., O'Malley, A.S. et al. (2017). Using the Consolidated Framework for Implementation Research (CFIR) to produce actionable findings: a rapid-cycle evaluation approach to improving implementation. *Implementation Science* 12: 15. https://doi.org/10.1186/s13012-017-0550-7.

Légaré, F. and Zhang, P. (2013). Barriers and facilitators: strategies for identification and measurement. In: *Knowledge Translation in Health Care: Moving from Evidence to Practice* (eds. S.E. Straus, J. Tetroe and I.D. Graham), 121–136. Chichester, UK: Wiley.

Légaré, F., Ratte, S., Gravel, K., and Graham, I.D. (2008). Barriers and facilitators to implementing shared decision-making in clinical practice: update of a systematic review of health professionals' perceptions. *Patient Education and Counseling* 73: 526–535. https://doi.org/10.1016/j.pec.2008.07.018.

Logan, J. and Graham, I.D. (1998). Toward a comprehensive interdisciplinary model of health care research use. *Science Communication* 20: 227–246. https://doi.org/10.1177/1075547098020002004.

Logan, J. and Graham, I.D. (2010). The Ottawa model of research use. In: *Models and Frameworks for Implementing Evidence-Based Practice: Linking Evidence to Action* (eds. J. Rycroft-Malone and T. Bucknall), 83–108. Oxford: Wiley Blackwell.

McCormack, B., McCarthy, G., Wright, J. et al. (2009). Development and testing of the Context Assessment Index (CAI). *Worldviews on Evidence-Based Nursing* 6: 27–35. https://doi.org/10.1111/j.1741-6787.2008.00130.x.

McEvoy, M.P., Williams, M.T., and Olds, T.S. (2010). Development and psychometric testing of a trans-professional evidence-based practice profile questionnaire. *Medical Teacher* 32: e373–e380. https://doi.org/10.3109/0142159x.2010.494741.

Melnyk, B.M., Fineout-Overholt, E., and Mays, M.Z. (2008). The evidence-based practice beliefs and implementation scales: psychometric properties of two new instruments. *Worldviews on Evidence-Based Nursing* 5: 208–216. https://doi.org/10.1111/j.1741-6787.2008.00126.x.

Menon, A., Cafaro, T., Loncaric, D. et al. (2010). Creation and validation of the PERFECT: a critical incident tool for evaluating change in the practices of health professionals. *Journal of Evaluation in Clinical Practice* 16: 1170–1175. https://doi.org/10.1111/j.1365-2753.2009.01288.x.

Michie, S., van Stralen, M.M., and West, R. (2011). The behaviour change wheel: a new method for characterising and designing behaviour change interventions. *Implementation Science* 6: 42. https://doi.org/10.1186/1748-5908-6-42.

Ready, Set, Change! online decision support tool (2014). [Online], Available: http://readiness.knowledgetranslation.ca – 1 (19 July 2019).

Registered Nurses' Association of Ontario (2012). *Toolkit: Implementation of Best Practice Guidelines*. Toronto, ON: Registered Nurses' Association of Ontario https://rnao.ca/sites/rnao-ca/files/RNAO_ToolKit_2012_rev4_FA.pdf.

Ritchie, K.C., Snelgrove-Clarke, E., and Murphy, A.L. (2019). The 23-item Evidence Based Practice-Knowledge Attitudes and Practices (23-item EBP-KAP) survey: initial validation among health professional students. *Health Professions Education* 5: 152–162. https://doi.org/10.1016/j.hpe.2018.09.004.

Rogers, E. (1995). *Diffusion of Innovations*. New York: Free Press.

Rye, M., Torres, E.M., Friborg, O. et al. (2017). The Evidence-based Practice Attitude Scale-36 (EBPAS-36): a brief and pragmatic measure of attitudes to evidence-based practice validated in US and Norwegian samples. *Implementation Science* 12: 44. https://doi.org/10.1186/s13012-017-0573-0.

Salbach, N.M. and Jaglal, S.B. (2011). Creation and validation of the evidence-based practice confidence scale for health care professionals. *Journal of Evaluation in Clinical Practice* 17: 794–800. https://doi.org/10.1111/j.1365-2753.2010.01478.x.

Salbach, N.M., Jaglal, S.B., Korner-Bitensky, N. et al. (2007). Practitioner and organizational barriers to evidence-based practice of physical therapists for people with stroke. *Physical Therapy* 87: 1284–1303. https://doi.org/10.2522/ptj.20070040.

Shea, C.M., Jacobs, S.R., Esserman, D.A. et al. (2014). Organizational readiness for implementing change: a psychometric assessment of a new measure. *Implementation Science* 9: 7. https://doi.org/10.1186/1748-5908-9-7.

Shi, Q., Chesworth, B.M., Law, M. et al. (2014). A modified evidence-based practice-knowledge, attitudes, behaviour and decisions/outcomes questionnaire is valid across multiple professions involved in pain management. *BMC Medical Education* 14: 263. https://doi.org/10.1186/s12909-014-0263-4.

Skolarus, T.A., Lehmann, T., Tabak, R.G. et al. (2017). Assessing citation networks for dissemination and implementation research frameworks. *Implementation Science* 12: 97. https://doi.org/10.1186/s13012-017-0628-2.

Squires, J.E., Linklater, S., Grimshaw, J.M. et al. (2014). Understanding practice: factors that influence physician hand hygiene compliance. *Infection Control and Hospital Epidemiology* 35: 1511–1520. https://doi.org/10.1086/678597.

Squires, J.E., Graham, I.D., Hutchinson, A.M. et al. (2015). Identifying the domains of context important to implementation science: a study protocol. *Implementation Science* 10: 135. https://doi.org/10.1186/s13012-015-0325-y.

Tabak, R.G., Khoong, E.C., Chambers, D.A., and Brownson, R.C. (2012). Bridging research and practice: models for dissemination and implementation research. *American Journal of Preventative Medicine* 43: 337–350. https://doi.org/10.1016/j.amepre.2012.05.024, https://www.ncbi.nlm.nih.gov/pmc/articles/PMC3592983/.

Timmings, C., Khan, S., Moore, J.E. et al. (2016). Ready, set, change! Development and usability testing of an online readiness for change decision support tool for healthcare organizations. *BMC Medical Informatics and Decision Making* 16: 24. https://doi.org/10.1186/s12911-016-0262-y.

Tornatzky, L.G. and Klein, K.J. (1982). Innovation characteristics and innovation adoption-implementation: a meta-analysis of findings. *IEEE Transactions on Engineering Management* EM-29: 28–45. https://doi.org/10.1109/TEM.1982.6447463.

10

Implementation Strategies

What Do We Know Works?

Introduction

The next stage of Roadmap is about selecting and tailoring (or modifying) implementation strategies that overcome the barriers to implementing the best practice and building on the drivers of change. However, before proceeding it is useful to review what is known about the effectiveness of implementation strategies as well as matching such strategies to the identified barriers and drivers for optimal success. At this juncture, Roadmap activity is about the integration of the science (what we know about effectiveness of implementation strategies) and the art of implementation (tailoring the strategies to the identified barriers). Understanding the state of the science around implementation strategies will provide information that can be used to optimize the chances of implementation success.

This chapter reviews taxonomies of implementation strategies, what is known about the effectiveness of implementation strategies, and finally, what is known about approaches to mapping implementation strategies to barriers and drivers of using best practice.

We have observed while working with groups and in giving implementation workshops that there can be a tendency to just want to get in there and implement the best practice. Because there is good evidence of the benefit of the best practice, there can be concern about individuals being denied it. While this sort of enthusiasm and eagerness are huge assets for any group, it can also work against the group's efforts if not properly bridled. There are lots of studies in the literature of well-meaning groups rushing to deploy implementation strategies to get their best practices used. Unfortunately, they are also highly susceptible to failure for two reasons: (i) not systematically assessing and planning for implementation and sustainability (rushing to the action/implementation phase without a plan), and (ii) selecting implementation strategies based largely on the principle- "It seemed like a good idea at the time" (ISLAGIATT)(Colquhoun et al. 2013; Powell et al. 2019). Roadmap will help with the first issue by providing a framework for action planning. If you have jumped to this chapter because you think your group is ready for implementation and/or the group believes that it intuitively knows how to implement the best practice, *please* consider reviewing the previous chapters before proceeding. We appreciate that there can be a natural tendency for practitioners to want to intervene clinically when presented with health issues and in a similar way there can be the tendency to want to implement and not get bogged down in a lot of planning. But without a plan informed by both a conceptual framework and solid local evidence, an ad hoc approach can fail to bring all the stakeholders together with a common approach and purpose, resulting in adopting misguided implementation efforts, and ultimately delaying the uptake of best practice.

The second point of intuitively knowing what is the best way forward should also not be dismissed lightly. This chapter is intended to provide some practical knowledge of what is currently known regarding implementation strategies. Historically, a lot of implementation effort that failed to result in practice or policy change, was due to the group's belief that they understood the implementation context and knew what needed to be done to bring about change. Those leading implementation projects need to demonstrate humility and rely on local evidence and data they collect from knowledge users and stakeholders to guide the process. We have often been surprised to find out what issues practitioners or patients and families think are barriers or drivers of change and how these factors may change over the course of an implementation initiative. Sometimes they align with each other, but they can also be quite different when considering what others think are the "real" barriers/drivers. If you do not ask, you do not learn these things which means potentially selecting the wrong, inappropriate, or ineffective implementation strategies for a given context.

A different issue that also needs to be raised because it sometimes causes confusion relates to the use of the term "intervention" which can have very different meanings depending on the audience (Eldh et al. 2017). For practitioners, the term is often considered synonymous with best practice or the evidence to be implemented (i.e. the innovation to be adopted). For implementation researchers, the term is often used to refer to the implementation intervention or strategy, i.e. what needs to be done to promote the uptake of the practice intervention/best practice. Throughout this book, we consistently use the term intervention to refer the practice or population health interventions that are to be implemented and reserve the term implementation strategy to refer to implementation interventions (the exception being when we cite others, as we use the term they use in their writings). Right from the beginning, as you are developing your implementation plan, decide on the terms you will use, define them and use them consistently so the entire group, as well as those beyond the group, understand what you mean. Confusion between what is meant by the practice intervention (what is being implemented) vs the implementation intervention (the strategy to implement it) has delayed the progress of many groups. For more information on implementation and knowledge translation (KT) terms see Curran's paper (Curran 2020).

Taxonomies of Implementation Strategies

When we speak about implementation strategies or implementation interventions, what exactly do we mean? We are referring to strategies or approaches that can be used to facilitate, promote, encourage the use of best practice. Historically in the health care field, the two most common implementation strategies used are education and audit and feedback. Educational approaches (e.g. course, interactive modules, presentations, written materials, academic detailing, role playing) are implementation strategies if they are designed to increase participants' knowledge and skills to perform the best practice. Audit and feedback, as an implementation strategy, involves the tracking of practitioners' performance, comparing it to others' practice or the gold standard/benchmark, and presenting it back to them so they can judge how their practice compares. There are however many more implementation strategies than these two. It can therefore be useful to have a sense of the breadth and nature of the totality of implementation strategies. A 2015 scoping review identified 51 classification schemes of implementation strategies, including 23 taxonomies, 15 frameworks, 8 intervention lists, 3 models, and 2 other formats (Lokker et al. 2015). These classification systems typically do not consider whether or not there is evidence for each listed strategy (we will discuss the evidence for the strategies in the next section of the chapter). However, the Lokker et al. (2015) review revealed that 55% of the classification schemes were based on a review of the literature and a third were based on theory.

We have tended to rely on a few taxonomies and will briefly discuss them now. The Effective Practice and Organisation of Care (EPOC) (Effective Practice and Organisation of Care (EPOC) Group 2020) of the international Cochrane Collaboration developed one of the first taxonomies to classify implementation strategies evaluated in their systematic reviews (Effective Practice and Organisation of Care (EPOC) 2015). As the title of the group indicates the focus of the group is on implementation strategies directed at influencing provider practice or the organization of care. They typically do not consider strategies directed at consumers or patients. The major categories of strategies are: Delivery of healthcare services, Financial arrangements, Governance arrangements, Implementation strategies and within each of these there are multiple subcategories. For the entire taxonomy please refer to Appendix 10.A.

The Cochrane Consumers and Communication Review Group (CCRG) (Cochrane Consumers and Communication Review Group 2020) similarly has a topic list which is essentially a classification of implementation strategies commonly directed at changing consumers' behavior or the clinical encounter (Cochrane Consumers and Communication Review Group 2012). This list comprises six categories: Interventions directed to the consumer, Interventions from the consumer, Interventions for communication exchange between providers and consumers, Interventions for communication between consumers, Interventions for communication to the healthcare provider from another source, Service delivery interventions with subcategories under each. See Appendix 10.B for the list.

More recently, Byron Powell and colleagues using a Delphi consensus method with over 70 implementation science and clinical practice experts set out to create a compilation of implementation strategies and their definitions (Powell et al. 2012, 2015). This compilation is known as the Expert Recommendations for Implementing Change (ERIC). ERIC comprises 73 implementation strategies and their definitions. See Appendix 10.C for the list. Perry et al. (2019) have used ERIC to compare implementation strategies used across seven large implementation initiatives.

Finally, Michie et al. (2013) wanting to improve the reporting of implementation strategies in research protocols and publications set out to create a taxonomy of behavior change techniques used in behavior change interventions. Also using a Delphi method as well as an open sort task, clustered 93 behavior change techniques into 16 groups. This taxonomy is derived largely from psychological theory about individual behavior change. For more information on implementation taxonomies please refer to Powell et al. (2019), Leeman et al. (2017) and Mazza et al. (2013).

What Is Known About the Effectiveness of Implementation Strategies?

Largely over the past two decades, there has been a growing body of literature on the effectiveness of strategies to promote implementation. Much of this literature has focused on implementation strategies tested on physicians but research studying effectiveness of implementation strategies used by nursing and allied health practice is growing.

The EPOC group of the international Cochrane Collaboration is an excellent source of systematic reviews on the effectiveness of implementation strategies directed at health care providers and policy makers. The group has conducted over 200 systematic reviews to date (Effective Practice and Organisation of Care (EPOC) Group 2020). The Cochrane CCRG has undertaken over 135 systematic reviews to date (Cochrane Consumers and Communication Review Group 2020). Cochrane reviews have a reputation for being of good quality, but it is always good to do your own critical appraisal of studies you come across. We always advise checking the Cochrane Library for systematic reviews on implementation strategies before making too many decisions. Another source of reviews of reviews of implementation strategies is the Canadian Agency for Drugs and Technology in Health (CADTH) Rx for change database (Canadian Agency for Drugs and Technologies in Health 2013). This database incorporates reviews from both EPOC and Cochrane CCRG and critically appraises the quality of the included reviews and uses the implementation strategy taxonomies from both these groups to classify their reviews of reviews. Although the database has not been updated since 2013, most of their reviews of reviews remain relevant and fairly accurate. However, we encourage anyone using this database to also search for more recent reviews since 2013 so as to not be caught off guard by more current information. In fact, it is advisable for any group planning an implementation initiative to search the literature for reviews on implementation strategies of interest. If the search does not turn up any reviews, then searching for primary studies testing the effectiveness of strategies of interest is called for. From an evidence-informed perspective, the key is to first understand the known effectiveness of implementation strategies being considered. After looking to see how effective a proposed implementation strategy is and finding no evidence or that it is of limited effectiveness, then our view is that it is appropriate to cautiously try or experiment with a novel strategy. This should be done in such a way that the findings can be shared with the implementation community to help reduce reinventing the implementation strategy wheel. The onus should always be on the implementors to justify why particular implementation strategies are selected, which includes reporting on what evidence might be available about it.

Because we feel it is essential for all those tasked with implementation to have a sense of the scientific basis of implementation strategies, we will first present a brief overview of what is generally known about the effectiveness of implementation strategies and then as it relates to nursing. Appendix 10.D draws on and updates a summary we developed for a chapter in Knowledge Translation in Health Care (Straus et al. 2013) which was based on the Rx for Change Database (Canadian Agency for Drugs and Technologies in Health 2013) and Grimshaw et al. (2012).

What should be evident from a quick scan of Appendix 10.D is that virtually all implementation strategies listed appear to work some of the time, but none work all the time. Also, the effect size (meaning the change in practice produced by the implementation strategy) is typically around 5–10%. Some interpret the small effect sizes for implementation strategies as proof changing practice and policy is notoriously difficult, time consuming, and expensive. On the other hand, changing the behavior of a healthcare provider population or group by 5–10% can translate into considerable impact when you appreciate each provider interacts with hundreds or even thousands of clients. Finally, for many implementation strategies there are dozens to hundreds of randomized controlled trials (RCTs) that have been conducted to determine their effectiveness. While more implementation trials may be justified if they are conducted with different patient or provider populations or different clinical settings, this does raise the question of how many trials are enough to demonstrate effectiveness, the need to better understand the mechanism of action of the implementation strategy, or focus on other implementation strategies.

We also know that counter to conventional wisdom, the deployment of more implementation strategies (sometimes referred to as multifaceted interventions), does not increase the likelihood of uptake of best practice. Squires et al. (2014) conducted an overview of systematic reviews to evaluate the effectiveness of multifaceted interventions in comparison to single-component interventions in changing health-care professionals' behavior in clinical settings. They included 25 systematic reviews in their overview and found no compelling evidence that multifaceted implementation interventions are more effective than single-component interventions.

On the other hand, there is evidence that tailoring or mapping implementation strategies to identified barriers to using best practice improves implementation success. Baker et al. (2010) conducted a Cochrane systematic review of studies that tailored implementation strategies to prospectively identified barriers to determine whether tailoring affected professional practice or healthcare outcomes. The review included 26 RCTs comparing an intervention tailored to address identified barriers to no intervention or an intervention(s) not tailored to the barriers. The effect sizes of these studies varied both across and within studies. Twelve studies provided enough data to be included in the quantitative analysis. They found that tailoring implementation strategies to prospectively identified barriers improved professional practice by about 1.5 times compared with no implementation strategy or simply disseminating guidelines. They also noted that the methods used to identify barriers and tailor interventions to them needed further development (more on this to come shortly).

Although much of the global evidence relates to the effectiveness of implementation strategies in influencing physician behavior, a number of systematic reviews of the effectiveness of implementation strategies have been undertaken in nursing over the past decade and a half. We now briefly describe the findings of these reviews that focus on the effectiveness of implementation strategies on nurses use of best practice.

Thompson et al. (2007) undertook a systematic review to assess the evidence on interventions aimed explicitly at increasing research use in nursing practice. Their search strategy included literature up to February 2006. Four studies (including five interventional cohorts) met the authors' inclusion criteria (three RCTs and one controlled before and after study design). The methodological quality of all four studies was rated low. The implementation strategies tested included educational meetings (three studies (one included opinion leader and education); and formation of multidisciplinary team (one study)). The strategies of multidisciplinary team and education meeting led by opinion leader had a significant effect on increasing nurses' research use, while educational meetings studied in the other two studies did not significantly change research use by nurses. They urged caution in interpreting the findings because of the generally low quality of the studies.

Yost et al. 2015 conducted a systematic review of implementation strategies (KT interventions) involving nurses in tertiary care to promote evidence informed decision-making knowledge, skills behaviors, and client outcomes. They searched the literature to November 2012. This review identified 30 articles "(18 quantitative, 10 qualitative, and 2 mixed methods studies). The quality of studies with quantitative data ranged from very low to high, and quality criteria was generally met for studies with qualitative data" (Yost et al. 2015). Most implementation strategies were multifaceted (20 studies), single strategies including educational meetings (7 studies), educational materials (2 studies) and a clinical decision support system (1 study). All included studies incorporated an educational aspect to strategies except one that implemented computerized decision support. The impact on knowledge and skills was not evaluated. The effectiveness of multifaceted KT strategies for promoting evidence-informed decision-making (EIDM) behaviors and improving client outcomes was primarily investigated. A meta-analysis of two studies revealed educational meetings and use of a mentor did not increase use of EIDM behaviors. The authors of the review declared that no definitive conclusions could be made about the relative effectiveness of the KT interventions because of differences in interventions and outcomes, as well as study limitations. Findings from qualitative studies revealed that organizational, individual, and interpersonal factors, as well as characteristics of the innovation were reported to influence implementation success. Again, there is nothing with good evidence to guide implementation strategy selection.

With colleagues, we have undertaken a systematic review of the effectiveness of implementation strategies to increase the use of practice guidelines by nurses in hospital and community settings. We searched the literature for RCTs through to January 2019. Of the 32004 citations screened, 38 RCTs met the criteria for inclusion. The methodological quality varied but the majority had low or moderate risk of bias. Most implementation strategies were multi-component (n = 31) and included a combination of educational materials and educational meetings (n = 30). Studies evaluating single implementation strategies focused on educational meetings alone (n = 6) or audit and feedback (with no education component) (n = 1).

Thirty-two RCTs compared guideline implementation strategies to usual approaches to guideline implementation. The majority of these (n = 31) evaluated education interventions using professional practice outcomes (n = 26), patient health outcomes (n = 11), professional knowledge (n = 6), and resource use/expenditure (n = 2). These studies consistently showed an effect on professional practice with effect sizes in the range of 2–13%. However, given the combination and permutations of implementation strategies and outcomes, we were limited in the comparisons we could analyze and thus, cannot make definitive conclusions. Although we cannot identify one strategy that was superior to others, education approaches appear to work in increasing the use of practice guidelines in nursing.

This review also reveals that the number of RCTs of implementation strategies in nursing continues to grow since the Yost et al. (2015) and Thompson et al. (2007) reviews were published; however, the scientific focus remains largely on evaluating educational implementation strategies. Unfortunately, the same educational strategies are not being evaluated making it difficult to truly understand what sort of educational strategies work better for what kinds of nurses (area of practice) under what circumstance. However, in this more current review we detailed the educational strategies so others could replicate and evaluate them. We also found that a number of studies employed implementation strategies that do not fit within the Cochrane EPOC taxonomy of implementation strategies, including theory-based approaches to implementation (n = 15), the use of external facilitation (n = 14), and adaptation of the guideline to local context (n = 10).

Historically, implementation trials in medicine have not been guided by implementation theory (Davies et al. 2010). So, we see the use of theory-based implementation strategies, implementation facilitation, and adaptation of guidelines to the local context as positive developments. These findings support the Roadmap approach that a theory-based implementation, alignment of the evidence to the context, and the role of facilitation may be critical components to success. Furthermore, we have found these components are all the more important when working with teams to bring about change. Keep in mind that these findings have yet to be peer reviewed or published so we urge caution in interpreting them.

Now that you have a sense of the range of implementation strategies and the evidence on their effectiveness (and gaps in the literature), we can turn to how to tailor implementation strategies to identified barriers and drivers. There are some published approaches for how to do this but for the most part, this is where the art of implementation comes into play. We next review some of these approaches.

Intervention and Implementation Mapping

Colquhoun et al. (2013) have an excellent chapter describing how to map barriers and drivers to implementation interventions (this is their term). Much of the literature they cite on intervention mapping was originally proposed for developing any sort of intervention (e.g. public health intervention) not specifically implementation interventions. Be aware that in the literature, the terms "intervention mapping to barriers and facilitators" and "tailoring interventions (or strategies) to barriers and drivers" are used to essentially mean the same thing- choosing interventions/strategies or components of them that are intended to target and overcome prospectively identified barriers to the use of best practice and optimize the drivers of the use of best practice.

As Colquhoun et al. (2013) describe, the key is to align specific components of the implementation strategies to identified barriers to address, alleviate, or reduce the impact of the barriers and thereby facilitate uptake of the best practice. Similarly, linking implementation strategy components to drivers is done to promote and maximize the impact of the strategy. Keep in mind that an implementation strategy (for example, education) usually includes multiple components to address the identified barriers and drivers (for example, a didactic session and/or printed materials to address knowledge gaps, problem based learning to develop and improve critical thinking skills, and role playing to practice new skills). Part of the rationale for explicitly mapping implementation strategy components to barriers and drivers is to understand if this leads to the change anticipated because of the strategy. It is only by understanding what causes change that we can then intervene to better influence change. Much of the literature related to testing implementation strategies has failed to provide any rationale for why a particular implementation strategy was chosen or whether it was in fact designed to address known barriers and drivers of the best practice. Without this information it is difficult to judge why an implementation strategy was or was not successful. We agree with Colquhoun et al. (2013) that when designing an implementation strategy it is critical to establish a hypothesized pathway with three elements: what barriers and facilitators or drivers the component of the strategy was intended to address, why the strategy component was selected, and how it is expected to create change (Michie et al. 2009). These concepts are foundational to Roadmap and the Action Map in charting an implementation. It is important to also keep in mind that barriers and drivers can exist at multiple levels and so the implementation strategy should consider how to address the barriers/drivers at the level of the patient, provider, team, or organization.

Approaches to Intervention Mapping

Methods for mapping interventions to barriers and drivers are in their infancy in the implementation field (Colquhoun et al. 2013). As Colquhoun et al. (2013) note, there are essentially two approaches to mapping implementation interventions/strategies to barriers/ drivers: (i) common sense approaches, and (ii) theory-based approaches. The evidence on the effectiveness of either approach is quite limited. The common-sense approaches rely on varying degrees of implicit theory and sound practical judgment to specify barriers/drivers, whereas the theory-based approaches explicitly use theory and their associated explanations and predictions to guide development of implementation strategies. Keep in mind that the common-sense approaches are often participatory or take an integrated KT approach by engaging and working collaboratively with the local stakeholders and knowledge users to develop the implementation strategy while the theory-based approaches tend to be more researcher driven but need not be.

In their chapter, Colquhoun et al. (2013) offer two example methods for each type of approach. For the common-sense approach to implementation strategy mapping, they describe the semi-structured interview method and the Plan-Do-Study-Act (PDSA) approach. They use intervention mapping and the behavior change technique matrix to illustrate the theory-based approach to implementation strategy development.

Semi-structured Interview Methods

With this approach the group uses individual interviews, brainstorming and/or focus groups to map strategy components to the barriers and drivers. This can be done by presenting the participants with the information on what are the identified barriers/drivers to using the best practice and then having them suggest implementation strategies (or components of strategies) they think would be helpful to overcome the barriers and build on the drivers (this is done through open interviews). Alternatively, or in addition, structured interview methods guided by checklists that summarize the barriers/drivers can be used to have participants link barriers to implementation strategy components more systematically. An advantage of the semi-structured interview approach is that the knowledge users' input is grounded in their understanding of the context and what is practical and feasible to do in their setting.

Plan-Do-Study-Act Approach

PDSA is a rapid cycle approach used in the field of continuous quality improvement. The emphasis is on continuous cycles of improvement within an organization involving multidisciplinary teams eliciting local input into what should be implementation components. The PDSA cycle starts by asking three questions: what is to be accomplished, how will we know that a change is an improvement, and what changes can we make that will result in improvement? The elements of the cycle are: Plan – set objectives, predictions, who will do what; Do – undertake the plan, document; Study – analyze, compare, summarize what happens; Act – what changes need to be made, what cycle should come next. While often not explicit, the multidisciplinary team leading the process and the knowledge users involved often consider barriers/drivers of change when selecting the actions to implement to improve quality of care. The process involves making small changes via rapid cycles each building on the last one. An advantage of this process is that PDSA approach is often already part of healthcare organization quality portfolios and familiar in many settings.

Intervention Mapping

This approach was initially developed for evidenced based health promotion programs and emphasizes the use of theories from social and behavioral sciences (Bartholomew et al. 2001; Kok et al. 2004, 2016). The process is comprised of five steps: (i) develop program objectives linked to their barriers (there can be multiple objectives for each barrier), (ii) select theory-based intervention methods and related practical strategies designed to meet the program objectives, (iii) operationalize the methods and strategies into a coherent feasible intervention, and (iv and v) anticipate the process adoption, implementation, sustainability and evaluation. Mapping implementation intervention components to barriers occurs in steps ii and iii. As Colquhoun et al. (2013) describe, this involves "selecting relevant intervention components that are supported by theory that is deemed by the participants as most relevant to the barriers or issues for behavior change, linking these techniques to practice strategies to change the barriers related to the targeted health behavior, and then integrating these techniques and strategies into a coherent intervention" (p. 143).

Approaches to choosing theory that will help explain a behavior change problem include: issue approach – search the literature for theories specific to the issues for behavior change; concept approach – start with a provisional list of explanatory factors from the literature related to the problem and then link to theories that appear useful; and general theories – consider general theories that may be important for the problem

(Kok et al. 2004). An advantage of the intervention mapping approach is the focus on determining objectives which encompasses the tailoring of intervention components to barriers. Actual guidance on how to select the best theory to guide intervention development remains general which can be challenging for those less familiar with relevant theories.

Behavior Change Technique Matrix

This approach was designed to facilitate development of theory-based interventions that have clearly articulated causal pathways between intervention components and the barriers and facilitators (Michie et al. 2008). The matrix contains a list of 53 effective behavior change techniques based on expert consensus and systematic review mapped to specific barriers and drivers. The barriers/drivers (determinants of behavior) are structured into 11 domains that make up the Theoretical Domains Framework (TDF) and comprise 33 constructs for 128 psychological theories. You will recall that the TDF was discussed in Chapter 9 as one method for carrying out a barriers' assessment. The matrix maps interventions to barriers. For example, if the barrier is related to social influences, the matrix offers interventions of encouragement, pressure, support, and modeling of the behavior by others. See Appendix 10.E for the matrix. The advantage of this approach it that it synthesizes the vast science of behavior change and neatly maps interventions to barriers/drivers and it heavily draws on psychological theories of behavior change.

Implementation Mapping

Fernandez et al. (2019) recently proposed another approach to developing implementation strategies called implementation mapping which they differentiate from intervention mapping. They describe their approach as a systematic process for planning or selecting implementation strategies. The process is based on intervention mapping but expands on the steps found in the intervention mapping process. Implementation mapping involves five tasks: (i) conduct an implementation needs assessment to identify program adopters and implementers; (ii) state adoption and implementation outcomes and performance objectives, identify determinants, and create matrices of change objectives; (iii) choose theoretical methods (mechanisms of change) and select or design implementation strategies; (iv) produce implementation protocols and materials; and (v) evaluate implementation outcomes. There are many similarities with the implementation mapping approach and elements of our Roadmap approach. While we do not have experience with this approach, we can see the potential usefulness of the implementation mapping logic model in helping implementors think through how to develop and evaluate implementation strategies. Figure 10.1 presents the implementation mapping logic model. As you read the logic model from left to right the causal pathways of change become evident, for example, the implementation strategies produce change by targeting determinants of the use of the best practice which leads to use of the best practice which then results in outcomes and impacts. The figure illustrates how the planning process goes from right to left starting with determining the desired outcomes and related performance objectives (Task 1), then identifying the determinants of use of the best practice and context influences (Task 2) which is then used to select and implement implementation strategies (Tasks 3 and 4).

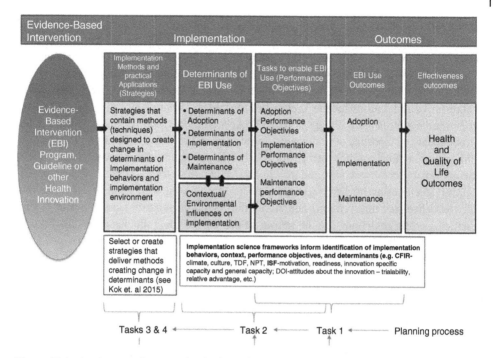

Figure 10.1   Implementation mapping logic model by Fernandez et al. 2019. *Source:* Reprinted with permission under the terms of the Creative Commons Attribution 4.0 International License (http://creativecommons.org/licenses/by/4.0) from Fernandez et al. (2019).

Reporting Guidelines for Interventions

One last topic that is useful to cover is how to report on implementation strategies so that there is transparency and it is possible to reproduce the implementation strategies should any group or organization want to do that. As we have discussed, part of Roadmap process is the drafting of an Action Map and Implementation Plan. What the strategies are and how they are operationalized is important to document, not only for the group and broader organization but also for those beyond who might want to implement the strategies in future.

There are several guidelines for how to report interventions or implementation studies. Historically, the description of implementation strategies (interventions) in the published literature has not been comprehensive making it difficult for the reader to really understand what comprised the intervention or how it was delivered. Often there was insufficient detail to replicate the intervention. The intent of these reporting guidelines is to improve the quality of the description of the intervention. In addition to promoting better description of interventions in the literature, the reporting elements can also be used to guide development of implementation strategies. The Template for Intervention Description and Replication (TIDieR) is a checklist comprising 12 items (brief name, why, what (materials), what (procedure), who provided, how, where, when and how much, tailoring, modifications, how well (planned), how well (actual)) (Hoffmann et al. 2014) (Appendix 10.F). The Standards for Reporting Implementation Studies (StaRI) initiative was developed to promote transparent and accurate reporting of implementation studies (Pinnock et al. 2017). StaRI is a 27-item checklist applicable to the broad range of study designs used in implementation science. The Workgroup for Intervention Development and Evaluation Research (WIDER) recommendations comprises a 20 item checklist to assess the quality of reporting of the essential components of behavior change interventions (KT interventions) (Albrecht et al. 2013) (Appendix 10.G). Finally, we would highlight the AIMD (Aims, Ingredients, Mechanism, Delivery) framework that reviewed and synthesized the 51 classification systems reported by Lokker et al. (2015) to produce a meta-framework (Bragge et al. 2017) (Appendix 10.H). AIMD was designed to guide development and reporting of implementation strategies. This validated and simplified framework comprises four components: (i) Aims: what do you want your intervention to achieve (including barriers to overcome) and for whom? (ii) Ingredients: what comprises the intervention? (iii) Mechanisms: how do you propose the intervention will work? and (iv) Delivery: how will you deliver the intervention? For more information on reporting guidelines or to find specific reporting guidelines, use the website of the EQUATOR (Enhancing the QUAlity and Transparency Of health research) Network (EQUATOR Network 2020).

Summary

This chapter has reviewed specific literature about categories of implementation strategies and what is known about the effectiveness of implementation strategies. Also covered were approaches to mapping implementation strategies to identified barriers and drivers of best practice. If you find some novel or promising strategies to potentially use, it would be pragmatic to make a note in the Action Map as you move forward with selection. In the next chapter we return to Roadmap and describe the matter of tailoring your implementation strategies and illustrate how we have usually gone about doing it.

Appendix 10.A: EPOC Taxonomy – Topics List

Source: Reprinted with permission from Effective Practice and Organisation of Care (EPOC) (2015) EPOC Taxonomy. Available at: https://epoc.cochrane.org/epoc-taxonomy.

Delivery Arrangements
Changes in **how**, **when** and **where** healthcare is organized and delivered, and **who** delivers healthcare.
Category:
How and when care is delivered

Subcategory	Definition	Notes
Group versus individual care	Comparisons of providing care to groups versus individual patients, for example intensive group therapy, group vs individual antenatal care.	
Queuing strategies	A reduction or increase in time to access a healthcare intervention, for example managed waiting lists, managing ER wait time.	

Subcategory	Definition	Notes
Coordination of care amongamongst different provider	Organizing different providers and services to ensure timely and efficient delivery of healthcare.	**See Category** 'Coordination of care and management of care processes' page 2
Quality and safety systems	Essential standards for quality of healthcare, and reduction of poor outcomes related to unsafe healthcare.	
Triage	Management of patients attending a healthcare facility, or contacting a healthcare professional by phone, and receiving advice or being referral to an appropriate service	

Category:
Where care is provided and changes to the healthcare environment

Subcategory	Definition	Notes
Environment	Changes to the physical or sensory healthcare environment, by adding or altering equipment or layout, providing music, art.	
Outreach services	Visits by health workers to different locations, for example involving specialists, generalists, mobile units	
Site of service delivery	Changes in where care is provided, for example home vs. healthcare facility, inpatient vs outpatient, specialized vs. non-specialized facility, walk in clinics, medical day hospital, mobile units	
Size of organizations	Increasing or decreasing the size of health service provider units	
Transportation services	Arrangements for transporting patients from one site to another	

Category:
Who provides care and how the healthcare workforce is managed
Changes in who provides care, to include the qualifications of who provides care; and the recruitment, distribution and retention of health workers

Subcategory	Definition	Notes
Role expansion or task shifting	Expanding tasks undertaken by a cadre of health workers or shifting tasks from one cadre to another, to include tasks not previously part of their scope of practice.	This may include substituting one cadre of healthcare work for another.
Self-management	Shifting or promoting the responsibility for healthcare or disease management to the patient and/or their family.	

(Continued)

Subcategory	Definition	Notes
Length of consultation	Changes in the length of consultations	
Staffing models	Interventions to achieve an appropriate level and mix of staff, recruitment and retention of staff, and transitioning of healthcare workers from one environment to another, for example interventions to increase the proportion of healthcare workers in underserved areas.	
Exit interviews	A verbal exchange or written questionnaire between employees' resignation and last working day	
Movement of health workers between public and private care	Strategies for managing the movement of health workers between public and private organizations	
Pre-licensure education	Changes in pre-licensure education of health professionals	
Recruitment and retention strategies for underserved areas	Strategies for recruiting and retaining health workers in underserved areas	
Recruitment and retention strategies for district health managers – LMIC	Interventions for hiring, retaining and training district health systems managers in LMIC	

Category:

Coordination of care and management of care processes

Changes in how health workers interact with each other or patients to ensure timely and efficient delivery of healthcare.

Subcategory	Definition	Notes
Care pathways	Aim to link evidence to practice for specific health conditions and local arrangements for delivering care.	
Case management	Introduction, modification or removal of strategies to improve the coordination and continuity of delivery of services i.e. improving the management of one "case" (patient)	
Communication between providers	Systems or strategies for improving the communication between health care providers, for example systems to improve immunization coverage in LMIC	
Comprehensive geriatric assessment	A multidimensional interdisciplinary diagnostic process focused on determining a frail older person's medical, psychological and functional capability to ensure that problems are identified, quantified and managed appropriately	

Subcategory	Definition	Notes
Continuity of care	Interventions to reduce fragmented care and undesirable consequences of fragmented care, for example by ensuring the responsibility of care is passed from one facility to another so the patient perceives their needs and circumstances are known to the provider.	
Discharge planning	An individualized plan of discharge to facilitate the transfer of a patient from hospital to a post-discharge setting.	
Disease management	Programs designed to manage or prevent a chronic condition using a systematic approach to care and potentially employing multiple ways of influencing patients, providers or the process of care	
Integration	Consolidating the provision of different healthcare services to one (or simply fewer) facilities.	
Packages of care	Introduction, modification, or removal of packages of services designed to be implemented together for a particular diagnosis/disease, e.g. tuberculosis management guidelines, newborn care protocols.	
Patient-initiated appointment systems	Systems that enable patients to make urgent appointments when they feel they cannot manage their condition or where something has changed unexpectedly	
Procurement and distribution of supplies	Systems for procuring and distributing drugs or other supplies	
Referral systems	Systems for managing referrals of patients between health care providers	
Shared care	Continuing collaborative clinical care between primary and specialist care physicians	
Shared decision-making	Sharing healthcare decision making responsibilities among different individuals, potentially including the patient.	
Teams	Creating and delivering care through a multidisciplinary team of healthcare workers.	
Transition of Care	Interventions to improve transition from one care provider to another, for example adolescents moving from child to adult health services.	

Category:

Information and communication technology (ICT)

ICT used by healthcare organizations to manage the delivery of healthcare, and to deliver healthcare

Subcategory	Definition	Notes
Health information systems	Health record and health management systems to store and manage patient health information, for example electronic patient records, or systems for recalling patients for follow-up or prevention, e.g. immunization.	
The use of information and communication technology	Technology based methods to transfer healthcare information and support the delivery of care.	
Smart home technologies	Electronic assistive technologies	
Telemedicine	Exchange of healthcare information from one site to another via electronic communication	

Financial Arrangements

Changes in how funds are collected, insurance schemes, how services are purchased, and the use of targeted financial incentives or disincentives

Category: Collection of funds

Mechanisms by which financial resources to pay for health care are obtained

Subcategory	Definition	Notes
User fees or out of pocket payments	Charges levied on any aspect of health services at the point of delivery.	
Caps and co-payments for drugs of health services	Direct patient payments for part of the cost of drugs or health services.	
Prepaid funding	Collection of funds through general tax revenues versus earmarked tax revenues versus employer payments versus direct payments.	
Community loan funds	Funds generated from contributions of community members that families can borrow to pay for emergency transportation and hospital costs.	
Health savings accounts	Prepayment schemes for individuals or families without risk pooling.	
External funding	Financial contributions such as donations, loans, etc. from public or private entities from outside the national or local health financing system.	

Category: Insurance schemes

Risk pooling to cover all or part of the costs of health care services

Subcategory	Definition	Notes
Social health insurance	Compulsory insurance that aims to provide universal coverage.	
Community based health insurance	A scheme managed and operated by an organization, other than a government or private for-profit company, that provides risk pooling to cover all or part of the costs of health care services.	
Private health insurance	Private for-profit health insurance.	

Category:

Mechanisms for the payment of health services

NB Pay for Performance mentioned in more than one category

Subcategory	Definition	Notes
Method of paying healthcare organisations	Global budgets, employer based insurance schemes, line- item budgets; case-based reimbursement; pay for performance; mixed payment	
Payment methods for health workers	Fee for services, capitation, salary	
Contracting out health services	Contracting is a strategy to use public sector funds to finance the provision of healthcare services.	
Voucher schemes	Provision of vouchers that can be redeemed for health services at specified facilities	
Conditional cash transfers	Monetary transfers to households on the condition that they comply with pre-defined requirements for healthcare	
Pricing and purchasing policies	Policies that determine the price that is paid or how commercial products are purchased, for example health technologies, drugs.	

Category:

Targeted financial incentives for health professionals and healthcare organisations.

NB Pay for Performance is mentioned in more than one category

Subcategory	Definition	Notes
Pay for performance – target payments	Transfer of money or material goods to healthcare providers conditional on taking a measurable action or achieving a predetermined performance target, for example incentives for lay health workers.	

(Continued)

Subcategory	Definition	Notes
Fund holding	Budgets allocated to a group or individual providers to purchase services with financial rewards for underspending or penalties for overspending (includes indicative budgets)	
Incentives for career choices	Financial or material rewards for career choices; e.g. choice of profession or primary care	

Governance Arrangements

Rules or processes that affect the way in which powers are exercised, particularly with regard to authority, accountability, openness, participation, and coherence

Category:
Authority and accountability for health policies

Subcategory	Definition	Notes
Decentralisation and centralisation	Decentralised versus centralised authority for health services. For example government regulation of health insurance; regional vs. national management of health budgets on efficiency and effectiveness of healthcare.	
Stakeholder involvement in policy decisions	Policies and procedures for involving stakeholders in decision-making	
Community mobilization	Processes that enable people to organize themselves	
Patients' rights	Policies that regulate patients' rights, including access to care and information (includes regulation of information provided to patients)	
Stewardship of private health services	Policies that regulate health services provided by the private sector	
Decision-making about what or who is covered	Processes for deciding what is reimbursed and who is covered by health insurance • Policies that regulate what drugs are reimbursed • Policies that regulate what services are reimbursed • Restrictions on reimbursement for health insurance • Strategies for expanding health insurance coverage	
Policies to reduce corruption	Regulations that are intended to reduce corruption in the health sector	
Policies to manage absenteeism	Regulations for managing absenteeism	

Category:
Authority and accountability for organisations

Subcategory	Definition	Notes
Ownership	Policies that regulate who can own health service organizations, for example for-profit vs not-for-profit; public vs private	
Insurance	Policies that regulate the provision of insurance, for example insurance coverage of essential drugs	
Accreditation	Processes for accrediting healthcare providers	
Multi-institutional arrangements	Policies for how multiple organizations work together • Policies that regulate interactions between donors and governments • Social Franchising • Governance arrangements for coordinating care across multiple providers • Mergers • Collaborations between local health and local government agencies for health improvement	
Liability of healthcare organisations	Policies that limit liability of healthcare organisations, for example risk management.	

Category:
Authority and accountability for commercial products

Subcategory	Definition	Notes
Registration	Procedures for registering or licensing commercial products, for example medical devices, drugs.	
Patents and profits	Policies that regulate patents and profits, for example medical devices, drugs.	
Marketing regulations	Policies that regulate marketing of commercial products, for example medical devices, drugs, the private provision of healthcare.	
Sales and dispensing	Policies that regulate sales and dispensing of commercial products, for example over the counter and prescription drugs.	
Liability for commercial products	Policies that regulate liability for commercial products	

Category:
Authority and accountability for health professionals

Subcategory	Definition	Notes
Training and licensing	Policies that regulate training, specialty certification and licensure requirements for health professionals	
Prescribing	Selection of a drug, by a suitably qualified healthcare worker, to treat a patient's health condition.	
Scope of practice	Policies that regulate what health professionals can do	
Emigration and immigration policies	Policies that regulate emigration and immigration of health professionals	
Dual practice	Policies that regulate dual practice, e.g., working in public and privately owned healthcare settings	
Authority and accountability for quality of practice	Policies that regulate authority and accountability for the quality of care or safety, for example implementation of clinical guidelines.	
Professional competence	Policies or procedures for assuring professional competence	
Professional liability	Policies that regulate liability for health professionals	

Implementation Strategies

Interventions designed to bring about changes in healthcare organizations, the behaviour of healthcare professionals or the use of health services by healthcare recipients

Category:

Interventions targeted at healthcare organisations

Subcategory	Definition	Notes
Organisational culture	Strategies to change organisational culture	

Category:

Interventions targeted at healthcare workers

Subcategory	Definition	Notes
Audit and feedback	A summary of health workers' performance over a specified period of time, given to them in a written, electronic or verbal format. The summary may include recommendations for clinical action.	
Clinical incident reporting	System for reporting critical incidents,	

Subcategory	Definition	Notes
Monitoring the performance of the delivery of healthcare	Monitoring of health services by individuals or healthcare organisations, for example by comparing with an external standard.	
Communities of practice	Groups of people with a common interest who deepen their knowledge and expertise in this area by interacting on an ongoing basis	
Continuous quality improvement	An iterative process to review and improve care that includes involvement of healthcare teams, analysis of a process or system, a structured process improvement method or problem solving approach, and use of data analysis to assess changes	
Educational games	The use of games as an educational strategy to improve standards of care.	
Educational materials	Distribution to individuals, or groups, of educational materials to support clinical care, i.e., any intervention in which knowledge is distributed. For example this may be facilitated by the internet, learning critical appraisal skills; skills for electronic retrieval of information, diagnostic formulation; question formulation	
Educational meetings	Courses, workshops, conferences or other educational meetings	
Educational outreach visits, or academic detailing.	Personal visits by a trained person to health workers in their own settings, to provide information with the aim of changing practice.	
Clinical Practice Guidelines	Clinical guidelines are systematically developed statements to assist healthcare providers and patients to decide on appropriate health care for specific clinical circumstances' (US IOM).	
Inter-professional **education**	Continuing education for health professionals that involves more than one profession in joint, interactive learning	
Local consensus processes	Formal or informal local consensus processes, for example agreeing a clinical protocol to manage a patient group, adapting a guideline for a local health system or promoting the implementation of guidelines.	
Local opinion leaders	The identification and use of identifiable local opinion leaders to promote good clinical practice.	

(Continued)

Subcategory	Definition	Notes
Managerial supervision	Routine supervision visits by health staff.	
Patient-mediated interventions	Any intervention aimed at changing the performance of healthcare professionals through interactions with patients, or information provided by or to patients.	
Public release of performance data	Informing the public about healthcare providers by the release of performance data in written or electronic form.	
Reminders	Manual or computerised interventions that prompt health workers to perform an action during a consultation with a patient, for example computer decision support systems.	
Routine patient-reported outcome measures	Routine administration and reporting of patient-reported outcome measures to providers and/or patients	
Tailored interventions	Interventions to change practice that are selected based on an assessment of barriers to change, for example through interviews or surveys.	

Category:
Interventions targeted at specific types of practice, conditions or settings

- Health conditions
  - Acute stroke
  - Acute surgery
  - Alcohol
- Practice and setting
  - Health promotion in dental settings

Appendix 10.B: Cochrane Consumers and Communication Group: Topics list

Reprinted with permission from Cochrane Consumers and Communication Review Group (2012) Topics list. https://cccrg.cochrane.org/sites/cccrg.cochrane.org/files/public/uploads/Topics.pdf

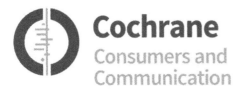

Cochrane
Consumers and
Communication

Topics list

Interventions directed to the consumer (Group 1)

Counselling
  Medication or genetic or diet counselling
  Cognitive behavioural counselling for coping
Cross-cultural communication
Health promotion
  Participation in screening programs
  Smoking cessation
  Vaccination programs
  Heart programs
  Healthy behaviour change
Information provision
  About trial participation
  About choices
  Patient-specific details
  About available health services
  Genetic risk assessment
Instruction
  About treatment
  About medication
  On discharge
  Prescriptions for screening or exercise
Marketing/advertising
  To participate in research
  Mass media campaigns
Consumer education
  About disease/condition
  About treatment/procedure
  About risk reduction
  Sex education

(Continued)

Topics list

Reminder systems directed to the consumer
    To attend screening
    To have vaccination
    To keep appointments
    To take medication
Skills training
    Relaxation techniques
    Self-examination methods
    Communication skills
    Self-care skills
Social support
    Emotional/psychosocial support
    Patient advocacy
Other

Interventions from the consumer (Group 2)
Consumer participation in reviews, committees, policy formulation
Feedback
    Consumer reporting of self-monitoring
    Reporting of consumer preferences
    Satisfaction with usual care
    Patient diaries
History taking or patient profiling
    Medical history
    Socio-economic factors
    Measurement of patient expectations
Information-seeking initiated by the consumer, or information given by the consumer
    to the provider
    During consultations
    Surveys of consumers
    Development or assessment of questionnaires
Provider education
Other
    Participation in trials

Interventions for communication exchange between providers and consumers (Group 3)
Discussion (individual, group)
Interview
    Motivational interview/therapy
    Consultation process
Negotiation or decision making
    Care plans
    Goal setting
    Compliance contracts
    Informed consent
    Shared decision making

Topics list

Patient-held medical record
   Health card or booklet
   Information sheet specific to particular patient
   Recording of consultation
   Patient summaries
   Medication record
Other

Interventions for communication between consumers (Group 4)

Focus groups
Peer support
   Self-help groups
   Learning together
   Sharing experiences
   Group education
   Group visits
   Buddy systems
Individual self-help
   Lay help
   Self-management learning by oneself
   Skills training
Support
   Family teamwork
   Presence of family member, carer or other person during education session, or consultation, or treatment, in support of patient
Other

Interventions for communication to the healthcare provider from another source (Group 5)

Education programs
   Skills training in communication or patient-centred care skills
Reminder systems for the clinician
Other

Service delivery interventions (Group 6)

Structure and delivery of care
   Family access to healthcare provider or to hospitalised patient
      Visiting hours
      Rooming-in
      Parent rooms
   Healthcare provision
      Specialist nurses or pharmacists providing the intervention
      Health plan choices
      Convenience of location of care
      Appointment choices
      Consumer as healthcare provider

(Continued)

Topics list

 Treatment or care changes/choices
  Administration or packaging of medication
  Extent of physical examination
 Coordination of care
  Discharge planning coordination
  Case management
  Team care
 Technology-based interventions
  Remote consultation by telephone or internet
  Interactive Health Communication Applications
 Other
Supportive environment

 Change in context of care
  Hospital versus home care
  Home visits
  Family care versus professional care
 Environmental effects
  Colours
  Background music
 Imagery
  Visual or psychological imagery as relaxation technique
 – Guided imagery
 Music
 Virtual reality
 Placebo effect
  Physical or psychological
 Other
 Touch

Appendix 10.C: ERIC discrete implementation strategy compilation (n = 73)

Source: Powell, B. J., Waltz, T. J., Chinman, M. J., Damschroder, L. J., Smith, J. L., Matthieu, M. M., Proctor, E. K. & Kirchner, J. E. (2015). Licensed under CC BY 4.0.

Strategy	Definitions
Access new funding	Access new or existing money to facilitate the implementation.
Alter incentive/allowance structures	Work to incentivize the adoption and implementation of the clinical innovation.
Alter patient/consumer fees	Create fee structures where patients/consumers pay less for preferred treatments (the clinical innovation) and more for less-preferred treatments.

Strategy	Definitions
Assess for readiness and identify barriers and facilitators	Assess various aspects of an organization to determine its degree of readiness to implement, barriers that may impede implementation, and strengths that can be used in the implementation effort.
Audit and provide feedback	Collect and summarize clinical performance data over a specified time period and give it to clinicians and administrators to monitor, evaluate, and modify provider behavior
Build a coalition	Recruit and cultivate relationships with partners in the implementation effort
Capture and share local knowledge	Capture local knowledge from implementation sites on how implementers and clinicians made something work in their setting and then share it with other sites
Centralize technical assistance	Develop and use a centralized system to deliver technical assistance focused on implementation issues
Change accreditation or membership requirements	Strive to alter accreditation standards so that they require or encourage use of the clinical innovation. Work to alter membership organization requirements so that those who want to affiliate with the organization are encouraged or required to use the clinical innovation
Change liability laws	Participate in liability reform efforts that make clinicians more willing to deliver the clinical innovation
Change physical structure and equipment	Evaluate current configurations and adapt, as needed, the physical structure and/or equipment (e.g., changing the layout of a room, adding equipment) to best accommodate the targeted innovation
Change record systems	Change records systems to allow better assessment of implementation or clinical outcomes
Change service sites	Change the location of clinical service sites to increase access
Conduct cyclical small tests of change	Implement changes in a cyclical fashion using small tests of change before taking changes system-wide. Tests of change benefit from systematic measurement, and results of the tests of change are studied for insights on how to do better. This process continues serially over time, and refinement is added with each cycle
Conduct educational meetings	Hold meetings targeted toward different stakeholder groups (e.g., providers, administrators, other organizational stakeholders, and community, patient/consumer, and family stakeholders) to teach them about the clinical innovation
Conduct educational outreach visits	Have a trained person meet with providers in their practice settings to educate providers about the clinical innovation with the intent of changing the provider's practice
Conduct local consensus discussions	Include local providers and other stakeholders in discussions that address whether the chosen problem is important and whether the clinical innovation to address it is appropriate
Conduct local needs assessment	Collect and analyze data related to the need for the innovation
Conduct ongoing training	Plan for and conduct training in the clinical innovation in an ongoing way
Create a learning collaborative	Facilitate the formation of groups of providers or provider organizations and foster a collaborative learning environment to improve implementation of the clinical innovation

(Continued)

Strategy	Definitions
Create new clinical teams	Change who serves on the clinical team, adding different disciplines and different skills to make it more likely that the clinical innovation is delivered (or is more successfully delivered)
Create or change credentialing and/or licensure standards	Create an organization that certifies clinicians in the innovation or encourage an existing organization to do so. Change governmental professional certification or licensure requirements to include delivering the innovation. Work to alter continuing education requirements to shape professional practice toward the innovation
Develop a formal implementation blueprint	Develop a formal implementation blueprint that includes all goals and strategies. The blueprint should include the following: 1) aim/purpose of the implementation; 2) scope of the change (e.g., what organizational units are affected); 3) timeframe and milestones; and 4) appropriate performance/progress measures. Use and update this plan to guide the implementation effort over time
Develop academic partnerships	Partner with a university or academic unit for the purposes of shared training and bringing research skills to an implementation project
Develop an implementation glossary	Develop and distribute a list of terms describing the innovation, implementation, and stakeholders in the organizational change
Develop and implement tools for quality monitoring	Develop, test, and introduce into quality-monitoring systems the right input—the appropriate language, protocols, algorithms, standards, and measures (of processes, patient/consumer outcomes, and implementation outcomes) that are often specific to the innovation being implemented
Develop and organize quality monitoring systems	Develop and organize systems and procedures that monitor clinical processes and/or outcomes for the purpose of quality assurance and improvement
Develop disincentives	Provide financial disincentives for failure to implement or use the clinical innovations
Develop educational materials	Develop and format manuals, toolkits, and other supporting materials in ways that make it easier for stakeholders to learn about the innovation and for clinicians to learn how to deliver the clinical innovation
Develop resource sharing agreements	Develop partnerships with organizations that have resources needed to implement the innovation
Distribute educational materials	Distribute educational materials (including guidelines, manuals, and toolkits) in person, by mail, and/or electronically
Facilitate relay of clinical data to providers	Provide as close to real-time data as possible about key measures of process/outcomes using integrated modes/channels of communication in a way that promotes use of the targeted innovation
Facilitation	A process of interactive problem solving and support that occurs in a context of a recognized need for improvement and a supportive interpersonal relationship
Fund and contract for the clinical innovation	Governments and other payers of services issue requests for proposals to deliver the innovation, use contracting processes to motivate providers to deliver the clinical innovation, and develop new funding formulas that make it more likely that providers will deliver the innovation
Identify and prepare champions	Identify and prepare individuals who dedicate themselves to supporting, marketing, and driving through an implementation, overcoming indifference or resistance that the intervention may provoke in an organization

Strategy	Definitions
Identify early adopters	Identify early adopters at the local site to learn from their experiences with the practice innovation
Increase demand	Attempt to influence the market for the clinical innovation to increase competition intensity and to increase the maturity of the market for the clinical innovation
Inform local opinion leaders	Inform providers identified by colleagues as opinion leaders or "educationally influential" about the clinical innovation in the hopes that they will influence colleagues to adopt it
Intervene with patients/ consumers to enhance uptake and adherence	Develop strategies with patients to encourage and problem solve around adherence
Involve executive boards	Involve existing governing structures (e.g., boards of directors, medical staff boards of governance) in the implementation effort, including the review of data on implementation processes
Involve patients/ consumers and family members	Engage or include patients/consumers and families in the implementation effort
Make billing easier	Make it easier to bill for the clinical innovation
Make training dynamic	Vary the information delivery methods to cater to different learning styles and work contexts, and shape the training in the innovation to be interactive
Mandate change	Have leadership declare the priority of the innovation and their determination to have it implemented
Model and simulate change	Model or simulate the change that will be implemented prior to implementation
Obtain and use patients/ consumers and family feedback	Develop strategies to increase patient/consumer and family feedback on the implementation effort
Obtain formal commitments	Obtain written commitments from key partners that state what they will do to implement the innovation
Organize clinician implementation team meetings	Develop and support teams of clinicians who are implementing the innovation and give them protected time to reflect on the implementation effort, share lessons learned, and support one another's learning
Place innovation on fee for service lists/formularies	Work to place the clinical innovation on lists of actions for which providers can be reimbursed (e.g., a drug is placed on a formulary, a procedure is now reimbursable)
Prepare patients/ consumers to be active participants	Prepare patients/consumers to be active in their care, to ask questions, and specifically to inquire about care guidelines, the evidence behind clinical decisions, or about available evidence-supported treatments
Promote adaptability	Identify the ways a clinical innovation can be tailored to meet local needs and clarify which elements of the innovation must be maintained to preserve fidelity
Promote network weaving	Identify and build on existing high-quality working relationships and networks within and outside the organization, organizational units, teams, etc. to promote information sharing, collaborative problem-solving, and a shared vision/goal related to implementing the innovation

(Continued)

Strategy	Definitions
Provide clinical supervision	Provide clinicians with ongoing supervision focusing on the innovation. Provide training for clinical supervisors who will supervise clinicians who provide the innovation
Provide local technical assistance	Develop and use a system to deliver technical assistance focused on implementation issues using local personnel
Provide ongoing consultation	Provide ongoing consultation with one or more experts in the strategies used to support implementing the innovation
Purposely reexamine the implementation	Monitor progress and adjust clinical practices and implementation strategies to continuously improve the quality of care
Recruit, designate, and train for leadership	Recruit, designate, and train leaders for the change effort
Remind clinicians	Develop reminder systems designed to help clinicians to recall information and/or prompt them to use the clinical innovation
Revise professional roles	Shift and revise roles among professionals who provide care, and redesign job characteristics
Shadow other experts	Provide ways for key individuals to directly observe experienced people engage with or use the targeted practice change/innovation
Stage implementation scale up	Phase implementation efforts by starting with small pilots or demonstration projects and gradually move to a system wide rollout
Start a dissemination organization	Identify or start a separate organization that is responsible for disseminating the clinical innovation. It could be a for-profit or non-profit organization
Tailor strategies	Tailor the implementation strategies to address barriers and leverage facilitators that were identified through earlier data collection
Use advisory boards and workgroups	Create and engage a formal group of multiple kinds of stakeholders to provide input and advice on implementation efforts and to elicit recommendations for improvements
Use an implementation advisor	Seek guidance from experts in implementation
Use capitated payments	Pay providers or care systems a set amount per patient/consumer for delivering clinical care
Use data experts	Involve, hire, and/or consult experts to inform management on the use of data generated by implementation efforts
Use data warehousing techniques	Integrate clinical records across facilities and organizations to facilitate implementation across systems
Use mass media	Use media to reach large numbers of people to spread the word about the clinical innovation
Use other payment schemes	Introduce payment approaches (in a catch-all category)
Use train-the-trainer strategies	Train designated clinicians or organizations to train others in the clinical innovation
Visit other sites	Visit sites where a similar implementation effort has been considered successful
Work with educational institutions	Encourage educational institutions to train clinicians in the innovation

Appendix 10.D: Summary of effectiveness of disseminating strategies

Meta-analyses	Number of studies/ individuals	Effect sizes
Distribution of educational materials (professional intervention)	Rx for Change Database (2013)	60 reviews that evaluated the effectiveness of distribution of educational materials were identified. Of these, 4/4 high quality/key reviews (Farmer et al. 2008; Blackwood et al. 2010; French et al. 2010; Nagendran et al. 2013) with a sufficient number of studies to draw conclusions found this intervention to be generally effective
	12 RCTs and 11 N-RCTs (Farmer et al. 2008)	Median absolute improvement on care of 4.3% (range − 8.0–9.6%)
	10 RCTs (Blackwood et al. 2010)	Mean duration of mechanical ventilation reduced by 25% (95% CI 9% to 39%, $P = 0.006$)
		Weaning duration from 6 trials was reduced by 78% (95% CI 31% to 93%, $P = 0.009$
	22 RCTs and 6 N-RCTs (French et al. 2010)	Absolute improvement in test ordering of 10.0% (IQR 0.0 to 27.7)
	8 RCTs (Nagendran et al. 2013)	MD in operating time − 11.76 (95% CI; −15.23 to −8.30) SMD in operative performance 1.6 (95% CI 0.72 to 2.58)
	Updated review (Farmer et al. 2008)	Median absolute RD in categorical practice outcomes of 2% (range 0–11%)
	Now 14 RCTs and 31 ITS (Giguère et al. 2012)	SMD for continuous practice outcomes of 13% (range − 16–36%)
Mass media (professional intervention)	Rx for Change Database (2013)	4 reviews that examined the effectiveness of mass media interventions were identified. Of these, 1/1 high quality/ key reviews (Grilli et al. 2002) with a sufficient number of studies to draw conclusions found this intervention to be generally effective.
	20 ITS (Grilli et al. 2002)	Direction of effect across studies was consistent suggesting mass media may be effective (range in effect size from 0.1 to −13.1)
Access to reviews and tailored messages	Rx for Change Database (2013)	Not listed an intervention on the Rx for Change Database
	1 RCT and 1 N-RCT (Perrier et al. 2011)	The first study utilized a non-experimental design to report an intervention where public health policy makers were offered the opportunity to receive five relevant reviews. At three months and two years, respectively, 23 and 63% of respondents reported using at least one of the systematic reviews to make a policy decision.
		The second study was a randomized trial where health departments received one of three interventions: access to an online registry of systematic reviews, tailored messages plus access to the online registry of systematic reviews, or tailored messages plus access to the registry along with a knowledge broker who worked one-on-one with decision makers over a period of one year.
		While none of the interventions showed a significant effect on global evidence-informed decision making, *tailored messages plus access to the online registry of systematic reviews showed a positive significant effect on public health policies and programs*

(Continued)

Meta-analyses	Number of studies/individuals	Effect sizes
Educational meetings (professional intervention)	Rx for Change Database (2013)	82 reviews that evaluated the effectiveness of educational meetings were identified. Of these, 2/9 high quality/key reviews (Jamtvedt et al. 2006; Forsetlund et al. 2009) with a sufficient number of studies to draw conclusions found this intervention to be generally effective.
	81 RCTs (involving more than 11 000 health professionals) (Forsetlund et al. 2009)	Mean absolute improvement in care of 6.0% (IQR = 1.8–15.9%)
	118 RCTs (Jamtvedt et al. 2006)	8/9 trials favored the intervention (audit and feedback with educational meetings versus no intervention)
		Adjusted risk ratio of compliance with desired practice ranged from 0.98 to 3.01 (median = 1.06, IQR = 1.03–1.09).
		Adjusted RD ranged from −1% to 24% (median = 1.5, IQR = 1.0–5.5).
		Adjusted percent change for the continuous outcomes ranged from 3 to 41% (median = 28.7, IQR = 14.3–36.5)
Educational outreach visits (academic detailing) (professional intervention)	**Rx for Change Database (2013)**	34 reviews that evaluated the effectiveness of educational outreach visits were identified. Of these, 2/3 high quality/key reviews (O'Brien et al. 2007; Nkansah et al. 2010) with a sufficient number of studies to draw conclusions found this intervention to be generally effective
	69 RCTs (Involving more than 15 000 health professionals) (O'Brien et al. 2007)	The median adjusted RD in compliance with desired practice was 5.6% (IQR = 3.0–9.0%).
		The adjusted RDs were highly consistent for prescribing behaviors [17 comparisons] median 4.8% (IQR = 3.0–6.5%), but varied for other types of professional performance (e.g. providing screening tests; 17 comparisons) – median 6.0% (IQR = 3.6 – 16.0%)
	43 RCTs (Nkansah et al. 2010)	Educational outreach visits by a pharmacist to promote guideline-based prescribing for two of four disease states (aspirin as antiplatelet therapy, angiotensin converting enzyme inhibitors [ACEIs] in heart failure, NSAIDs in osteoarthritis pain, antidepressants for depression) resulted in a statistically significant 5.2% increase (OR = 1.24; 95% CI 1.07–1.42) in overall guideline adherence (Freemantle et al. 2002).
		Pharmacist provided academic detailing related to cholesterol treatment significantly increased the number of lipid-treatment prescriptions in females (Diwan et al. 1995).
	140 RCTs (Ivers et al. 2012)	Audit and feedback with educational outreach compared to audit and feedback alone
		24 comparisons from 19 studies that compared audit and feedback alone to the combination of audit and feedback and educational outreach (also known as academic detailing).

Meta-analyses	Number of studies/individuals	Effect sizes
		For the 15 studies with dichotomous outcomes focusing on professional practice, the weighted median adjusted RD for audit and feedback with outreach versus feedback alone was a 0.7% increase in desired practice (IQR = −1.1–5.1%).
		For the four studies with continuous outcomes, the median adjusted change relative to baseline control was 27% (IQR = 0–40.5%).
Providing information or education (consumer intervention)	**Rx for Change Database (2013)**	4 reviews (Gibson et al. 2002; Johnson et al. 2003; Nicolson et al. 2009; Li et al. 2011) were identified. Overall there is insufficient evidence to support the use of interventions that provide information or education as a single component to improve adherence, knowledge or clinical outcomes – they are generally ineffective.
		There is evidence that decision aids improve knowledge about treatments, accuracy of risk perception, and congruence between informed values and care choices (Stacey et al. 2017).
	12 RCTs (Gibson et al. 2002)	Limited asthma education did not reduce hospitalization for asthma (WMD −0.03 average hospitalizations per person per year, 95% CI -0.09 to 0.03), but in two studies, perceived asthma symptoms did improve (OR = 0.44, 95% CI 0.26 to 0.74).
		Limited asthma education was associated with reduced emergency department visits (reduction of −2.76 average visits per person per year, 95% CI -4.34 to 1.18).
	2 studies, RCT, CCT (Johnson et al. 2003)	Written plus verbal information at discharge reduced return to the emergency department, when compared with verbal information alone (combined intervention groups 3.1% and control 10.1%, p < 0.05 by Fisher's exact test).
		There was no significant change in need to call a physician for advice when written and verbal discharge information was compared to verbal information alone (standardized verbal information group 11.1%, interventions group [written information in addition to verbal information] 15.1% and control 22.8%).
		There is some evidence that verbal and written health information, when compared to verbal information only, increases knowledge of medicines post discharge – it is generally effective (average knowledge score for the intervention group 0.902, no SD provided and the average knowledge score for the control group 0.765 no SD provided, p < 0.05)
		There is some evidence that verbal and written health information, when compared to verbal information only, may improve satisfaction with discharge instructions (intervention group 0.96, standardized verbal information group 0.96 and control group 0.85, no SD given, p < 0.0001).

(Continued)

Meta-analyses	Number of studies/ individuals	Effect sizes
	25 RCTs involving 4788 participants (Nicolson et al. 2009)	Written information – 25 RCTs, the combined evidence was insufficient to say whether written medicines information is effective in changing knowledge, attitudes and behaviors related to medicine taking.
	2 RCTs involving 207 patients (Li et al. 2011)	Compared with no educational programs, educational programs for patients with diabetes on dialysis improved patients' knowledge for the following outcomes: • diagnosis (SMD 1.14, 95% CI 0.93 to 1.90); • monitoring (SMD 1.51, 95% CI 1.0 to 2.01); • hypoglycemia (SMD 1.67, 95% CI 1.16 to 2.17), • hyperglycemia (SMD 0.80, 95% CI 0.35 to 1.25); • medication with insulin (SMD 1.21, 95% CI 0.74 to 1.68); • oral medication (SMD 0.98, 95% CI 0.52 to1.43); • personal health habits (SMD 1.84, 95% CI 1.33 to 2.36); • diet (SMD 0.53, 95% CI 0.09 to 0.97); • exercise (SMD 1.13, 95% CI 0.67 to 1.60); • chronic complications (SMD 1.28, 95% CI 0.80 to1.75) • living with diabetes and coping with stress (SMD 0.71, 95% CI 0.26 to 1.15). However, with only two studies with small sample sizes and inadequate quality included in this review, there is inadequate evidence to support the beneficial effects of education programs.
	105 RCTs involving 31 043 participants (Stacey et al. 2017)	With regard to the attributes of the choice made, decision aids increased participants' knowledge (MD 13.27/100; 95% CI 11.32 to 15.23; 52 studies; N = 13 316; high-quality evidence), accuracy of risk perceptions (RR 2.10; 95% CI 1.66 to 2.66; 17 studies; N = 5096; moderate-quality evidence), and congruency between informed values and care choices (RR 2.06; 95% CI 1.46 to 2.91; 10 studies; N = 4626; low-quality evidence) compared to usual care.
Acquiring skills and competencies (consumer intervention)	**Rx for Change Database (2013)**	31 reviews focusing on the acquisition of skills relevant to medicines use were identified; 20 were of high quality. There is some evidence that strategies which focus on the acquisition of skills and competencies (self-monitoring and self-management) may improve adherence, medicines use and clinical outcomes, but results are mixed
	Self-management programs – 17 RCTs involving 7442 participants (Foster et al. 2007)	Foster et al. (2007) was referenced in Grimshaw et al. (2012) but not included as one of the 20 high quality reviews listed in the Rx for Change Database summary referred to above – however we have included it here as an example: Small (clinically insignificant) short-term improvements in pain, disability, fatigue and depression were found. Positive effects on confidence to manage and self-rated health were found. There was no effect on quality of life or use of health services

Meta-analyses	Number of studies/ individuals	Effect sizes
		Health status: There was a small, statistically-significant reduction in: pain (11 studies, SMD −0.10 [95% CI -0.17 to −0.04]); disability (8 studies, SMD −0.15 (95% CI -0.25 to −0.05); and fatigue (7 studies, SMD −0.16 (95% CI -0.23 to −0.09); and a small, statistically-significant improvement in depression (6 studies, SMD −0.16 95% CI -0.24 to −0.07).
		There was a small (but not statistically- or clinically-significant) improvement in: psychological well-being (5 studies; SMD −0.12 [95% CI -0.33 to 0.09]); but no difference between groups for health-related quality of life (3 studies; WMD −0.03 (95% CI -0.09 to 0.02).
		Six studies showed a statistically-significant improvement in self-rated general health (WMD −0.20 (95% CI -0.31 to −0.10).
		Health behaviors: 7 studies showed a small, statistically-significant increase in self-reported aerobic exercise (SMD −0.20 [95% CI -0.27 to −0.12]) and a moderate increase in cognitive symptom management (4 studies, WMD −0.55 [95% CI -0.85 to −0.26]).
		Healthcare use: There were no statistically-significant differences between groups in physician or general practitioner attendance (9 studies; SMD −0.03 [95% CI -0.09 to 0.04]). There were also no statistically-significant differences between groups for days/nights spent in hospital (6 studies; WMD −0.32 [95% CI -0.71 to 0.07]).
		Self-efficacy: (confidence to manage condition) showed a small statistically-significant improvement (10 studies): SMD −0.30, 95% CI -0.41 to −0.19.
Local opinion leaders (OLs) (professional intervention)	**Rx for Change Database (2013)**	6 reviews that evaluated the effectiveness of local opinion leaders were identified. Of these, 2/2 high quality/key reviews (Thomas et al. 2000; Flodgren et al. 2011) with a sufficient number of studies to draw conclusions found this intervention to be generally effective.
	18 RCTs (involving more than 296 hospitals and 318 primary care physicians) (Flodgren et al. 2011)	The use of local opinion leaders alone or combined with other interventions was generally effective for improving appropriate care outcomes – median absolute improvement of care of 12% across studies (IQR = 6.0–14.5%).
	18 RCTs (involving more than 467 healthcare professionals (Thomas et al. 2000)	Insufficient evidence exists for local opinion leaders compared to educational meetings to draw any conclusions about the effectiveness of the intervention on appropriate care.
	Updated Cochrane SR (Flodgren et al. 2019) 24 RCTs (involving more than 337 hospitals, 350 primary care practices, 3005 healthcare professionals, and 29 167 patients)	18 studies contributed to the median adjusted RD for the main comparison • The results suggested that the OL interventions probably improve healthcare professionals' compliance with evidence-based practice (10.8% absolute improvement in compliance, IQR = 3.5–14.6%; moderate-certainty evidence). • Results for the secondary comparisons also suggested that OLs probably improve compliance with evidence-based practice (moderate-certainty evidence):

(Continued)

Meta-analyses	Number of studies/ individuals	Effect sizes
		• OLs alone versus no intervention: RD (IQR): 9.15% (−0.3–15%);
		• OLs alone versus a single intervention: RD (range): 13.8% (12–15.5%);
		• OLs, with a single or more intervention(s) versus the same single or more intervention(s): RD (IQR): 7.1% (−1.4–9%);
		• OLs with a single or more intervention(s) versus no intervention: RD (IQR): 10.25% (0.6–15.75%).
		Local OLs alone, or in combination with other interventions, can be effective in promoting evidence-based practice, but the effectiveness varies both within and between studies.
Local consensus process (professional intervention)	Rx for Change Database (2013)	8 reviews that evaluated the effectiveness of local consensus process were identified and none were assessed as being of high quality or a key review therefore no conclusions drawn.
	New SR found 6 RCTs (Wolfenden et al. 2018)	All studies used multiple strategies to improve the implementation of policies and practices, including: educational meetings, interventions tailored to the specific needs of the workplace, and workplace consensus processes to implement a policy or practice.
		Of the five trials comparing implementation strategies with a no intervention control, pooled analysis was possible for three RCTs reporting continuous score-based measures of implementation outcomes. The meta-analysis found no difference in standardized effects (SMD −0.01, 95% CI−0.32 to 0.30; 164 participants; 3 studies; low certainty evidence), suggesting no benefit of implementation support in improving policy or practice implementation, relative to control.
Linkage and exchange (professional intervention)	Rx for Change Database (2013)	Not listed an intervention on the Rx for Change Database
	1 SR including 17 studies (Lavis et al. 2005)	Two factors emerged from the systematic review as being important to policy makers' and appear to increase the prospects for research use among policymakers:
		• interactions between researchers and health care policy-makers and,
		• timing/timeliness of the information
		Interviews with health care managers and policy-makers suggest that they would benefit from:
		• having information that is relevant for decisions highlighted for them (e.g. contextual factors that affect a review's local applicability and information about the benefits, harms/risks and costs of interventions) and
		• having reviews presented in a way that allows for rapid scanning for relevance and then graded entry (such as one page of take-home messages, a three-page executive summary and a 25-page report).

Meta-analyses	Number of studies/ individuals	Effect sizes
	8 studies – 2 C-RCTs, 3 RCTs, 3 ITS (Murthy et al. 2012)	Eight studies were included evaluating the effectiveness of different interventions designed to support the uptake of systematic review evidence. The overall quality of the evidence was very low to moderate. Two RCTs tested an intervention that can be characterized as a linkage and exchange activity (Wyatt et al. 1998; Dobbins et al. 2009).
		Dobbins et al. 2009 (Knowledge broker + targeted messages + access to health evidence web site versus access to health evidence web site)
		Intervention: n = 36 public health departments
		Control: n = 36 public health departments
		Utilization of research
		There was no statistically significant effect of tailored messages on evidence-informed decision making (mean change −0.42; 95% CI -1.10 to 0.26, P < 0.45). There was no statistically significant effect (mean change −0.09; 95% CI -0.78 to 0.60) of having access to a knowledge broker (in conjunction with delivery of tailored messages and access to Health Evidence) compared to access to Health Evidence on evidence informed decision-making.
		A statistically significant effect of tailored messages on the number of public health policies and programs being implemented from baseline to follow-up immediately after the intervention (mean change 1.67; 95% CI 0.37 to 2.97, P < 0.01) was reported.
		Wyatt et al. 1998 (A single education visit, access to Cochrane Pregnancy and Childbirth Reviews and a short video outlining evidence-based medicine to enhance the use of systematic review evidence in practice)
		Intervention – n = 12 obstetric units
		Control – n = 13 obstetric units
		There was a statistically significant difference between randomized groups at baseline for two of the four selected clinical practices, with a significantly higher use of ventouse and polyglycolic acid sutures in the control units. This makes it difficult to interpret changes at follow-up. The median effect size for the four clinical marker practices was RR 0.92 (range RR 0.57 to RR 1.01).
		If the intention is to develop awareness and knowledge of systematic review evidence, and the skills for implementing this evidence, a multifaceted intervention that addresses each of these aims may be required, though there is insufficient evidence to support this approach.
Consumer system participation (consumer intervention)	Rx for Change Database (2013)	A single high-quality review (Nilsen et al. 2006) which assessed the effectiveness of consumer participation in different system-level roles indicates there is some evidence that medicine information materials developed with consumer involvement can increase knowledge and side-effect recognition, without increasing anxiety – they are generally effective. However, results were based on a single study and so are limited; and may not apply to consumer participation in other systems-level roles.

(Continued)

Meta-analyses	Number of studies/individuals	Effect sizes
	5 RCTs involving 1031 participants (Nilsen et al. 2006)	There is moderate quality evidence that involving consumers in the development of patient information material results in material that is more relevant, readable and understandable to patients, without affecting their anxiety. This "consumer-informed" material can also improve patients' knowledge.

Anxiety:

- small differences in the proportions of patients who were worried about becoming addicted (P = 0.68), about getting too much drug (P = 0.21), or about giving themselves too much drug (P = 0.26) with patient controlled analgesia (PCA).

- 80 and 90% of participants were not at all or only slightly worried in both groups for all three questions evaluating worries.

- measure of anxiety, ranging from "completely calm" to "terrified," for various aspects of endoscopic procedures. For anxiety level, there was a small, statistically significant difference in favor of the leaflet developed with consumers (P = 0.04).

Relevance, readability, understandability of information:

- more patients rated the information given in leaflets developed following consumer consultation as being very or extremely clear (84%), compared with patients who received leaflets which had no consumer consultation in their preparation (48%, P < 0.001).

- 30% of those who read the leaflet developed following consumer consultation required no more information about the "painkiller," compared with 8% of those who read the leaflet developed without consumer consultation (P = 0.002).

- patients were significantly more satisfied with leaflets developed following consumer consultation compared with leaflets developed without consumer consultation (P = 0.04).

Knowledge Improvement:

- 58% of those who read the leaflet developed following consumer consultation recognized that all the side effects listed could be caused by PCA, whereas none of those who read the leaflet developed without consumer consultation gave the correct answer (P < 0.001)

- 49 of those who read the leaflet developed following consumer consultation knew that morphine was used in PCA compared with seven of those who read the leaflet developed without consumer consultation (P < 0.001).

Meta-analyses	Number of studies/individuals	Effect sizes
Audit and feedback (professional intervention)	Rx for Change Database (2013)	A single high-quality review (Jamtvedt et al. 2006) showed that audit and feedback used alone or in combination with other interventions to be generally effective for improving appropriate care and prescribing outcomes.
	118 RCTs (Jamtvedt et al. 2006)	Thirty new studies were added to this update, and a total of 118 studies are included. In the primary analysis 88 comparisons from 72 studies were included that compared any intervention in which audit and feedback is a component compared to no intervention.
		For dichotomous outcomes the adjusted RD of compliance with desired practice varied from − 0.16 (a 16% absolute decrease in compliance) to 0.70 (a 70% increase in compliance) (median absolute improvement = 5%, IQR = 3% to 11%).
		For continuous outcomes the adjusted percent change relative to control varied from −0.10 (a 10% absolute decrease in compliance) to 0.68 (a 68% increase in compliance) (median = 0.16, IQR = 0.05 to 0.37).
		Low baseline compliance with recommended practice and higher intensity of audit and feedback were associated with larger adjusted risk ratios (greater effectiveness) across studies.
	Newer SR found 140 RCTs (Ivers et al. 2012)	A total of 108 comparisons from 70 studies compared any intervention in which audit and feedback was a core, essential component to usual care and evaluated effects on professional practice.
		After excluding studies at high risk of bias, there were 82 comparisons from 49 studies featuring dichotomous outcomes, and the weighted median adjusted RD was a 4.3% (IQR = 0.5–16%) absolute increase in healthcare professionals' compliance with desired practice.
		Across 26 comparisons from 21 studies with continuous outcomes, the weighted median adjusted percent change relative to control was 1.3% (IQR = 1.3–28.9%).
		For patient outcomes, the weighted median RD was −0.4% (IQR −1.3–1.6%) for 12 comparisons from six studies reporting dichotomous outcomes and the weighted median percentage change was 17% (IQR 1.5–17%) for eight comparisons from five studies reporting continuous outcomes.
		Multivariable meta-regression indicated that feedback may be more effective when baseline performance is low, the source is a supervisor or colleague, it is provided more than once, it is delivered in both verbal and written formats, and when it includes both explicit targets and an action plan. In addition, the effect size varied based on the clinical behavior targeted by the intervention.

(Continued)

Meta-analyses	Number of studies/ individuals	Effect sizes
Reminders (professional intervention)	Rx for Change Database (2013)	71 reviews evaluating the effectiveness of general reminders were identified. Of these, 5/5 high quality/key reviews (Shojania et al. 2009; French et al. 2010; Boyle et al. 2011; Laliberte et al. 2011; Arditi et al. 2012) with a sufficient number of studies to draw conclusions found this intervention to be generally effective.
	27 RCT, C-RCT (Arditi et al. 2012)	Computer-generated reminders delivered on paper (n = 37 comparisons) to healthcare professionals had a median improvement of 7.0% (IQR: 3.9–16.4%) in processes of care outcomes;
		Implementing reminders alone (n = 24 comparisons) improved care by 11.2% (IQR 6.5–19.6%) compared with usual care; and
		Implementing reminders in addition to another intervention (n = 13 comparisons) improved care by 4.0% (IQR 3.0–6.0%) compared with other intervention.
	11 studies – 3 RCTs and 8 N-RCTs (Boyle et al. 2011)	Documentation of tobacco status and increased referral to cessation counseling do appear to increase following the introduction of an expectation to use the electronic health record (EHR) to record and treat patient tobacco use at medical visits.
	28 studies – 22 RCTs, 6 N-RCTs (French et al. 2010)	Reminders were found to be generally effective for improving screening (n = 2) and test ordering (n = 2), but there was insufficient evidence to determine its effectiveness for improving procedures (adherence to guidelines).
		To improve the use of imaging in the management of osteoporosis, the effect of any type of intervention compared to no-intervention controls was modest (absolute improvement in bone mineral density [BMD] test ordering + 10%, IQR 0.0 to + 27.7). Patient mediated, reminder, and organizational interventions appeared to have most potential for improving imaging use in osteoporosis.
	13 studies (Laliberte et al. 2011)	The majority of studies were multifaceted and involved patient educational material, physician notification, and/ or physician education. Absolute differences in the incidence of BMD testing ranged from 22–51% for high-risk patients only and from 4–18% for both at-risk and high-risk patients.
		Absolute differences in the incidence of osteoporosis treatment initiation ranged from 18–9% for high-risk patients only and from 2–4% for at-risk and high-risk patients.
		Pooling the results of six trials showed an increased incidence of osteoporosis treatment initiation (RD = 20%; 95% CI: 7–33%) and of BMD testing and/or osteoporosis treatment initiation (RD = 40%; 95% CI: 32–48%) for high-risk patients following intervention.
		Multifaceted interventions targeting high-risk patients and their primary care providers may improve the management of osteoporosis, but improvements are often clinically modest.

Meta-analyses	Number of studies/individuals	Effect sizes
	28 RCTs (Shojania et al. 2009)	Median absolute improvement in adherence of 4.2% (IQR: 0.8% to 18.8%) across all reported process outcomes.
		Point of care computer reminders generally achieve small to modest improvements in provider behavior
		• 3.3% (IQR: 0.5–10.6%) for medication ordering
		• 3.8% (IQR: 0.5–6.6%) for vaccinations, and
		• 3.8% (IQR: 0.4–16.3%) for test ordering.
	Newer SR found	Tested the use of EHR reminders to improve clinicians' documentation or treatment of tobacco use.
	16 studies – 6 C-RCTs involving 98 clinics, 1 P-RCT, 9 observational studies (Boyle et al. 2014)	In 1 C-RCT involving 26 clinics – more intervention clinic than control clinic smokers quit (5.3% vs 1.9%, $p < 0.001$)
		Overall the studies showed modest improvements in some of the recommended clinician actions on tabaco use – documenting smoking status, giving advice to quit, assessing interest in quitting, and providing assistance including referral. Studies did not all assess the same outcomes. Non randomized and uncontrolled studies also showed positive effects
	Newer SR found	Median improvement 6.8% (IQR: 3.8–17.5%);
	30 RCTs and 5 N-RCTs (Arditi et al. 2017)	Computer-generated reminders delivered on paper to healthcare professionals, alone or in addition to co-intervention(s), probably improves quality of care slightly compared with usual care or the co-intervention(s) without the reminder component moderate-certainty evidence).
		Median improvement 11.0% (IQR 5.4–20.0%);
		Computer-generated reminders delivered on paper to healthcare professionals alone (single-component intervention) probably improves quality of care compared with usual care moderate-certainty evidence).
		Median improvement 4.0% (IQR 3.0–6.0%);
		Computer-generated reminders delivered on paper to healthcare professionals to one or more co-interventions (multi-component intervention) probably improves quality of care slightly compared with the co-intervention(s) without the reminder component
Patient mediated (professional intervention)	Rx for Change Database (2013)	16 reviews that evaluated the effectiveness of patient-mediated interventions were identified. Of these, 1/3 high quality/key reviews (Grimshaw et al. 2004) with a sufficient number of studies to draw conclusions found this intervention to be generally effective to improve appropriate care.

(Continued)

Meta-analyses	Number of studies/ individuals	Effect sizes
	6 studies – RCTs, C-RCTs (Grimshaw et al. 2004)	Patient-mediated interventions: new clinical information (not previously available) collected directly from patients and given to the provide (e.g. depression scores from an instrument).
		Patient-mediated interventions compared with no interventions (n = 6), were found to be effective for improving appropriate care with medium effect sizes. Overall median RD 9.5% (0.8–25.4%): medium effect size.
		All three C-RCT comparisons observed improvements in care; the median effect size was + 20.8% (range + 10.0 to + 25.4%) absolute improvement in performance (however, all three comparisons had potential unit of analysis errors). All three P-RCT comparisons reporting dichotomous process of care variables observed improvements in care. The median effect size was + 1.0% (range 0.8 to + 9.0%) absolute improvement in performance.
	New SR found 25 studies involving 12 268 patients (Fonhus et al. 2018)	*Patient-reported health information interventions,* probably improve professional practice by increasing healthcare professionals' adherence to recommended clinical practice (moderate-certainty evidence). For every 100 patients consulted or treated, 26 (95% CI 23 to 30) are in accordance with recommended clinical practice compared to 17 per 100 in the comparison group (no intervention or usual care).
		Patient information interventions, probably improve professional practice by increasing healthcare professionals' adherence to recommended clinical practice (moderate-certainty evidence). For every 100 patients consulted or treated, 32 (95% CI 24 to 42) are in accordance with recommended clinical practice compared to 20 per 100 in the comparison group (no intervention or usual care).
		Patient education interventions may also improve professional practice (low-certainty evidence). For every 100 patients consulted or treated, 46 (95% CI 39 to 54) are in accordance with recommended clinical practice compared to 35 per 100 in the comparison group (no intervention or usual care).
		Patient decision aid interventions may make little or no difference to the number of healthcare professionals' adhering to recommended clinical practice (low-certainty evidence). For every 100 patients consulted or treated, 32 (95% CI 24 to 43) are in accordance with recommended clinical practice compared to 37 per 100 in the comparison group (usual care).

Meta-analyses	Number of studies/ individuals	Effect sizes
Facilitating communication and decision making (consumer intervention)	**Rx for Change Database (2013)**	20 reviews – with strategies to improve communication skills and/or decision making were identified, 16 of high quality. While some individual strategies are promising, the evidence on strategies to promote communication and/ or decision making is mixed overall. Some example studies are summarized below
	86 RCTs involving 20 209 participants (Stacey et al. 2011)	Decision aids – 31 studies are new in this update. Decision aids improved knowledge and accuracy of risk perception; reduced the proportion of people who were passive in decision making; resulted in higher proportion of patients achieving decisions informed and consistent with their values; reduced the number of people remaining undecided; reduced decisional conflict; decreased the choice of major elective surgery in favor of conservative options.
		A) Criteria involving decision attributes
		Decision aids performed better than usual care interventions by increasing knowledge (MD 13.77 out of 100; 95% CI 11.40 to 16.15; n = 26).
		When more detailed decision aids were compared to simpler decision aids, the relative improvement in knowledge was significant (MD 4.97 out of 100; 95% CI 3.22 to 6.72; n = 15).
		Exposure to a decision aid with expressed probabilities resulted in a higher proportion of people with accurate risk perceptions (RR 1.74; 95% CI 1.46 to 2.08; n = 14).
		The effect was stronger when probabilities were expressed in numbers (RR 1.93; 95% CI 1.58 to 2.37; n = 11) rather than words (RR 1.27; 95% CI 1.09 to 1.48; n = 3).
		Exposure to a decision aid with explicit values clarification compared to those without explicit values clarification resulted in a higher proportion of patients achieving decisions that were informed and consistent with their values (RR 1.25; 95% CI 1.03 to 1.52; n = 8).
		B) Criteria involving decision process attributes:
		Decision aids compared to usual care interventions resulted in:
		a) lower decisional conflict related to feeling uninformed (MD −6.43 of 100; 95% CI -9.16 to −3.70; n = 17);
		b) lower decisional conflict related to feeling unclear about personal values (MD −4.81; 95% CI -7.23 to −2.40; n = 14);
		c) reduced the proportions of people who were passive in decision making (RR 0.61; 95% CI 0.49 to 0.77; n = 11); and
		d) reduced proportions of people who remained undecided post-intervention (RR 0.57; 95% CI 0.44 to 0.74; n = 9).

(Continued)

Meta-analyses	Number of studies/individuals	Effect sizes
		Decision aids appear to have a positive effect on patient-practitioner communication in the four studies that measured this outcome.
		For satisfaction with the decision (n = 12) and/or the decision-making process (n = 12), those exposed to a decision aid were either more satisfied or there was no difference between the decision aid versus comparison interventions.
		Secondary outcomes:
		Exposure to decision aids compared to usual care continued to demonstrate reduced choice of major elective invasive surgery in favor of conservative options (RR 0.80; 95% CI 0.64 to 1.00; n = 11).
		Exposure to decision aids compared to usual care also resulted in reduced choice of prostate-specific antigen (PSA) screening (RR 0.85; 95% CI 0.74 to 0.98; n = 7).
		When detailed compared to simple decision aids were used, there was reduced choice of menopausal hormones (RR 0.73; 95% CI 0.55 to 0.98; n = 3).
		The effect of decision aids on length of consultation varied from −8 minutes to +23 minutes (median 2.5 minutes).
	22 RCTs (Edwards et al. 2006)	Personalized risk communications – 22 RCTs (weak evidence), consistent with a small effect that personalized risk communication increases uptake of screening tests.
		Personalized risk communication (whether written, spoken or visually presented) increases uptake of screening tests (OR 1.31 (random effects, 95% CI 0.98 to 1.77).
		In three studies the interventions showed a trend toward more accurate risk perception (OR 1.65 (95% CI 0.96 to 2.81), and three other trials with heterogenous outcome measures showed improvements in knowledge with personalized risk interventions.
		More detailed personalized risk communication which used and presented numerical calculations of risk may be associated with a smaller increase in uptake of tests – OR for test uptake was 0.82 (95% CI 0.65 to 1.03).
		For risk estimates or calculations which were categorized into high, medium or low strata of risk, the OR was 1.42 (95% CI 1.07 to 1.89). For risk communication that simply listed personal risk factors the OR was 1.42 (95% CI 0.95 to 2.12).
		The five studies examining risk communication in high risk individuals (individuals at higher risk due to, for example, a family history of breast cancer or other conditions) showed larger ORs for uptake of tests than the other studies (random effects OR 1.74; 95% CI 1.05 to 2.88).

Meta-analyses	Number of studies/ individuals	Effect sizes
	33 RCTs involving 8244 participants (Kinnersley et al. 2007)	Communications before consultations – The most common interventions were question checklists and patient coaching delivered immediately before the consultations. They may increase patient participation in consultation and improve patient satisfaction.
		Meta-analyses, showed small and statistically significant increases for question asking (SMD 0.27 [95% CI 0.19 to 0.36]) and patient satisfaction (SMD 0.09 [95% CI 0.03 to 0.16]).
		There was a notable but not statistically significant decrease in patient anxiety before consultations (WMD −1.56 [95% CI -7.10 to 3.97]).
		There were small and not statistically significant changes in patient anxiety after consultations (reduced) (SMD −0.08 [95%CI -0.22 to 0.06]), patient knowledge (reduced) (SMD −0.34 [95% CI -0.94 to 0.25]), and consultation length (increased) (SMD 0.10 [95% CI -0.05 to 0.25]).
		Further analyses showed that both coaching and written materials produced similar effects on question asking but that coaching produced a smaller increase in consultation length and a larger increase in patient satisfaction.
		Interventions immediately before consultations led to a small and statistically significant increase in consultation length, whereas those implemented some time before the consultation had no effect.
	Updated SR 105 RCTs involving 31 043 participants (Stacey et al. 2017)	Decision aids – This update added 18 studies and removed 28 previously included studies comparing detailed versus simple decision aids.
		Compared to usual care across a wide variety of decision contexts, people exposed to decision aids feel more knowledgeable, better informed, and clearer about their values, and they probably have a more active role in decision making and more accurate risk perceptions.
		New for this update is evidence indicating improved knowledge and accurate risk perceptions when decision aids are used either within or in preparation for the consultation.
		Attributes of the choice made
		Decision aids compared to usual care increased participants':
		• knowledge (MD 13.27/100; 95% CI 11.32 to 15.23; 52 studies; N = 13 316; high-quality evidence),
		• accuracy of risk perceptions (RR 2.10; 95% CI 1.66 to 2.66; 17 studies; N = 5096; moderate-quality evidence), and
		• congruency between informed values and care choices (RR 2.06; 95% CI 1.46 to 2.91; 10 studies; N = 4626; low-quality evidence)
		Attributes related to the decision-making process
		Decision aids compared to usual care decreased:
		• decisional conflict related to feeling uninformed (MD − 9.28/100; 95% CI −12.20 to −6.36; 27 studies; N = 5707; high-quality evidence),

(Continued)

Meta-analyses	Number of studies/ individuals	Effect sizes
		• indecision about personal values (MD −8.81/100; 95% CI −11.99 to −5.63; 23 studies; N = 5068; high-quality evidence), and
		• the proportion of people who were passive in decision making (RR 0.68; 95% CI 0.55 to 0.83; 16 studies; N = 3180; moderate-quality evidence).
		Decision aids compared to usual care also reduced the number of people choosing major elective invasive surgery in favor of more conservative options (RR 0.86; 95% CI 0.75 to 1.00; 18 studies; N = 3844), but this reduction reached statistical significance only after removing the study on prophylactic mastectomy for breast cancer gene carriers (RR 0.84; 95% CI 0.73 to 0.97; 17 studies; N = 3108).
		Compared to usual care, decision aids reduced the number of people choosing prostate-specific antigen screening (RR 0.88; 95% CI 0.80 to 0.98; 10 studies; N = 3996) and increased those choosing to start new medications for diabetes (RR 1.65; 95% CI 1.06 to 2.56; 4 studies; N = 447).
		The median effect of decision aids on length of consultation was 2.6 minutes longer (24 versus 21; 7.5% increase).
		The costs of the decision aid group were lower in two studies and similar to usual care in four studies.
		People receiving decision aids do not appear to differ from those receiving usual care in terms of anxiety, general health outcomes, and condition-specific health outcomes.
	Updated SR 41 studies involving 28 700 people (Edwards et al. 2013)	Personalized risk communication – 19 new studies were identified in this update, adding to the 22 studies included in the previous two iterations of the review.
		There is strong evidence from three trials that personalized risk estimates incorporated within communication interventions for screening programs enhance informed choices.
		Overall 45.2% (592/1309) of participants who received personalized risk information made informed choices, compared to 20.2% (229/1135) of participants who received generic risk information.
		The overall ORs for informed decision were 4.48 (95% CI 3.62 to 5.53 for fixed effect) and 3.65 (95% CI 2.13 to 6.23 for random effects).
		Our results (OR 1.15 [95% CI 1.02 to 1.29]) constitute low quality evidence, consistent with a small effect, that personalized risk communication in which a risk score was provided (6 studies) or the participants were given their categorized risk (6 studies), increases uptake of screening tests.

Meta-analyses	Number of studies/ individuals	Effect sizes
	65 RCTs involving 9021 patients (Kinnersley et al. 2013)	Studies used written materials, audio-visual materials and decision aids. Some interventions were delivered before admission to hospital for the procedure while others were delivered on admission.
		Outcomes – individual components of informed consent such as knowledge, anxiety, and satisfaction with the consent process. Important but less commonly-measured outcomes were deliberation, decisional conflict, uptake of procedures and length of consultation.
		Meta-analyses showed statistically-significant improvements in:
		• Knowledge when measured immediately after interventions (SMD 0.53 [95% CI 0.37 to 0.69] I^2 73%), shortly afterwards (between 24 hours and 14 days) (SMD 0.68 [95% CI 0.42 to 0.93] I^2 85%) and at a later date (15 days or more) (SMD 0.78 [95% CI 0.50 to 1.06] I^2 82%).
		• Satisfaction with decision making was also increased (SMD 2.25 [95% CI 1.36 to 3.15] I^2 99%) and
		• Decisional conflict was reduced (SMD −1.80 [95% CI -3.46 to −0.14] I^2 99%).
		• No statistically-significant differences were found for generalized anxiety (SMD −0.11 [95% CI -0.35 to 0.13] I^2 82%), anxiety with the consent process (SMD 0.01 [95% CI -0.21 to 0.23] I^2 70%) and satisfaction with the consent process (SMD 0.12 [95% CI -0.09 to 0.32] I^2 76%).
		• Consultation length was increased in those studies with continuous data (mean increase 1.66 minutes [95% CI 0.82 to 2.50] I^2 0%) and in the one study with non-parametric data (control 8.0 minutes versus intervention 11.9 minutes, IQR of 4–11.9 and 7.2–5.0 respectively).
		In general, sensitivity analyses removing studies at high risk of bias made little difference to the overall results.
Tailored interventions (Professional intervention)	**Rx for Change Database (2013)**	2 reviews that evaluated the effectiveness of tailored interventions were identified. Of these, 2/2 high quality/ key reviews (Cheater et al. 2005; Baker et al. 2010), with a sufficient number of studies to draw conclusions found this intervention to be generally effective for improving appropriate care and prescribing outcomes.
	26 RCTs (Baker et al. 2010)	Studies comparing an intervention tailored to address identified barriers to change to no intervention or an intervention(s) not tailored to the barriers were included.
		Twelve studies provided enough data to be included in the quantitative analysis. A meta-regression model was fitted adjusting for baseline odds by fitting it as a covariate, to obtain the pooled OR of 1.54 (95% CI, 1.16 to 2.01) from Bayesian analysis and 1.52 (95% CI, 1.27 to 1.82, P < 0.001) from classical analysis.
		The heterogeneity analyses found that no study attributes investigated were significantly associated with effectiveness of the interventions.

(Continued)

Meta-analyses	Number of studies/individuals	Effect sizes
	15 RCTs (Cheater et al. 2005)	Compared an intervention tailored to address identified barriers to change compared to no intervention or an intervention(s) not tailored to the barriers.
		A meta-regression of a subset of the included studies, using a classical approach estimated a combined OR of 2.18 (95% CI: 1.09, 4.34), p = 0.026 in favor of tailored interventions. However, when a Bayesian approach was taken, meta-regression gave a combined OR of 2.27 (95% Credible Interval: 0.92, 4.75), which was not statistically significant.
		Interventions tailored to prospectively identify barriers may improve care and patient outcomes. However, from the studies included in this review, it wasn't possible to determine whether the barriers were valid, which were the most important barriers, whether all barriers were identified and if they had been addressed by the intervention chosen. Based on the evidence presented in this review, the effectiveness of tailored interventions remains uncertain and more rigorous trials (including process evaluations) are needed.
	Updated SR 32 RCTs (15 studies included in the meta-analysis) (Baker et al. 2015)	Nine studies were added to this review to bring the total number of included studies to 32 comparing an intervention tailored to address identified determinants of practice to no intervention or an intervention(s) not tailored to the determinants.
		Meta-regression using 15 randomized trials – the pooled OR was 1.56 (95% CI, 1.27–1.93, $p < 0.001$).
		Tailored interventions can change professional practice, although they are not always effective and, when they are, the effect is small to moderate.
Multifaceted interventions (Professional intervention)	**Rx for Change Database (2013)**	134 reviews that evaluated the effectiveness of multiple interventions were identified. Of these, 8/16 high quality/key reviews (Pirkis et al. 1998; Lewin et al. 2001; Davey et al. 2005; Jamtvedt et al. 2006; O'Brien et al. 2007; Smith et al. 2007; French et al. 2010; Baskerville et al. 2012) with a sufficient number of studies to draw conclusions found this intervention to be generally effective.
	23 RCTs involving 1398 practices (Baskerville et al. 2012)	Intervention(s): Outreach, Practice facilitation, Audit and feedback, Educational materials and guidelines, Reminders, Practice consensus building, Goal setting, Meetings, Quality circles, Learning collaboratives.
		An overall effect size of 0.56 (95% CI, 0.43–0.68) favored practice facilitation (z = 8.76; P < 0.001), and publication bias was evident.
		Primary care practices are 2.76 (95% CI, 2.18–3.43) times more likely to adopt evidence-based guidelines through practice facilitation.
		Meta-regression analysis indicated that tailoring (P = 0.05), the intensity of the intervention (P = 0.03), and the number of intervention practices per facilitator (P = 0.004) modified evidence-based guideline adoption.

Meta-analyses	Number of studies/individuals	Effect sizes
	66 RCT, CCT, CBA and ITS studies (Davey et al. 2005)	Intervention(s): Organizational (provider) – other, Educational outreach visits, Formulary, Professional – other, Revision of professional roles – pharmacy, Reminders – general, Distribution of educational materials, Audit and feedback, Multifaceted.
		To estimate the effectiveness of professional interventions that alone, or in combination, are effective in promoting prudent antibiotic prescribing to hospital inpatients.
		Of the six interventions that aimed to increase treatment, five reported a significant improvement in drug outcomes and one a significant improvement in clinical outcome. Of the 60 interventions that aimed to decrease treatment 47 reported drug outcomes of which 38 (81%) significantly improved, 16 reported microbiological outcomes of which 12 (75%) significantly improved and nine reported clinical outcomes of which two (22%) significantly deteriorated and 3 (33%) significantly improved. Due to differences in study design and duration of follow up it was only possible to perform meta-regression on a few studies.
	28 RCT, CT, ITS studies (French et al. 2010)	Intervention(s): Patient mediated, reminder, and organizational interventions
		The effect of any type of intervention to improve the use of imaging in the management of osteoporosis compared to no-intervention controls was modest (absolute improvement in bone mineral density test ordering +10%, IQR 0.0 to +27.7).
		For low back pain studies, the most common intervention evaluated was distribution of educational materials and this showed varying effects. Other interventions in low back pain studies also showed variable effects. For other musculoskeletal conditions, distribution of educational materials, educational meetings and audit and feedback were not shown to be effective for changing imaging ordering behavior. Across all conditions, increasing the number of intervention components did not increase effect.
	118 RCTs (Jamtvedt et al. 2006)	Intervention(s): Audit and feedback, educational meetings, multifaceted
		Thirty new studies were added to this update. In the primary analysis 88 comparisons from 72 studies were included that compared any intervention in which audit and feedback is a component compared to no intervention.
		For dichotomous outcomes the adjusted RD of compliance with desired practice varied from – 0.16 (a 16% absolute decrease in compliance) to 0.70 (a 70% increase in compliance) (median absolute improvement = 5%, IQR = 3% to 11%).
		For continuous outcomes the adjusted percent change relative to control varied from −0.10 (a 10% absolute decrease in compliance) to 0.68 (a 68% increase in compliance) (median = 0.16, IQR = 0.05 to 0.37).
		Low baseline compliance with recommended practice and higher intensity of audit and feedback were associated with larger adjusted risk ratios (greater effectiveness) across studies.

(Continued)

Meta-analyses	Number of studies/ individuals	Effect sizes
	17 RCT, CT, CBA studies (Lewin et al. 2001)	Intervention(s): Multifaceted, Educational meetings, Distribution of educational materials.
		Of the included studies, 11 were RCT's. Multifaceted educational interventions (n = 6) were found to be generally ineffective with a number of the studies reporting mixed results for appropriate care.
	69 RCTs involving more than 15 000 health care providers (O'Brien et al. 2007)	Intervention(s): Multifaceted, Educational outreach visits, Distribution of educational materials, Educational meetings, Reminders – general.
		The median adjusted RD in compliance with desired practice was 5.6% (IQR = 3.0–9.0%).
		The adjusted RDs were highly consistent for prescribing (median 4.8%, IQR = 3.0–6.5% for 17 comparisons), but varied for other types of professional performance (median 6.0%, IQR = 3.6%–16.0% for 17 comparisons).
		Multifaceted interventions (that include educational outreach and distribution of educational materials) compared to a control group, multifaceted interventions (including educational outreach) compared to distribution of educational materials and educational outreach visits alone compared to a control group were all effective for improving appropriate care outcomes.
		Educational outreach visits with or without the addition of other interventions can be effective in improving practice in the majority of circumstances, but found the effect to be small to moderate. The effects on prescribing are small and consistent (median 4.8%, IQR = 3.0–6.5%) whereas the effect on other professional behaviors is more variable (median adjusted RD 6%, IQR = 3.6–16%).
	20 RCT, CBA studies (Smith et al. 2007)	Intervention(s): Multifaceted, Clinical multidisciplinary teams, Educational meetings, Continuity of care.
		The majority of studies examined complex multifaceted interventions and were of relatively short duration. The results were mixed. Overall there were no consistent improvements in physical or mental health outcomes, psychosocial outcomes, psychosocial measures including measures of disability and functioning, hospital admissions, default or participation rates, recording of risk factors and satisfaction with treatment. However, there were clear improvements in prescribing in the studies that considered this outcome.
	10 RCTs (Pirkis et al. 1998)	Intervention(s): Reminders – general, Multifaceted (General practitioner [GP] and patient directed reminders)
		Based on meta-analysis in seven studies where women whose GPs had been prompted to remind them to have a Pap test were significantly more likely to do so than were control women (TRD 6.6%, 95% CI 5.2%–8.0%).
		Sensitivity analysis revealed that a single study stood out as an exceptional result. When this study was omitted, the remaining studies were homogeneous, with a RD of 7.9% (95% CI 6.5%–9.4%).

Meta-analyses	Number of studies/ individuals	Effect sizes
	Updated SR 89 RCT, C-RCT, CCT, CBA and ITS studies included (Davey et al. 2013)	Interventions to reduce excessive antibiotic prescribing to hospital inpatients can reduce antimicrobial resistance or hospital-acquired infections, and interventions to increase effective prescribing can improve clinical outcome
		For the persuasive interventions, the median change in antibiotic prescribing was 42.3% for the ITSs, 31.6% for the controlled ITSs, 17.7% for the CBAs, 3.5% for the C-RCTs and 24.7% for the RCTs.
		The restrictive interventions had a median effect size of 34.7% for the ITSs, 17.1% for the CBAs and 40.5% for the RCTs.
		The structural interventions had a median effect of 13.3% for the RCTs and 23.6% for the C-RCTs.
		Meta-analysis of 52 ITS studies was used to compare restrictive versus purely persuasive interventions. Restrictive interventions had significantly greater impact on prescribing outcomes at 1 month (32%, 95% CI 2% to 61%, $P = 0.03$) and on microbial outcomes at 6 months (53%, 95% CI 31% to 75%, $P = 0.001$) but there were no significant differences at 12 or 24 months.
		Meta-analysis of clinical outcomes showed that four interventions intended to increase effective prescribing for pneumonia were associated with significant reduction in mortality (RR 0.89, 95% CI 0.82 to 0.97), whereas nine interventions intended to decrease excessive prescribing were not associated with significant increase in mortality (RR 0.92, 95% CI 0.81 to 1.06)
	Updated SR (Lewin et al. 2001) 43 RCTs (Dwamena et al. 2012)	29 RCTs are new in this update.
		Descriptive and pooled analyses showed generally positive effects on consultation processes on a range of measures relating to clarifying patients' concerns and beliefs; communicating about treatment options; levels of empathy; and patients' perception of providers' attentiveness to them and their concerns as well as their diseases. A new finding for this update is that short-term training (less than 10 hours) is as successful as longer training.
		The analyses showed mixed results on satisfaction, behavior and health status. Studies using complex interventions that focused on providers and patients with condition-specific materials generally showed benefit in health behavior and satisfaction, as well as consultation processes, with mixed effects on health status.
		Pooled analysis of the fewer than half of included studies with adequate data suggests moderate beneficial effects from interventions on the consultation process; and mixed effects on behavior and patient satisfaction, with small positive effects on health status.

(Continued)

Meta-analyses	Number of studies/ Individuals	Effect sizes
	Updated SR 42 RCTs, NRCTs, CBA and ITS studies involving 18 859 participants (Smith et al. 2017)	41 studies examined complex multi-faceted interventions and lasted from six to 24 months.
		Results showed probably few or no differences in clinical outcomes overall with a tendency toward improved blood pressure management in the small number of studies on shared care for hypertension, chronic kidney disease and stroke (MD 3.47, 95% CI 1.68 to 5.25) (based on moderate-certainty evidence).
		Mental health outcomes improved, particularly in response to depression treatment (RR 1.40, 95% CI 1.22 to 1.62; six studies, N = 1708) and recovery from depression (RR 2.59, 95% CI 1.57 to 4.26; 10 studies, N = 4482) in studies examining the "stepped care" design of shared care interventions (based on high-certainty evidence).
		Investigators noted modest effects on mean depression scores (SMD −0.29, 95% CI -0.37 to −0.20; six studies, N = 3250). Differences in patient-reported outcome measures (PROMs), processes of care and participation and default rates in shared care services were probably limited (based on moderate-certainty evidence). Studies probably showed little or no difference in hospital admissions, service utilization and patient health behaviors (with evidence of moderate certainty).

Abbreviations: C-RCTs = cluster randomized control trial; CBA = controlled before and after (study); CCT = controlled clinical trial; CI = confidence interval; IQR = interquartile range; ITS = interrupted time series (study); MD = mean difference; N-RCT = non-randomized controlled trial; OR = odds ratio; P-RCT = patient randomized control trial; RCT = randomized control trial; RD = risk difference; RR = risk ratio; SD = standard deviation; SMD = standardized mean difference; SR = systematic review; TRD = typical risk difference; =WMD = weighted mean difference.

Source: Summary of effectiveness of disseminating strategies is based on:
- Rx for Change Database (last update 2013): Canadian Agency for Drugs and Technologies in Health (2013) Rx for Change, (Online), Available: https://www.cadth.ca/rx-change (May 20, 2020);
- Grimshaw et al. (2012); and
- Updated Cochrane Systematic Reviews.

Appendix 10.E: Behaviour Change Techniques and Labels Identified in Three Stages: (a) Reviews; (b) Brainstorming; (c) Textbook Consultation[1]

Reprinted with permission from Michie, S., Johnston, M., Francis, J., Hardeman, W. & Eccles, M. (2008) From Theory to Intervention: Mapping Theoretically Derived Behavioural Determinants to Behaviour Change Techniques. Applied Psychology 57, 660-680. © 2008 The Authors. Journal compilation © 2008 International Association of Applied Psychology. Published by Blackwell Publishing, 9600 Garsington Road, Oxford OX4 2DQ, UK and 350 Main Street, Malden, MA 02148, USA.

Stage	Technique number	Technique label and definition
(a) Review identified techniques	1.	**Goal**: set behavioural goal
	2.	**Standard**: decide target standard of behaviour (specified and observable)
	3.	**Monitoring**: record specified behaviour (person has access to recorded data of behavioural performance e.g. from diary)
	4.	**Record antecedents and consequences of behaviour** (social and environmental situations and events, emotions, cognitions)
	5.	**Feedback**: of monitored (inc. self-monitored) behaviour
	6.	**Comparison**: provide comparative data (cf. standard, person's own past behaviour, others' behaviour)
	7.	**Social comparison**: provide opportunities for social comparison e.g. contests and group learning
	8.	**Discrepancy assessment**: highlight nature of discrepancy (direction, amount) between standard, own or others' behaviour (goes beyond simple self-monitoring)
	9.	**Contract**: of agreed performance of target behaviour with at least one other, written and signed
	10.	**Planning**: identify component parts of behaviour and make plan to execute each one *or* consider when and/or where a behaviour will be performed, i.e. schedule behaviours (not including coping planning—see 11)
	11.	**Coping planning**: identify and plan ways of overcoming barriers (note, this must include identification of specific barriers e.g. "problem-solving how to fit into weekly schedule" would not count)
	12.	**Goal review**: assess extent to which the goal/target behaviour is achieved, identify the factors influencing this and amend goal if appropriate
	13.	**Discriminative (learned) cue**: environmental stimulus that has been repeatedly associated with contingent reward for specified behaviour

(Continued)

Stage	Technique number	Technique label and definition
	14.	**Prompt**: stimulus that elicits behaviour (inc. telephone calls or postal reminders designed to prompt the behaviour)
	15.	**Reward**: contingent valued consequence, i.e. if and only if behaviour is performed (inc. social approval, exc. general non-contingent encouragement or approval)
	16.	**Punishment**: contingent aversive consequence, i.e. if and only if behaviour is not performed
	17.	**Omission**: contingent removal of valued consequence, i.e. if and only if behaviour is not performed
	18.	**Negative reinforcement**: contingent removal of aversive consequence, i.e. if and only if behaviour is performed
	19	**Threat**: offer future punishment or removal of reward contingent on performance
	20.	**Fear arousal**: induce aversive emotional state associated with the behaviour
	21.	**Anticipated regret**: induce expectations of future regret about non-performance of behaviour
	22.	**Graded tasks**: set easy tasks to perform, making them increasingly difficult until target behaviour performed
	23.	**Instruction**: teach new behaviour required for performance of target behaviour (not as part of graded hierarchy or as part of modelling) e.g. give clear instructions
	24.	**Shaping**: build up behaviour by initially reinforcing behaviour closest to required behaviour and systematically altering behaviour required to achieve contingent reinforcement
	25.	**Chaining**: build up behaviour by starting with final component; gradually add components earlier in sequence
	26.	**Behavioural rehearsal**: perform behaviour (repeatedly)
	27.	**Mental rehearsal**: imagine performing the behaviour repeatedly
	28.	**Habit formation**: perform same behaviour in same context
	29.	**Role play**: perform behaviour in simulated situation
	30.	**Behavioural experiments**: testing hypotheses about the behaviour, its causes and consequences, by collecting and interpreting data
	31.	**Modelling**: observe the behaviour of others
	32.	**Vicarious reinforcement**: observe the consequences of others' behaviour
	33.	**Self talk**: planned self-statements (aloud or silent) to implement behaviour change techniques
	34.	**Imagery**: use planned images (visual, motor, sensory) to implement behaviour change techniques (inc. mental rehearsal)
	35.	**Cognitive restructuring**: changing cognitions about causes and consequences of behaviour

Stage	Technique number	Technique label and definition
(b) Brain-stormed techniques	36.	**Relapse prevention**: identify situations that increase the likelihood of the behaviour not being performed and apply coping strategies to those situations
	37.	**Behavioural information**: provide information about antecedents or consequences of the behaviour, or connections between them, or behaviour change techniques
	38.	**Personalised message**: tailor techniques or messages from others to individual's resources and context (includes stages of change-based information; does not include personal plans and feedback)
	39.	**Verbal persuasion/persuasive communication**: credible source presents arguments in favour of the behaviour. Note, there must be evidence of presentation of arguments; general pro-behaviour communication does not count.
	40.	**Social support (instrumental)**: others perform component tasks of behaviour or tasks that would compete with behaviour e.g. offering childcare
	41.	**Social support (emotional)**: others listen, provide empathy and give generalised positive feedback
	42.	**Decision-making**: generate alternative courses of action, and pros and cons of each, and weigh them up
	43.	**Coping strategies**: behaviours undertaken to avoid or reduce stressors
	44.	**Stress management**: behaviours undertaken to reduce stressors or impact of stressors
	45.	**Relaxation**: systematic instruction in physical and cognitive strategies to reduce sympathetic arousal, and to increase muscle relaxation and a feeling of calm
(c) Textbook identified techniques	46.	**Desensitisation**: exposure to threatening experiences
	47.	**Systematic desensitisation**: graded exposure to increasingly threatening experiences
	48.	**Time management**: action planning applied to the perceived problem of shortage of time
	49.	**Motivational interviewing**: elicit self-motivating statements and evaluation of own behaviour to reduce resistance to change
	50.	**Environmental change**: change the environment in order to facilitate the target behaviour (other than prompts, rewards, and punishments e.g. choice of food provided)
	51.	**Set homework tasks**
	52.	**Non-specific social support** (only if additional to 40 and 41)
	53.	**General information** about the behaviour and behaviour change (other than 37)
	54.	**General problem-solving**

[1] This Appendix presents work in progress. Further work is needed to agree the final definitions for the techniques.

Stage	Technique number	Technique label	Technique number	Technique label
	55.	Anti-depression skills training	86.	Token economy
	56.	Biofeedback	87.	Activity scheduling
	57.	Differential reinforcement	88.	Adventitious reinforcement/ superstitious conditioning
	58.	Escape	89.	Altering antecedent chains
	59.	Extinction	90.	Anger control training
	60.	Flooding	91.	Assertion training
	61.	Group contingencies	92.	Buddy system
	62.	Implosive therapy	93.	Clarification (supportive therapy)
	63.	Avoidance	94.	Classical conditioning
	64.	Counter-conditioning	95.	Community reinforcement
	65.	Distraction	96.	Covert conditioning
	66.	Exposure	97.	Covert sensitisation
	67.	Fading; thinning	98.	Deflection techniques
	68.	Flooding in imagination	99.	Discrimination training
	69.	Habit reversal	100.	Emetic therapy
	70.	Negative punishment	101.	Encounter (existential analysis)
	71.	Non-contingent delivery of reinforcing stimuli	102.	Fishbowl
	72.	Overcorrection	103.	Fogging
	73.	Peer-administered contingencies	104.	Functional communication training
	74.	Problem identification	105.	Functional family therapy
	75.	Rational emotive therapy	106.	Identification (psychoanalysis)
	76.	Reinforcer sampling	107.	Instigation
	77.	Response cost	108.	Interpretation (psychoanalysis)
	78.	Response priming	109.	Least-to-most prompting
	79.	Satiation	110.	Lottery
	80.	Screening	111.	Most to least prompt sequences
	81.	Social skills training	112.	Motivational techniques
	82.	Stress inoculation program	113.	Multiple exemplar training (generalisation)
	83.	Symbolic desensitisation	114.	Natural maintaining contingencies (generalisation)
	84.	Thought stopping	115.	Negotiation training
	85.	Time out	116.	Paradoxical instructions

Stage	Technique number	Technique label	Technique number	Technique label
	117.	Paradoxical intention (behaviour therapy)	128.	Rule release
	118.	Positive reinforcement	129.	Self-exploration
	119.	Positive scanning	130.	Self-help
	120.	Premackian reinforcers	131.	Small group exercises
	121.	Rate reduction	132.	Stimulus generalisation
	122.	Reassurance (supportive therapy)	133.	Stimulus narrowing
	123.	Recapitulation	134.	Systematic rational conditioning
	124.	Reframing	135.	Thinning
	125.	Reinforcer displacement	136.	Turtle technique
	126.	Response priming	137.	Vicarious punishment
	127.	Restitution		

Appendix 10.F: TIDieR Checklist

Reprinted with permission from Hoffmann, T. C., Glasziou, P. P., Boutron, I., Milne, R., Perera, R., Moher, D., Altman, D. G., Barbour, V., Macdonald, H., Johnston, M., Lamb, S. E., Dixon-Woods, M., McCulloch, P., Wyatt, J. C., Chan, A. W. & Michie, S. (2014) Better reporting of interventions: template for intervention description and replication (TIDieR) checklist and guide. BMJ 348, g1687. © Georg Thieme Verlag KG

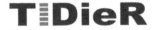

Template for Intervention Description and Replication

The TIDieR (Template for Intervention Description and Replication) Checklist[*]

Information to include when describing an intervention and the location of the information

Item number	Item	Where located[**] Primary paper (page or appendix number)	Other[†] (details)
	BRIEF NAME		
1.	Provide the name or a phrase that describes the intervention.	_____	_____
	WHY		
2.	Describe any rationale, theory, or goal of the elements essential to the intervention.	_____	_____
	WHAT		
3.	Materials: Describe any physical or informational materials used in the intervention, including those provided to participants or used in intervention delivery or in training of intervention providers. Provide information on where the materials can be accessed (e.g. online appendix, URL).	_____	_____
4.	Procedures: Describe each of the procedures, activities, and/or processes used in the intervention, including any enabling or support activities.	_____	_____
	WHO PROVIDED		
5.	For each category of intervention provider (e.g. psychologist, nursing assistant), describe their expertise, background and any specific training given.	_____	_____
	HOW		
6.	Describe the modes of delivery (e.g. face-to-face or by some other mechanism, such as internet or telephone) of the intervention and whether it was provided individually or in a group.	_____	_____
	WHERE		
7.	Describe the type(s) of location(s) where the intervention occurred, including any necessary infrastructure or relevant features.	_____	_____

Item number	Item	Where located**	
		Primary paper (page or appendix number)	Other† (details)
	WHEN and HOW MUCH		
8.	Describe the number of times the intervention was delivered and over what period of time including the number of sessions, their schedule, and their duration, intensity or dose.	_____	_____
	TAILORING		
9.	If the intervention was planned to be personalised, titrated or adapted, then describe what, why, when, and how.	_____	_____
	MODIFICATIONS		
10.‡	If the intervention was modified during the course of the study, describe the changes (what, why, when, and how).	_____	_____
	HOW WELL		
11.	Planned: If intervention adherence or fidelity was assessed, describe how and by whom, and if any strategies were used to maintain or improve fidelity, describe them.	_____	_____
12.‡	Actual: If intervention adherence or fidelity was assessed, describe the extent to which the intervention was delivered as planned.	_____	_____

** **Authors** – use N/A if an item is not applicable for the intervention being described. **Reviewers** – use '?' if information about the element is not reported/not sufficiently reported.

† If the information is not provided in the primary paper, give details of where this information is available. This may include locations such as a published protocol or other published papers (provide citation details) or a website (provide the URL).

‡ If completing the TIDieR checklist for a protocol, these items are not relevant to the protocol and cannot be described until the study is complete.

* We strongly recommend using this checklist in conjunction with the TIDieR guide (see *BMJ* 2014;348:g1687) which contains an explanation and elaboration for each item.

* The focus of TIDieR is on reporting details of the intervention elements (and where relevant, comparison elements) of a study. Other elements and methodological features of studies are covered by other reporting statements and checklists and have not been duplicated as part of the TIDieR checklist. When a **randomized trial** is being reported, the TIDieR checklist should be used in conjunction with the CONSORT statement (see www.consort-statement.org) as an extension of **Item 5 of the CONSORT 2010 Statement.** When a **clinical trial protocol** is being reported, the TIDieR checklist should be used in conjunction with the SPIRIT statement as an extension of **Item 11 of the SPIRIT 2013 Statement** (see www.spirit-statement.org). For alternate study designs, TIDieR can be used in conjunction with the appropriate checklist for that study design (see www.equator-network.org).

Appendix 10.G: WIDER recommendations to improve reporting of the content of behavior change interventions

Reprinted by permission from Springer Nature: Implementation Science from Albrecht, L., Archibald, M., Arseneau, D. & Scott, S. D. (2013) Development of a checklist to assess the quality of reporting of knowledge translation interventions using the Workgroup for Intervention Development and Evaluation Research (WIDER) recommendations. Implementation Science 8, 52. © 2013 Albrecht et al.; licensee BioMed Central Ltd.

WIDER recommendations	Supplementary recommendations
Detailed description of interventions in published papers	1) Characteristics of those delivering the intervention
	2) Characteristics of the recipients
	3) The setting
	4) The mode of delivery
	5) The intensity
	6) The duration
	7) Adherence/fidelity to delivery protocols
	8) Detailed description of the intervention content provided for each study group
Clarification of assumed change process and design principles	1) The intervention development
	2) The change techniques used in the intervention
	3) The causal processes targeted by these change techniques
Access to intervention manuals/protocols,	Submit protocols or manuals for publication to make these supplementary materials easily accessible (i.e., online).
Detailed description of active control conditions	1) Characteristics of those delivering the control
	2) Characteristics of the recipients
	3) The setting
	4) The mode of delivery
	5) The intensity
	6) The duration
	7) Adherence/fidelity to delivery protocols
	8) Detailed description of the control content provided

Appendix 10.H: The AIMD Framework

Source: Bragge, P., Grimshaw, J. M., Lokker, C., Colquhoun, H. & Aimd Writing/Working Group (2017) AIMD – a validated, simplified framework of interventions to promote and integrate evidence into health practices, systems, and policies. BMC Medical Research Methodology 17, 38. https://bmcmedresmethodol.biomedcentral.com/articles/10.1186/s12874-017-0314-8. Licensed under CC BY 4.0.

Component	Description	Definition and considerations
Aims	What do you want your intervention to achieve and for whom?	This component relates to the objective and outcome of the intervention. Based on your endpoint, what are you measuring in whom? It could include consideration of proximal and intermediate outcomes, and process outcomes related to implementation.
Ingredients	What comprises the intervention?	These are the observable, replicable, and irreducible aspects of the intervention. To increase the detail specified, other taxonomies could be used in conjunction with the AIMD framework. This might include intervention taxonomies or reporting guidance.
Mechanism	How do you propose the intervention will work?	This refers to the pathways or processes by which it is proposed that an intervention effects change or which change comes into effect. As with ingredients, other taxonomies could be used in conjunction with AIMD to add detail. The proposed mechanism could be based on either theory or empirical evidence, and be made specific to the setting. The use of mechanism may change depending on if the framework is used for reporting or designing: why was the ingredient selected (design) and what is the pathway in which it worked (reporting).
Delivery	How will you deliver the intervention?	This encompasses logistical and practical information pertaining to intervention delivery, including mode (e.g. video, brochure); level (e.g. individual, team, population); dose, frequency, intensity; who's delivering; and size of target group.

References

Albrecht, L., Archibald, M., Arseneau, D., and Scott, S.D. (2013). Development of a checklist to assess the quality of reporting of knowledge translation interventions using the Workgroup for Intervention Development and Evaluation Research (WIDER) recommendations. *Implementation Science* 8: 52. https://doi.org/10.1186/1748-5908-8-52.

Arditi, C., Rege-Walther, M., Wyatt, J.C. et al. (2012). Computer-generated reminders delivered on paper to healthcare professionals; effects on professional practice and health care outcomes. *Cochrane Database of Systematic Reviews* (12): CD001175. https://doi.org/10.1002/14651858.CD001175.pub3.

Arditi, C., Rege-Wlther, M., Durieux, P., and Burnand, B. (2017). Computer-generated reminders delivered on paper to healthcare professionals: effects on professional practice and healthcare outcomes. *Cochrane Database of Systematic Reviews* Version published: 06 July 2017 (7): CD001175. https://doi.org/10.1002/14651858.CD001175.pub4.

Baker, R., Camosso-Stefinovic, J., Gillies, C. et al. (2010). Tailored interventions to overcome identified barriers to change: effects on professional practice and health care outcomes. *Cochrane Database of Systematic Reviews* (3): CD005470. https://doi.org/10.1002/14651858.CD005470.pub2, https://www.ncbi.nlm.nih.gov/pmc/articles/PMC4164371/.

Baker, R., Camosso-Stefinovic, J., Gillies, C. et al. (2015). Tailored interventions to address identified determinants of practice. *Cochrane Database of Systematic Reviews* (4): CD005470. https://doi.org/10.1002/14651858.CD005470.pub3.

Bartholomew, L.K., Parcel, G.S., Kok, G., and Gottlieb, N.H. (2001). *Intervention Mapping: Designing Theory- and Evidence-Based Health Promotion Programs*. Mountain View: Mayfield Publishing Company.

Baskerville, N.B., Liddy, C., and Hogg, W. (2012). Systematic review and meta-analysis of practice facilitation within primary care settings. *Annals of Family Medicine* 10 (1): 63–74. https://doi.org/10.1370/afm.1312.

Blackwood, B., Alderdice, F., Burns, K.E. et al. (2010). Protocolized versus non-protocolized weaning for reducing the duration of mechanical ventilation in critically ill adult patients. *Cochrane Database of Systematic Reviews* (5): CD006904. https://doi.org/10.1002/14651858. CD006904.pub2.

Boyle, R., Solberg, L., and Fiore, M. (2011). Use of electronic health records to support smoking cessation. *Cochrane Database of Systematic Reviews* (12): CD008743.

Boyle, R., Solberg, L., and Fiore, M. (2014). Use of electronic health records to support smoking cessation. *Cochrane Database of Systematic Reviews* (12): CD008743. https://doi. org/10.1002/14651858.CD008743.pub2.

Bragge, P., Grimshaw, J.M., Lokker, C. et al. (2017). AIMD – a validated, simplified framework of interventions to promote and integrate evidence into health practices, systems, and policies. *BMC Medical Research Methodology* 17: 38. https://doi.org/10.1186/ s12874-017-0314-8.

Canadian Agency for Drugs and Technologies in Health (2013). *Rx for Change*, [Online], Available: https://www.cadth.ca/rx-change [May 20, 2020].

Cheater, F., Baker, R., Gillies, C. et al. (2005). Tailored interventions to overcome identified barriers to change: effects on professional practice and health care outcomes. *Cochrane Database of Systematic Reviews* (3): CD005470. https://doi.org/10.1002/14651858.CD005470.

Cochrane Consumers and Communication Review Group (2012). *Topics List*, [Online], Available: https://cccrg.cochrane.org/sites/cccrg.cochrane.org/files/public/uploads/Topics. pdf [February 28, 2020].

Cochrane Consumers and Communication Review Group (2020). *About us*, [Online], Available: https://cccrg.cochrane.org/about [February 28, 2020].

Colquhoun, H., Grimshaw, J., and Wensing, M. (2013). Chapter 3.3b Mapping KT interventions to barriers and facilitators. In: *Knowledge Translation in Health Care. Moving from Evidence to Practice*, 2e (eds. S. Straus, J. Tetroe and I.D. Graham), 137–149. Chichester: Wiley-Blackwell.

Curran, G.M. (2020). Implementation science made too simple: a teaching tool. *Implementation Science Communications* 1 https://doi.org/10.1186/s43058-020-00001-z.

Davey, P., Brown, E., Fenelon, L. et al. (2005). Interventions to improve antibiotic prescribing practices for hospital inpatients. *Cochrane Database of Systematic Reviews* (4): CD003543. https://doi.org/10.1002/14651858.CD003543.pub2.

Davey, P., Brown, E., Charani, E. et al. (2013 Apr 30). Interventions to improve antibiotic prescribing practices for hospital inpatients. *Cochrane Database of Systematic Reviews* (4): CD003543. https://doi.org/10.1002/14651858.CD003543.pub3.

Davies, P., Walker, A.E., and Grimshaw, J.M. (2010). A systematic review of the use of theory in the design of guideline dissemination and implementation strategies and interpretation of the results of rigorous evaluations. *Implementation Science* 5: 14. https://doi.org/10.1186/1748-5908-5-14.

Diwan, V.K., Wahlström, R., Tomson, G. et al. (1995). Effects of "group detailing" on the prescribing of lipid-lowering drugs: a randomized controlled trial in Swedish primary care. *Journal of Clinical Epidemiology* 48 (5): 705–711. https://doi.org/10.1016/0895-4356(94)00221-b.

Dobbins, M., Hanna, S.E., Ciliska, D. et al. (2009). A randomized controlled trial evaluating the impact of knowledge translation and exchange strategies. *Implementation Science* 4 (61) https://doi.org/10.1186/1748-5908-4-61.

Dwamena, F., Holmes-Rovner, M., Gulden, C. et al. (2012 Dec 12). Interventions for providers to promote a patient-centered approach in clinical consultations. *Cochrane Database of Systematic Reviews* (12): CD003267. https://doi.org/10.1002/14651858.cd003267.pub2.

Edwards, A.G., Evans, R., Dundon, J. et al. (2006). Personalised risk communication for informed decision making about taking screening tests. *Cochrane Database of Systematic Reviews* (4): CD001865. https://doi.org/10.1002/14651858.CD001865.pub2.

Edwards, A.G.K., Naik, G., Ahmed, H. et al. (2013). Personalised risk communication for informed decision making about taking screening tests. *Cochrane Database of Systematic Reviews* published: 28 February 2013 (2): CD001865. https://doi.org/10.1002/14651858.CD001865.pub3.

Effective Practice and Organisation of Care (EPOC) (2015). *EPOC Taxonomy*. Available at: https://epoc.cochrane.org/epoc-taxonomy.

Effective Practice and Organisation of Care (EPOC) Group (2020). *About us*, [Online], Available: https://epoc.cochrane.org/about-us [February 28, 2020].

Eldh, A.C., Almost, J., DeCorby-Watson, K. et al. (2017). Clinical interventions, implementation interventions, and the potential greyness in between -a discussion paper. *BMC Health Services Research* 17: 16. https://doi.org/10.1186/s12913-016-1958-5.

EQUATOR Network (2020). *Enhancing the QUAlity and Transparency Of health Research*, [Online], Available: https://www.equator-network.org [February 28, 2020].

Farmer, A.P., Légaré, F., Turcot, L. et al. (2008). Printed educational materials: effects on professional practice and health care outcomes. *Cochrane Database of Systematic Reviews* (3): CD004398. https://doi.org/10.1002/14651858.CD004398.pub2.

Fernandez, M.E., Ten Hoor, G.A., van Lieshout, S. et al. (2019). Implementation mapping: using intervention mapping to develop implementation strategies. *Frontiers in Public Health* 7: 158. https://doi.org/10.3389/fpubh.2019.00158.

Flodgren, G., Parmelli, E., Doumit, G. et al. (2011). Local opinion leaders: effects on professional practice and health care outcomes. *Cochrane Database of Systematic Reviews* (8): CD000125. https://doi.org/10.1002/14651858.CD000125.pub4.

Flodgren, G., O'Brien, M., Parmelli, E., and Grimshaw, J. (2019). Are local opinion leaders effective in promoting best practice of healthcare professionals and improving patient outcomes? *Cochrane Database of Systematic Reviews* 2019 (6): CD000125. https://doi.org/10.1002/14651858.CD000125.pub5.

Fonhus, M.S., Dalsbo, T.K., Johansen, M. et al. (2018). Patient-mediated interventions to improve professional practice. *Cochrane Database of Systematic Reviews* (9): CD012472. https://doi.org/10.1002/14651858.CD012472.pub2.

Forsetlund, L., Bjorndal, A., Rashidian, A. et al. (2009). Continuing education meetings and workshops: effects on professional practice and health care outcomes. *Cochrane*

Database of Systematic Reviews (2): CD003030.1. https://doi.org/10.1002/14651858. CD003030.pub2.

Foster, G., Taylor, S.J., Eldridge, S.E. et al. (2007). Self-management education programmes by lay leaders for people with chronic conditions. *Cochrane Database of Systematic Reviews* (4): CD005108. https://doi.org/10.1002/14651858.CD005108.pub2.

Freemantle, N., Nazareth, I., Eccles, M. et al. (2002). A randomised controlled trial of the effect of educational outreach by community pharmacists on prescribing in UK general practice. *The British Journal of General Practice: The Journal of the Royal College of General Practitioners* 52 (477): 290–295. https://bjgp.org/content/52/477/290.long.

French, S.D., Green, S., Buchbinder, R., and Barnes, H. (2010). Interventions for improving the appropriate use of imaging in people with musculoskeletal conditions. *Cochrane Database of Systematic Reviews* (1): CD006094. https://doi.org/10.1002/14651858.CD006094.pub2.

Gibson, P.G., Powell, H., Coughlan, J. et al. (2002). Limited (information only) patient education programs for adults with asthma. *Cochrane Database of Systematic Reviews* (2): CD001005. https://doi.org/10.1002/14651858.CD001005.

Giguère, A., Légaré, F., Grimshaw, J. et al. (2012). Printed educational materials: effects on professional practice and health care outcomes. *Cochrane Database of Systematic Reviews* (10): CD004398. https://doi.org/10.1002/14651858.CD004398.pub3.

Grilli, R., Ramsey, C., and Minozzi, S. (2002). Mass media interventions: effects on health service utilization. *Cochrane Database of Systematic Reviews* (1): CD000389. https://doi.org/10.1002/14651858.CD000389.

Grimshaw, J.M., Thomas, R.E., MacLennan, G. et al. (2004). Effectiveness and efficiency of guideline dissemination and implementation strategies. *Health Technology Assessment* 8 (6): iii–72. https://doi.org/10.3310/hta8060.

Grimshaw, J.M., Eccles, M.P., Lavis, J.N. et al. (2012). Knowledge translation of research findings. *Implementation Science* 7: 50. https://doi.org/10.1186/1748-5908-7-50.

Nagendran, M., Gurusamy, K.S., Aggarwal, R. et al. (2013). Virtual reality training for surgical trainees in laparoscopic surgery. *Cochrane Database of Systematic Reviews* (8): CD006575. https://doi.org/10.1002/14651858.CD006575.pub3.

Hoffmann, T.C., Glasziou, P.P., Boutron, I. et al. (2014). Better reporting of interventions: template for intervention description and replication (TIDieR) checklist and guide. *BMJ* 348: g1687. https://doi.org/10.1136/bmj.g1687.

Ivers, N., Jamtvedt, G., Flottorp, S. et al. (2012). Audit and feedback: effects on professional practice and healthcare outcomes. *Cochrane Database of Systematic Reviews* (6): CD000259. https://doi.org/10.1002/14651858.CD000259.pub3.

Jamtvedt, G., Young, J.M., Kristoffersen, D.T. et al. (2006). Audit and feedback: effects on professional practice and health care outcomes. *Cochrane Database of Systematic Reviews* (2): CD000259. https://doi.org/10.1002/14651858.CD000259.pub2.

Johnson, A., Sandford, J., and Tyndall, J. (2003). Written and verbal information versus verbal information only for patients being discharged from acute hospital settings to home. *Cochrane Database of Systematic Reviews* (4): CD003716. https://doi.org/10.1002/14651858.CD003716.

Kinnersley, P., Edwards, A., Hood, K. et al. (2007). Interventions before consultations for helping patients address their information needs. *Cochrane Database of Systematic Reviews* (3): CD004565. https://doi.org/10.1002/14651858.CD004565.pub2.

Kinnersley, P., Phillips, K., Savage, K. et al. (2013). Interventions to promote informed consent for patients undergoing surgical and other invasive healthcare procedures. *Cochrane Database of Systematic Reviews* Version published: 06 July 2013 (7): CD009445. https://doi. org/10.1002/14651858.CD009445.pub2.

Kok, G., Schaalma, H., Ruiter, R.A. et al. (2004). Intervention mapping: protocol for applying health psychology theory to prevention programmes. *Journal of Health Psychology* 9: 85–98. https://doi.org/10.1177/1359105304038379.

Kok, G., Gottlieb, N.H., Peters, G.J. et al. (2016). A taxonomy of behaviour change methods: an intervention mapping approach. *Health Psychology Review* 10: 297–312. https://doi.org/ 10.1080/17437199.2015.1077155.

Laliberte, M.C., Perreault, S., Jouini, G. et al. (2011). Effectiveness of interventions to improve the detection and treatment of osteoporosis in primary care settings: a systematic review and meta-analysis. *Osteoporosis International* 22 (11): 2743–2768. https://doi.org/10.1007/s00198-011-1557-6.

Lavis, J., Davies, H., Oxman, A. et al. (2005). Towards systematic reviews that inform health care management and policy-making. *Journal of Health Services Research & Policy* 10 (Suppl1): 35–48. https://doi.org/10.1258/1355819054308549.

Leeman, J., Birken, S.A., Powell, B.J. et al. (2017). Beyond "implementation strategies": classifying the full range of strategies used in implementation science and practice. *Implementation Science* 12: 125. https://doi.org/10.1186/s13012-017-0657-x.

Lewin, S.A., Skea, Z.C., Entwistle, V. et al. (2001). Interventions for providers to promote a patient-centred approach in clinical consultations. *Cochrane Database of Systematic Reviews* (4): CD003267. https://doi.org/10.1002/14651858.CD003267.

Li, T., Wu, H.M., Wang, F. et al. (2011). Education programmes for people with diabetic kidney disease. *Cochrane Database of Systematic Reviews* (6): CD007374. [PubMed] DOI: https:// doi.org/10.1002/14651858.CD007374.pub2.

Lokker, C., McKibbon, K.A., Colquhoun, H., and Hempel, S. (2015). A scoping review of classification schemes of interventions to promote and integrate evidence into practice in healthcare. *Implementation Science* 10: 27. https://doi.org/10.1186/s13012-015-0220-6.

Mazza, D., Bairstow, P., Buchan, H. et al. (2013). Refining a taxonomy for guideline implementation: results of an exercise in abstract classification. *Implementation Science* 8: 32. https://doi.org/10.1186/1748-5908-8-32.

Michie, S., Johnston, M., Francis, J. et al. (2008). From theory to intervention: mapping theoretically derived behavioural determinants to behaviour change techniques. *Applied Psychology* 57: 660–680. https://doi.org/10.1111/j.1464-0597.2008.00341.x.

Michie, S., Fixsen, D., Grimshaw, J.M., and Eccles, M.P. (2009). Specifying and reporting complex behaviour change interventions: the need for a scientific method. *Implementation Science* 4: 40. https://doi.org/10.1186/1748-5908-4-40.

Michie, S., Richardson, M., Johnston, M. et al. (2013). The behavior change technique taxonomy (v1) of 93 hierarchically clustered techniques: building an international consensus for the reporting of behavior change interventions. *Annals of Behavioral Medicine* 46: 81–95. https://doi.org/10.1007/s12160-013-9486-6.

Murthy, L., Shepperd, S., Clarke, M.J. et al. (2012). Interventions to improve the use of systematic reviews in decision-making by health system managers, policy makers and clinicians. *Cochrane Database of Systematic Reviews* (9): CD009401. https://doi. org/10.1002/14651858.CD009401.pub2.

Nicolson, D., Knapp, P., Raynor, D.K., and Spoor, P. (2009). Written information about individual medicines for consumers. *Cochrane Database of Systematic Reviews* (2): CD002104. https://doi.org/10.1002/14651858.CD002104.pub3.

Nilsen, E.S., Mryhaug, H.T., Johansen, M. et al. (2006). Methods of consumer involvement in developing healthcare policy and research, clinical practice guidelines and patient information material. *Cochrane Database of Systematic Reviews*, version published: 19 July 2006 (3): CD004563. https://doi.org/10.1002/14651858.CD004563.pub2.

Nkansah, N., Mostovetsky, O., Yu, C. et al. (2010). Effect of outpatient pharmacists' non-dispensing roles on patient outcomes and prescribing patterns. *Cochrane Database of Systematic Reviews* (7): CD000336. https://doi.org/10.1002/14651858.CD000336.pub2.

O'Brien, M.A., Rogers, S., Jamtvedt, G. et al. (2007). Educational outreach visits: effects on professional practice and health care outcomes. *Cochrane Database of Systematic Reviews* (4): CD000409. https://doi.org/10.1002/14651858.CD000409.pub2.

Perrier, L., Mrklas, K., Lavis, J., and Straus, S. (2011). Interventions encouraging the use of systematic reviews by health policymakers and managers: a systematic review. *Implementation Science* 6 https://doi.org/10.1186/1748-5908-6-43.

Perry, C.K., Damschroder, L.J., Hemler, J.R. et al. (2019). Specifying and comparing implementation strategies across seven large implementation interventions: a practical application of theory. *Implementation Science* 14: 32. https://doi.org/10.1186/s13012-019-0876-4.

Pinnock, H., Barwick, M., Carpenter, C.R. et al. (2017). Standards for Reporting Implementation Studies (StaRI): explanation and elaboration document. *BMJ Open* 7: e013318. https://doi.org/10.1136/bmjopen-2016-013318.

Pirkis, J.E., Jolley, D., and Dunt, D.R. (1998). Recruitment of women by GPs for pap tests: a meta-analysis. *British Journal of General Practice* 48 (434): 1603–1607. https://bjgp.org/content/48/434/1603.long.

Powell, B.J., McMillen, J.C., Proctor, E.K. et al. (2012). A compilation of strategies for implementing clinical innovations in health and mental health. *Medical Care Research and Review* 69: 123–157. https://doi.org/10.1177/1077558711430690.

Powell, B.J., Waltz, T.J., Chinman, M.J. et al. (2015). A refined compilation of implementation strategies: results from the Expert Recommendations for Implementing Change (ERIC) project. *Implementation Science* 10: 21. https://doi.org/10.1186/s13012-015-0209-1.

Powell, B.J., Fernandez, M.E., Williams, N.J. et al. (2019). Enhancing the impact of implementation strategies in healthcare: a research agenda. *Frontiers in Public Health* 7: 3. https://doi.org/10.3389/fpubh.2019.00003.

Shojania, K.G., Jennings, A., Mayhew, A. et al. (2009). The effects of on-screen, point of care computer reminders on processes and outcomes of care. *Cochrane Database of Systematic Reviews* (3): CD001096. https://doi.org/10.1002/14651858.CD001096.pub2.

Smith, S.M., Allwright, S., and O'Dowd, T. (2007). Effectiveness of shared care across the interface between primary and specialty care in chronic disease management. *Cochrane Database of Database of Systematic Reviews* (3): CD004910. https://doi.org/10.1002/14651858.CD004910.pub2.

Smith, S.M., Grainne, C., Clyne, B. et al. (2017). Shared care across the interface between primary and specialty care in management of long-term conditions. *Cochrane Database of*

Systematic Reviews Version published: 23 February 2017 (2): CD004910. https://doi. org/10.1002/14651858.CD004910.pub3.

Squires, J.E., Sullivan, K., Eccles, M.P. et al. (2014). Are multifaceted interventions more effective than single-component interventions in changing health-care professionals' behaviours? An overview of systematic reviews. *Implementation Science* 9: 152. https://doi. org/10.1186/s13012-014-0152-6.

Stacey, D., Bennett, C.L., Barry, M.J. et al. (2011). Decision aids for people facing health treatment or screening decisions. *Cochrane Database of Systematic Reviews* (10): CD001431. https://doi.org/10.1002/14651858.CD001431.pub3.

Stacey, D., Légaré, F., Lewis, K. et al. (2017). Decision aids for people facing health treatment or screening decisions. *Cochrane Database of Systematic Reviews* Version published: 12 April 2017 (4): CD001431. https://doi.org/10.1002/14651858.CD001431.pub5.

Straus, S., Tetroe, J., and Graham, I.D. (eds.) (2013). *Knowledge Translation in Health Care. Moving from Evidence to Practice*, 2e. Chichester: Wiley Blackwell.

Thomas, L., Cullum, N., McColl, E. et al. (2000). Guidelines in professions allied to medicine. *Cochrane Database of Systematic Reviews* (2): CD000349. https://doi.org/10.1002/14651858. CD000349.

Thompson, D.S., Estabrooks, C.A., Scott-Findlay, S. et al. (2007). Interventions aimed at increasing research use in nursing: a systematic review. *Implementation Science* 2: 15. https://doi.org/10.1186/1748-5908-2-15.

Wolfenden, L., Goldman, S., Stacey, F.G. et al. (2018). Strategies to improve the implementation of workplace-based policies or practices targeting tobacco, alcohol, diet, physical activity and obesity. *Cochrane Database of Systematic Reviews* (11): CD012439. https://doi. org/10.1002/14651858.CD012439.pub2.

Wyatt, J.C., Paterson-Brown, S., Johanson, R. et al. (1998). Randomised trial of educational visits to enhance use of systematic reviews in 25 obstetric units. *BMJ* 317 (7165): 1041–1046. https://doi.org/10.1136/bmj.317.7165.1041.

Yost, J., Ganann, R., Thompson, D. et al. (2015). The effectiveness of knowledge translation interventions for promoting evidence-informed decision-making among nurses in tertiary care: a systematic review and meta-analysis. *Implementation Science* 10: 98. https://doi. org/10.1186/s13012-015-0286-1.

11

Tailor Implementation Strategies

In the last chapter, we concentrated on the available evidence about specific implementation strategies and gaps in our knowledge about what strategies work. Also covered was the business of tailoring implementation strategies to barriers and drivers and guidelines for reporting on implementation strategies. In this chapter, the focus is on sharing our experience with using these strategies and some newer ones we have uncovered during our implementation initiatives. This stage is about prioritizing the barriers to implementation that need to be targeted, carefully tailoring interventions to those barriers and developing an implementation strategies delivery fidelity checklist.

To summarize the journey following Roadmap to this point, you will have identified the evidence-practice gap, measured its magnitude, and determined that there is a need to address the issue. You will have selected and customized the best practice to the local context and importantly identified potential barriers and drivers to the use of the best practice. The way we think of tailoring is comprised of two components. The first is mapping the potential implementation strategies to barriers and then adjusting the proposed strategies to the local context. The output of this activity will be the selection of the implementation strategies the group will activate to facilitate the uptake of the best practice.

Goal: At this stage of Roadmap, the purpose is to select and tailor implementation strategies to the identified barriers and drivers of best practice. Pertinent questions include:

- What exactly is the decision making or behavior (best practice) that is to be promoted?
- Which barriers and drivers to the use of the best practice should be targeted by the implementation strategies?
- How will tailoring of the strategies be done for your setting/context?
  - What potential implementation strategies map to the prioritized barriers and drivers?
  - What are the adjustments that need to be made to the potential strategies to make them practical and feasible to deliver in your context?
  - What resources will be required to deliver the implementation strategies?
- How will the fidelity of the delivery of the implementation strategies be assessed?

In much of our work, our approach to tailoring and mapping implementation strategies would fall under the common-sense approach (described in the previous chapter), although we do have experience with the behavior change techniques matrix (Michie et al. 2008).

Knowledge Translation in Nursing and Healthcare: A Roadmap to Evidence-informed Practice, First Edition. Margaret B. Harrison and Ian D. Graham.

Our approach to tailoring starts back at the customization stage with the group clearly defining the best practice (behaviors) to be undertaken, by whom, how, under what circumstances, and when, which we put into the Action Map (see Chapter 8). This is the foundation of the Action Map and Implementation Plan. Then during the barriers' assessment stage, barriers and drivers to each of the elements of best practice are identified and added to the Action Map (see Chapter 9). These are the data which are the groundwork for the group's discussion on tailoring and mapping implementation strategies to the local context. We then share these data with our knowledge users. Often this has been the core implementation group. Other times we have also engaged a broader group of individuals and patients from the setting. Repeating advice we have already provided, the key is to be inclusive (involve individuals from all the knowledge user and stakeholder groups that will be affected by the change or have a vested interest in the change) to ensure you receive input from all perspectives. It is important to remember that the science around how to effectively and efficiently tailor implementation strategies is emerging. There is no one right way to do it. Much of the work now involves combining both the art and science of implementation.

The Decision-Making Process for Tailoring Implementation Strategies

We usually obtain input about tailoring implementation strategies by meeting with our knowledge users in a focus group like session or town hall meeting over coffee, and/or sometimes we have one-to-one discussions. We always establish ground rules for these meetings that includes the session being a safe place for discussion, and that all perspectives from those of managers, point-of-care staff, individuals/families (including dissenting views) are valued and respected. No questions or comments are inappropriate. Depending on the context, we have held separate meetings with managers, staff, and individuals/families, while at other times we have brought them all together. Sometimes we have done both: held separate meetings with knowledge users and stakeholder groups followed by joint meetings of these groups so everyone can hear each other's perspectives. If we have a sense that the proposed change or the barriers to change may be controversial or there may be issues between management and staff, we may have separate meetings for the two groups so that they feel comfortable expressing their views. Depending on the culture of the organization in which the change is occurring (especially more hierarchical structures where questioning may not be commonplace), it may be necessary to work at convincing participants that they can safely speak up. Now and then we have invoked the "what happens in Vegas stays in Vegas" rule which means that what is discussed in the room stays in the room. Sometimes this strategy is helpful when there has been controversy about the proposed change and we wanted participants to be completely candid and not worry about word getting back to others (e.g. staff concerned about what managers might think of their views).

It can also happen that during in-camera sessions that other organizational practices possibly related to the proposed change (e.g. safety issues, scopes of practice, that may be violating organizational policy) are brought up. Depending on the severity and nature of these issues that emerge and the potential risk they pose to the organization, it may be necessary to bring them to the attention of appropriate individuals in the organizations. This needs to be done delicately while respecting the confidentiality of the participants. It also means that the working group should discuss among themselves before the sessions what their process would be to deal with safety or other serious issues that might become known during their sessions. They should consider the criteria the group would use to decide when to escalate an issue to others in the organization. This type of situation has occurred very rarely during this stage of the implementation process, but we think it is important that implementation groups or those responsible for leading implementation be prepared should it happen. Finding safety, risk, and other significant issues is much more common during the evidence-practice gap assessment stage and easier to deal with then, as it only requires briefing the relevant parties on the findings of the assessment (which they are usually interested in).

Box 11.1   Hidden challenges

With one project, while discussing implementation interventions, we became aware that many units were not following the organization's policy on when to document certain observations in the health record. This was a significant breach in policy with implications for patient safety. The facilitator of the meeting spoke with a senior manager in the organization alerting the manager to the possibility that the charting on some units might not be policy compliant. The manager discretely investigated and confirmed adherence to the policy was lacking and took steps to address it.

The objective of these meetings is to come up with ideas of strategies that might mitigate barriers or strengthen drivers of using best practice. Much care must be taken in running these meetings. Ideally the facilitators of these meetings should be respected, nonjudgmental, and good working with people and eliciting their views. Sometimes the facilitators have been completely neutral about the change (and perceived to be neutral by participants). In other cases, the manager leading the change has facilitated the meeting. Both approaches have worked for us. What is critical is that those participating in the meeting feel that the input they provide will be considered. No one wants to be spending time at meetings providing advice to later find it was ignored. It may not always be taken up but has to be considered. For this reason, we also encourage that all views, positive and negative about implementation strategies be included in the reporting of the discussion. This ensures that the implementation plan will be completely transparent and will increase the credibility of the process, especially if this is not usual practice in the setting.

Turning to the actual business of the meeting, there are two related goals. The first is to reflect on barriers and drivers to the best practice and select the ones the group is going to focus on. The second is to suggest implementation strategies or components of strategies that they believe would be particularly useful (and ideally successful) in addressing the barriers and drivers in their setting. We also remind those participating in this exercise that tailoring of implementation strategies needs to result in strategies that are feasible and practical to implement and ones for which there are available resources to deliver them and that they should consider these issues in their deliberations.

Prioritize Barriers to Implementation Strategies

To get started, the group needs to review the proposed best practice and the barriers and drivers identified to each component of the best practice. We have found walking through the Action Map (refer to Action Map document completed in Chapter 8) and ensuring all understand the customized best practice to be adopted. The identified barriers and drivers is a good way to start. Next, the group will need to prioritize the barriers as there may be too many to try to address. This can be done through open discussion or by using a modified nominal group technique (NGT) (Pokorny et al. 1988). The modified NGT involves listing the barriers on paper placed around the room and giving participants a pre-determined number of stickers (e.g. 3, 5, 10) that they can use to essentially vote for the barriers that they think are most important to address. A quick tally of the number of stickers per barrier gives the group the barriers they will focus on. Once the short list of barriers and drivers has been identified, the group can move on to the task of tailoring the implementation strategies to the barriers and drivers.

Questions guiding this activity include:

• What are the most important barriers and drivers to focus on?
• Have barriers at the level of the individual, team, unit, or organization been considered?

Tailor Implementation Strategies to Barriers and Drivers to Use of Best Practice

To help the group shift its focus to implementation strategies that might be appropriate to consider, we often start by summarizing for the group what is known about the effectiveness of different implementation strategies and present taxonomies or lists of implementation strategies as background information to ground discussions such as those described in Chapter 10.

We have also found it useful when the group is starting to think about tailoring strategies to review the Ottawa Model of Research Use (OMRU) classification of implementation strategies (Graham and Logan 2004). OMRU directs attention to three distinct categories of implementation strategies.

1) *Barriers management strategies:* these are typically focused at organizational or system level barriers. They comprise strategies that use a top-down approach and could include such strategies as revising professional roles, integrating the best practice implementation into quality improvement processes, modifying the electronic health record or charting process, changing staffing arrangements or modifying team composition, procurement of equipment or supplies, altering remuneration, creating an audit and feedback process, etc. Once these types of barriers are addressed, they are removed for all (or many) potential adopters. To deploy these types of strategies requires active engagement and support by managers and senior leaders in the organization as they almost always have resource implications. If the leaders are not onside, the strategies will not happen.

2) *Knowledge transfer strategies:* These are strategies that target barriers related specifically to potential adopters of the best practice and can address lack of awareness and

knowledge of, and poor attitudes toward the best practice. They may also target the barrier of lack of necessary skills to perform and use the best practice including lack of confidence in being able to perform best practice. These strategies typically fall under educational strategies, both passive ones (e.g. guideline documents and pocket cards, didactic lectures and conferences) and active ones (e.g. interactive hands on workshops, use of opinion leaders or local influencers, educational outreach visits, development of quality circles, etc.). Patient-directed implementation strategies would also fall within this category as they are intended to activate patients to adopt best practice (can affect their knowledge, attitudes and decision making) or prompt their health care providers to do so (e.g. patient decision aids, health literacy interventions).

3) *Follow-up strategies:* These can be considered sustainability strategies or maintenance "booster shots" to augment earlier implementation strategies, especially if the implementation period is lengthy as it can be with complex large-scale changes. The follow-up strategies are also used to prompt continued use of the best practice when the process evaluation reveals adherence to the best practice starts falling off, as often happens the further you get away from the active implementation period. The follow-up sustainability strategies can include more or the same barrier management and knowledge transfer strategies.

Box 11.2   Complex solutions sometimes needed

We found that the OMRU classification of interventions was most helpful to groups. They told us it facilitated a systematic approach to their Building Solutions phase. Most barriers required an integrated combination of solutions aimed at both the practice, managerial and system level, e.g. a guideline which changes the management of wound care in the community typically involves expenditures and procurement of new bandaging, prescriptions and dressing supplies, changes in home and clinic schedules, adjustments to patient referral patterns, revisions to professional scopes of practice, skills training and education for practitioners and patients, a communications strategy, and a means to monitor the delivery of care across multiple regional sites.

The OMRU provides a comprehensive guide through all these aspects.

Thinking in terms of these three categories can assist the group in making sure it considers all the determinants of using best practice, not just focus on barriers related to the potential adopter of the best practice (in particular education strategies – but more on this later in the chapter).

Turning again to the actual business of the meeting, the goal is to have those participating reflect on the practice change, the barriers and drivers of it and suggest implementation strategies or components of strategies that they believe will be particularly useful (and ideally successful) in addressing them in their setting. Having reviewed the literature on effectiveness of implementation strategies and keeping in mind the need to consider barriers and implementation strategies at multiple levels (individual, team, unit, organization), the group is ready to start mapping implementation strategies to barriers and drivers.

In Chapter 9 we described the method for doing a stakeholder analysis that takes into consideration the support and influence of the stakeholder groups revealing potential barriers and drivers to implementation. A potential exercise to warm up the group to thinking about implementation strategies mapping, is to reintroduce the results of the stakeholder analysis. Ask the group to brainstorm about what implementation strategies might be useful for each type of stakeholder in the table. In Figure 11.1, implementation strategies have been added to the stakeholder analysis presented initially in Chapter 9. The cell containing influential but unsupportive stakeholders pose the greatest threat to implementation and strategies. We point out that it is critical to bring them on side or

STAKEHOLDER INFLUENCE & SUPPORT GRID		
	Low ← **INFLUENCE** → **High**	
SUPPORT ↑↓ Low	• Least able to influence dissemination and adoption • Could have negative impact on plans • Some attention to obtain support &/or maintain neutrality • Work towards project buy-in Strategies • Consensus • Build relationships • Recognize needs • Use external stakeholders and consultants • Involve at some level • Monitor	• Can negatively affect dissemination and adoption in a big way • Need great amount of attention to obtain support &/or neutrality • Work towards buy-in Strategies • Consensus • Build relationships • Recognize needs • Use external stakeholders & consultants • Involve at some level • Stress how BPGs are developed • Don't provoke into action • Monitor
	Low Support Low Influence	High Support Low Influence
	High Support Low Influence	High Support High Influence
High	• Can positively affect dissemination and adoption if given attention • Need attention to maintain buy-in and prevent development of neutrality Strategies • Collaborate • Encourage feedback • Empower with professional status • Encourage participation • Prepare for change management • Involve at some level	• Will positively affect dissemination and adoption • Need a great deal of attention and information to maintain their buy-in Strategies • Collaborate • Involve &/or provide opportunities where they can be supportive • Support and nurture • Encourage feedback • Prepare for change management • Empower

Figure 11.1 Stakeholder influence and support grid. *Source:* Reprinted with permission from Registered Nurses' Association of Ontario (2012).

neutralize any negativity they may express about the implementation of the best practice and ask how this might be brought about.

Turning to the stakeholders that are not supportive and have low influence, they also need to be encouraged to buy-in even though they may not have the influence to scuttle implementation. We ask the group for suggestions for strategies to encourage these stakeholders to be more supportive. Finally, we ask the working group to suggest ways to keep highly influential and supportive stakeholders and supportive but not influential stakeholders onside and continuing to be supportive. After letting the group come up with implementation strategies and adding them to their stakeholder analysis table, we have sometimes shown them the completed table (Figure 11.1) and discuss each of the cells and the implementation strategies mapping process.

Next, we move to the list of prioritized barriers and drivers and ask the group as a whole or in small groups to brainstorm about each barrier and what might be done to overcome the identified barriers and why. Sometimes we need to remind the group about the evidence for specific implementation strategies they suggest. We also remind those participating in this exercise that tailoring of implementation strategies needs to result in strategies that are feasible and practical to implement and ones for which there are available resources to deliver them and that they should consider these issues in their deliberations.

If the group is large enough and the prioritized list of barriers long, different tables can be assigned different barriers to work on. If there is an abundance of implementation strategies or components suggested, they can be winnowed down via open discussion or another modified NGT can be used by the group to prioritize strategies. This time it involves listing the barriers and proposed strategies on paper placed around the room and giving participants stickers that they can use to vote for the strategies they think will be most successful. Again, a quick tally of the number of stickers by barrier identifies how the group might tailor strategies to barriers. Keep in mind, that the same strategy may be able to address multiple barriers so it may not be necessary to have a different strategy for each barrier. If the Theoretical Domains Framework was used to identify the barriers then the Behavior Change Techniques associated with the barriers (Appendix 11.A) can be used to narrow down the candidate implementation strategies (Michie et al. 2008; Cane et al. 2015). Again, if there is a need to prioritize the strategies, the modified NGT or other consensus processes described above can be used.

A slightly different approach that can also work involves a few members of the working group doing this task and then meeting with the full group to validate the proposed suggestions or modifying what is proposed by adding additional strategies or removing/modifying some of the proposed ones. This seems to work the best when it becomes difficult to get the whole group scheduled for a session.

Guiding questions for this activity include:

- What is the evidence for the implementation strategies being proposed?
- Can the same strategy address multiple barriers?
- Do the proposed strategies collectively address barriers found at all levels?
- Are the implementation strategies feasible to use?
- Are there adequate resources to support using the implementation strategies?

Some Thoughts on Educational Implementation Strategies

Educational interventions as they are often referred to in the literature, are the most common implementation strategies used in nursing and the most common strategies tested in implementation studies in nursing. For this reason, we think it useful to describe education interventions that have been evaluated and to show the great variation in the types and nature of these interventions, the differences in how they are delivered and the resources required to deliver them.

In virtually every implementation with which we have been involved, education interventions have been selected. This is also evident in the overabundance of different education interventions seen in the research literature (see EPOC) (Effective Practice and Organisation of Care (EPOC) 2015). However, an educational intervention can vary greatly in the type (didactic, interactive), how delivered (hands-on, virtually), duration, and frequency and related cost and resource use. To illustrate and assist in selecting educational strategies for the local context we have developed a detailed grid of educational implementation strategies tested in randomized controlled trials.

As you can see from Table 11.1 there are many approaches to education and it will be important once your group tailors implementation strategies to the identified barriers and drivers, that if the group decides to employ an educational strategy, they carefully consider the time involved, expertise available and resources required.

In our experience we have used both in-house and external educational approaches. Depending on the topic, needed learning can entail both theoretical and a practical component for experience. The modality for delivery could be delivered in-house, remotely through other agencies, e.g. local college or as we have often seen "train-the-trainer" approach to develop local expertise and make it possible to continue with peer teaching.

When designing educational implementation strategies, it is also important to consider the key ingredients that make educational interventions work in a continuing education approach for practitioners. Van Hoof and Meehan (2011) have identified five key ingredients that are necessary to optimize the success of education interventions, they are:

- Relevant-based on educational needs assessment
- Intensiveness-multifaceted
- Logical-sequencing
- Engagement-interactive
- Commitment to change of participants.

When thinking of educational strategies, we also find it helpful to also think of the goals of the education sessions in terms of cognitive domains of thinking or knowledge. Bloom's taxonomy is a useful framework (Bloom 1956; Anderson and Krathwohl 2001).

Is the objective of the strategy to generate:

- Knowledge – define, identify, list, recall
- Comprehension – describe, discuss, explain
- Application – apply, demonstrate, use, solve
- Analysis – analyze, compare, contrast, categorize
- Evaluate – appraise, argue, defend, judge, select, support, value
- Create – design, assemble, formulate, develop

Note the verbs related to each category. Once we identify the category we are hoping the educational strategy is to address, we then use the verbs in writing up the learning objectives for the sessions. If the group does not include a member with formal pedagogical training, it may want to seek out such a person to assist with designing the education intervention.

Table 11.1 Methods and approaches used in interventions classified as "educational sessions."

Method/Approach	Duration	Frequency	Author/Year (n = 30)
Instructional meeting + recommendations and supplementary documents (both hardcopy and PDF formats)	1 hour	Once	Hodl (2019)
A 36-hour pre-intervention training program was conducted in this study to enhance the nurses' decision-making. The training contents included knowledge and skills for nurse-led hypertension management.	3 hours	Not reported	Zhu (2018)
Tailored educational training for nurses + feedback discussions (from clinical managers and head nurses) (intervention); Clean Hands Campaign (ASH) training (control)	Not reported	Not reported	Von Lengerke (2017)
Human patient simulation (HPS) education with scenario (both intervention and control) + verbal feedback + structured debriefing (intervention only)	human patient simulation (HPS) education for 20 minutes with 10-minute scenario + verbal feedback + 60-minute structured debriefing	Once	Jansson (2016a, b)
Distribution of guidelines for both intervention and control; 4 educational meetings for the implementation leaders (two nurses in each ICU were chosen as the implementation leaders), each lasting 1 day, over 9 months (intervention only). A fifth day was organized for both the intervention and control group to share experiences, best practices and results.	4 meetings, each lasting 1 day, over 9 months	4 meetings over 9 months	Noome et al. (2017)
Education program (seminar with oral presentations, exercises and discussions) + printed short summary of the clinical practice guideline (intervention); basic information on pain management (control)	6 hours of education program	Once	Kalinowski (2015)
Delirium training sessions with educational material	30-minute training sessions	2 sessions	Moon and Lee (2015)

Educational meetings and personalized feedback by individualized coaching. This included 2-hour monthly educational meetings + individualized coaching at least once between monthly meetings.	2 hours per month, for 6 months (total 6 meetings): first introductory meeting is 4 hours, then 5 more 2 hours meetings	Once per month for 6 months: 6 meetings (monthly)	Snelgrove-Clark et al. (2015)
Human patient simulation (HPS) education with scenario (both intervention and control) + verbal feedback + structured debriefing (intervention only)	human patient simulation (HPS) education for 20 minutes with 10-minute scenario + verbal feedback + 60-minute structured debriefing	Once	Jansson (2014)
Structured education program for all nursing staff + external structured 1-day intensive training workshop for nominated key nurses from different nursing homes + printed supportive material (guidelines 16-page short version, flyer for relatives, posters) (intervention); standard information (control)	90-minute information program for all nursing staff + structured 1-day intensive training workshop for nominated key nurses	Once	Kopke (2012)
Educational meeting for nurses and educational materials (CD ROMs with educational material). The feedback system included small-scale educational meetings for all nurses (1.5 hours) + two case discussions on every ward (30 minutes) + A CD-ROM with education material + computerized feedback on the process and outcome indicators.	Educational meetings, 1.5 hours; two case discussions, 30 minutes	The frequency of educational meetings and case discussions are unclear	Van Gaal (2011a, b)
Education of nursing and medical staff via a web-based course, and provision of resource texts, videotapes, and training manuals. The TRIP intervention included a 60-minute continuing education program for senior administrative leaders to discuss their role in promoting adoption of EB pain management practices and foster support for revision of institution-specific documents (e.g. documentation forms, policies, and procedures).	3 days – nurse opinion leaders; 60 minutes-physician opinion leaders	Not reported	Titler (2009)

(Continued)

Table 11.1 (Continued)

Method/Approach	Duration	Frequency	Author/Year (n = 30)
Lecture with discussion, video presentation, observed role-play with individual and peer feedback, written materials, and self-study	2 half-day workshops	Not reported	Cheater (2006)
Limited didactic presentations, interactive case study discussions, hands-on exercises through small group teams for the development of action plans for patient self-care, exercises in how to teach patients to use peak flow meters, metered dose inhalers and MIDI spacers	Half day increments	2 duplicate sessions	Daniels (2005)
Lectures, group discussions, role-play and presentations. Interactive training targeted four clinical guidelines and other related areas including the conduct of the physical examination, rational drug use, and the use of effective communication skills	3-day training workshop	Once	Pagaiya and Gamer (2005)
Interactive training utilized experienced facilitators, as well as role-playing and audiotaping, to help nurses increase their skills in communicating with an motivating their patients to adhere to treatment instructions	Not reported	Not reported	Feldman (2004)
Asthma nurses – trained in EPR2 and self-management support techniques Nurses – motivational enhancement and problem-solving techniques Conference calls – to review written materials	Asthma nurses – 2 workshops; Nurses – full day training session	Weekly or every other week for 10 weeks – 1 hour conference calls	Lozano (2004)
APNs – orientation and training program to develop competencies related to early recognition and treatment of acute episodes of heart failure in elders	2 months	Not reported	Naylor (2004)
Lecture and discussion on pain and pain management Advanced session incorporated role-playing and assertiveness training to enhance the nurses' role as patient advocates and improve their communication with physicians, patients, and caregivers	4 hours	Twice	Vallerand (2004)

Nurses – session on screening for high blood cholesterol and training on how to give the intervention On-site coordinator – tutorial	Nurses – 2 hours On-site coordinator 4 hours	Not reported	Ammerman (2003)
Individualized intervention consisting of information, discussion of worries and negotiating agreement on goals, and cognitive behavioral advice about how to achieve them.	Not reported	Once	Mayou (2002)
Education done in small groups. For each programme, a detailed plan, learning outcomes and practice outcomes were identified. A variety of teaching methods were utilized, including both didactic and interactive approaches, and practical bedside demonstrations.	2 hours	Once	Day (2001)
Training programme modeled on a curriculum developed by the Provincial Health Department. Participants used a problem-solving exercise to define objectives to improve the quality of STD management in their clinics, which they then carried out. 3 follow-up sessions were held in each clinic	2-day workshop	4	Harrison (2000)
Teaching sessions on core elements of asthma care	Not reported	6	Premaratne (1999)
Mini-fellowship provided at the start of the intervention period to provide state-of-the-art CPM attitudes and behavior among 27 opinion leader clinicians. The mini-fellowship consisted of didactic presentations and clinical preceptorships with experiential clinical rounds in oncology inpatient units and hospice visits. Educational methods included lectures, small group discussions, case studies, and practicum	2 days	Once	Elliott (1997)

(*Continued*)

Table 11.1 (Continued)

Method/Approach	Duration	Frequency	Author/Year (n = 30)
Learning groups of no more than 30 to 35 staff members. All clinic staff, including clerical workers, participated in each session to ensure that everyone in the clinics understood the program and how they could contribute to it. Special emphasis on defining the role of clerks, public health assistants, and laboratory technicians, and teaching them how they could contribute to the program by answering questions, encouraging compliance, and, if families expressed doubts or concerns, encouraging them to resolve them with the doctor or nurse. Sessions included: a skit written by the faculty and performed by clinic staff to model how the program would work and introduced an interactive exercise called force field analysis to help clinic teams plan how to start the program in their clinics. Introduction of prevention and treatment protocols based on the NAEPP Guidelines.	3 hours	5 sessions over a 5-month period 2 additional 3-hour sessions at end of first follow-up year	Evans (1997)
Modeling of optimal communication skills for medical interviews and family education using videotapes showing a faculty doctor and nurse conducting an initial visit for asthma with a patient. A tutorial session in which each BCH physician spent 3 hours observing a Columbia faculty physician treating children with asthma at Columbia-Presbyterian Medical Center			
Computer assisted intervention presented several patient scenarios. Nurses had to respond by identifying appropriate barrier equipment for situation, and were given immediate feedback on their answers.	3 hours	Twice	Wright (1997)
A variety of approaches used: including lectures, panel discussions, role playing, small group discussions, and audiovisual exhibits. Other strategies included play-acting and role modeling.	2 days	Not reported	Hodnett (1996)
Nurses presented the innovation via role playing of how to conduct a baseline nursing assessment	30 minutes	Not reported	Dufault (1995)
Short sessions were expected to enhance learning. Sessions were in lecture format followed by a question-and-answer period	20 minutes	7 sessions conducted 2 weeks apart. Entire program took 12 weeks to complete	Parker et al. (1995)

Box 11.3   Covering Your Bases

In our Leg Ulcer implementation example, we employed multiple education strategies that involved remote and in-house delivery, train-the-trainer and peer teaching, theory as well as practical hands-on sessions.

A limited number of specialized enterostomal nurses assessed and delivered care to the venous leg ulcer (VLU) population. However, this was becoming impractical with the numbers of community cases. As community nurses assumed more of the care of people with VLUs, the agency and home care authority as well as associated physicians, needed to have the confidence they could carry out the evidence-informed protocol. Two care aspects were key: the use of a Doppler to calculate the ankle brachial index and the knowledge and skill to manage compression bandaging treatments.

At the time, there were no courses in VLU care, thus we contracted with colleagues in the UK to deliver a well-established program remotely. The instructors for the course flew in for master class sessions at the beginning and end of the course. Hands-on sessions were organized at our local blood flow lab and peer teaching followed by those who had been trained. On-going continuing education programs were developed for orientation of new team members and review of new research.

In the best practice for hospital discharge of those with heart failure two educational strategies were used: in-house sessions and an educational booklet.

The challenge here was that on discharge home, best practice was to counsel about medications, diet, exercise and rest, fluid management, etc. Hospital discharges often happened quickly and nurses on general medical units did not necessarily have specialized knowledge. We therefore developed a self-management guide for the nurse to use in counseling patients and families about these aspects and it was in plain language in order to be sent home with them and the teaching picked up by the home care nurse. It was also made available on our national Heart and Stroke website for free download: Heart and Stroke Foundation Canada (2002) Managing Congestive Heart Failure. Copyright transferred from Harrison, M.B., Toman C., & Logan, J., formerly Partners in Care for Congestive Heart Failure, Ottawa.

A Note on Fidelity

Fidelity is the integrity or adherence of an intervention. Another way to think about it is to consider whether the intervention is being delivered as intended. With evidence-informed practice and implementation of best practice, it will be important to consider the fidelity of delivering both the implementation strategy as well as the fidelity in delivering the new care (evidence informed practice). If the implementation strategy has been less than effective because it was not delivered as intended, then moving on to launch an implementation will produce less than anticipated results. If new skills or different processes are required, the fidelity of these to the evidence recommendation becomes critical to attain the desired result.

Murphy and Gutman (2012) outlined five fidelity aspects. Albeit intended for research interventions, they are equally applicable to KT strategies and implementation. The elements include intervention (or strategy) design, the training, the delivery, the receipt of intervention, and the enactment of skills gained from the intervention (pg. 387). To develop a fidelity checklist the group could consider the elements described by Carroll et al. (2007): (i) adherence (content, coverage, frequency, and duration); (ii) moderators (complexity, facilitation, and quality of delivery and participant responsiveness); (iii) identification of essential elements.

Develop Implementation Strategy Delivery Fidelity Checklist

You will know that you have completed this stage of Roadmap when the working group has tailored implementation strategies to the prioritized prospective barriers to implementing the best practice and produced the implementation delivery fidelity checklist. We have found groups generally find this exercise interesting and can see how it should lead to more successful implementation (perhaps because this stage is often not done in implementation projects in the real world). We have also observed that during the exercise, as is the case for much of the group or collective work required by Roadmap, the members of the group further embrace their commitment to the proposed change. We have not studied this phenomenon specifically to know the mechanism of action but we expect that the team-based approach to problem solving contributes to giving the group ownership and control over how to reduce the identified evidence-practice gap. It also provides a natural opportunity for learning about knowledge uptake and change which might be applied to other practice issues.

Lastly, because the entire process is about finding and tailoring practical solutions to the group's identified barriers and local context, it reinforces that the implementation is all about them and their context. They are guiding and driving implementation which further promotes group ownership and common vision when the group is inclusive (something that is not as common as it should be in healthcare because of long standing traditional disciplinary divides).

Summary

The group will know the implementation strategies stage is complete when the Action Map (Table 11.2) identifies the practice to be implemented, barriers and drivers to it, implementation strategies tailored to each of the barriers and drivers, with a rationale for how the strategies should work. Also, the group will have drafted an implementation strategies section of the Implementation Plan.

Table 11.2 Part 2: ACTION MAP for Solution Building (*with Wound Example*).

Customized best practice recommendations	Barriers and facilitating factors (drivers)	Implementation Strategies and Field Testing
	Factors related to each recommendation, potential adopters, or context. *What would aid or prevent implementation?*	Implementation strategies are mapped, tailored and field tested.
1. Evening shift RN to daily conduct head to toe skin assessment during HS care and document in flow chart	Most nurses familiar with head-to-toe skin assessment	On unit education briefing during evening shifts to ensure all staff are aware of best practice
	Not in orientation for new staff	Add best practice to Staff Orientation
	HS routine happens with every patient so will be incremental extra	Chart audit for assessment. Indicator: 90% of patients should be assessed on evening shift
2. Braden Risk assessment conducted with head to toe skin assessment by attending RN on evening shift daily and documented in nursing notes	Staff on several units not familiar with risk assessment scale (6 sub-scales), questioning total score, perceived as a lot of work	On-unit education in identified areas plus handout materials (flyer, pocket cards). Clinical shadowing with someone trained
	Not in orientation for new staff	Add education module to Staff Orientation
		Hold consultation on how to make it even more easy to chart and use subscale deficit(s) and to decide on clinical interventions to address patient deficits identified by subscales
		Chart audit for assessment. Indicator: 90% of patients should be assessed on evening shift
3. etc.		
Sustainability thinking continues here. . .	Barriers assessment conducted such that it can be redone in future, if necessary.	Implementation strategies selected in part based on being able to continue them in future.
	Target implementation strategies to known barriers and drivers to improve the uptake and ongoing maintenance.	Use all data and info for ongoing maintenance, planning and evaluation.
Chapter 8	Chapter 8 and 9	Chapter 10 (+ appendix), 11, 12

At this point the group should have clarity about the questions you began with:

- The decision making or behavior (best practice) that is being promoted is outlined
- Barriers and drivers have been prioritized for attention
- Implementation strategies have been tailored for your setting/context
  - Effectiveness of the potentially relevant implementation strategies were analyzed and selected
  - The practicality for your setting assessed
  - The needed resources were acquired to deliver the implementation strategies
- An implementation strategies checklist for fidelity has been developed

Writing Up the Description of the Implementation Strategy

As you will recall from the section of reporting guidelines for implementation strategies in the previous Chapter, there are several reporting guidelines that can be used as templates. The simplest one is the AIMD (Aims, Ingredients, Mechanism, Delivery) framework (Bragge et al. 2017) which was designed to guide development and reporting of implementation strategies. This framework comprises four components: (i) Aims: what do you want your intervention to achieve and for whom? (ii) Ingredients: what comprises the intervention? (iii) Mechanisms: how do you propose the intervention will work? and (iv) Delivery: how will you deliver the intervention? When tailoring the implementation strategies, have the group consider each of these questions. Use the questions to challenge everyone's thinking and assumptions about the strategies being proposed. When the group reaches consensus on the answer, document the deliberations and decisions. Include this information in the Implementation Plan either in prose or in a table. This information provides transparency and the rationale for the group's choice and tailoring of implementation strategies which can be useful for gaining staff and management's support for the implementation strategies.

In the next Chapter, we discuss going "live" with the implementation. This includes field testing the implementation strategies, planning the evaluation, and preparing to fully launch the implementation strategies.

Appendix 11.A: Data from Consensus Process for Linking behavior Change Techniques with Determinants of behavior

Reproduced with permission from Michie, S., Johnston, M., Francis, J., Hardeman, W. & Eccles, M. (2008) From Theory to Intervention: Mapping Theoretically Derived Behavioural Determinants to Behaviour Change Techniques. Applied Psychology 57, 660–680. © 2008 The Authors. Journal compilation © 2008 International Association of Applied Psychology. Published by Blackwell Publishing, 9600 Garsington Road, Oxford OX4 2DQ, UK and 350 Main Street, Malden, MA 02148, USA.

Technique for behavior change	Techniques judged to be effective in changing each construct domain										
	1	2	3	4	5	6	7	8	9	10	11
Goal/target specified: behavior or outcome											
Monitoring											
Self-monitoring											
Contract											
Rewards; incentives (inc. self-evaluation)											
Graded task, starting with easy tasks											
Increasing skills: problem-solving, decision-making, goal-setting											
Stress management											
Coping skills											
Rehearsal of relevant skills											
Role-play											
Planning, implementation											
Prompts, triggers, cues											
Environmental changes (e.g. objects to facilitate behavior)											
Social processes of encouragement, pressure, support											
Persuasive communication											
Information regarding behavior, outcome											
Personalized message											
Modelling/demonstration of behavior by others											
Homework											
Personal experiments, data collection (other than self-monitoring of behavior)											
Experiential: tasks to gain experiences to change motivation											
Feedback											

Self talk											
Use of imagery											
Perform behavior in different settings											
Shaping of behavior											
Motivational interviewing											
Relapse prevention											
Cognitive restructuring											
Relaxation											
Desensitisation											
Problem-solving											
Time management											
Identify/ prepare for difficult situation/problems											

Techniques judged to be effective in changing each construct domain

1 Social/Professional role and identity
2 Knowledge
3 Skills
4 Beliefs about capabilities
5 Beliefs about consequences
6 Motivation and goals
7 Memory, attention, decision processes
8 Environmental context and resources
9 Social influences
10 Emotion
11 Action planning

KEY[a]:

	Agreed use
	Uncertain
	Disagreement
	Agreed non-use

[a] In the study to map behavior change techniques on to behavioral determinants, four expert judges independently answered the following question by placing numbers in the cells of the matrix: "Whcih techniques would you use as part of an intervention to change each construct domain?" Response options were "blank" = No; 1 = Possibly; 2 = Probably; 3 = Definitely. Responses were collated and coded as indicated in the key to identify agreement between the four judges, or disagreement, or uncertainty (see text for further detail).

References

Ammerman, A.S., Keyserling, T.C., Atwood, J.R. et al. (2003). A randomized controlled trial of a public health nurse directed treatment program for rural patients with high blood cholesterol. *Preventive Medicine* 36: 340–351. https://doi.org/10.1016/s0091-7435(02)00042-7.

Anderson, L.W. and Krathwohl, D.R. (eds.) (2001). *A Taxonomy for Learning, Teaching, and Assessing: A Revision of Bloom's Taxonomy of Educational Objectives*. New York: Addison Wesley Longman, Inc.

Registered Nurses' Association of Ontario (2012). *Toolkit: Implementation of best practice guidelines*, 2e. Toronto, ON: Registered Nurses' Association of Ontario https://rnao.ca/sites/rnao-ca/files/RNAO_ToolKit_2012_rev4_FA.pdf.

Bloom, B.S. (1956). *Taxonomy of Educational Objectives: The Classification of Educational Goals*. New York, NY: Longmans, Green.

Bragge, P., Grimshaw, J.M., Lokker, C. et al. (2017). AIMD – a validated, simplified framework of interventions to promote and integrate evidence into health practices, systems, and policies. *BMC Medical Research Methodology* 17: 38. https://doi.org/10.1186/s12874-017-0314-8.

Cane, J., Richardson, M., Johnston, M. et al. (2015). From lists of behavior change techniques (BCTs) to structured hierarchies: comparison of two methods of developing a hierarchy of BCTs. *British Journal of Health Psychology* 20: 130–150. https://doi.org/10.1111/bjhp.12102.

Carroll, C., Patterson, M., Wood, S. et al. (2007). A conceptual framework for implementation fidelity. *Implementation Science* 2: 40. https://doi.org/10.1186/1748-5908-2-40.

Cheater, F.M., Baker, R., Reddish, S. et al. (2006). Cluster randomized controlled trial of the effectiveness of audit and feedback and educational outreach on improving nursing practice and patient outcomes. *Medical Care* 44: 542–551. https://doi.org/10.1097/01.mlr.0000215919.89893.8a.

Daniels, E.C., Bacon, J., Denisio, S. et al. (2005). Translation squared: improving asthma care for high-disparity populations through a safety net practice-based research network. *Journal of Asthma* 42: 499–505. https://doi.org/10.1081/JAS-67598.

Day, T., Wainwright, S.P., and Wilson-Barnett, J. (2001). An evaluation of a teaching intervention to improve the practice of endotracheal suctioning in intensive care units. *Journal of Clinical Nursing* 10: 682–696. https://doi.org/10.1046/j.1365-2702.2001.00519.x.

Dufault, M.A., Bielecki, C., Collins, E., and Willey, C. (1995). Changing nurses' pain assessment practice: a collaborative research utilization approach. *Journal of Advanced Nursing* 21: 634–645. https://doi.org/10.1046/j.1365-2648.1995.21040634.x.

Effective Practice and Organisation of Care (EPOC) (2015). *EPOC Taxonomy*. Available at: https://epoc.cochrane.org/epoc-taxonomy.

Elliott, T.E., Murray, D.M., Oken, M.M. et al. (1997). Improving cancer pain management in communities: main results from a randomized controlled trial. *Journal of Pain and Symptom Management* 13: 191–203. https://doi.org/10.1016/s0885-3924(96)00275-8.

Evans, D., Mellins, R., Lobach, K. et al. (1997). Improving care for minority children with asthma: professional education in public health clinics. *Pediatrics* 99: 157–164. https://doi.org/10.1542/peds.99.2.157.

Feldman, P.H., Peng, T.R., Murtaugh, C.M. et al. (2004). A randomized intervention to improve heart failure outcomes in community-based home health care. *Home Health Care Services Quarterly* 23: 1–23. https://doi.org/10.1300/J027v23n01_01.

Graham, I.D. and Logan, J. (2004). Innovations in knowledge transfer and continuity of care. *The Canadian Journal of Nursing Research* 36: 89–103.

Harrison, A., Karim, S.A., Floyd, K. et al. (2000). Syndrome packets and health worker training improve sexually transmitted disease case management in rural South Africa: randomized controlled trial. *AIDS* 14: 2769–2779. https://doi.org/10.1097/00002030-200012010-00017.

Hodl, M., Halfens, R.J.G., and Lohrmann, C. (2019). Effectiveness of conservative urinary incontinence management among female nursing home residents-A cluster RCT. *Archives of Gerontology and Geriatrics* 81: 245–251. https://doi.org/10.1016/j.archger.2019.01.003.

Hodnett, E.D., Kaufman, K., O'Brien-Pallas, L. et al. (1996). A strategy to promote research-based nursing care: effects on childbirth outcomes. *Research in Nursing and Health* 19: 13–20. https://doi.org/10.1002/(SICI)1098-240X(199602)19:1<13::AID-NUR2>3.0.CO;2-O.

Jansson, M.M., Ala-Kokko, T.I., Ohtonen, P.P. et al. (2014). Human patient simulation education in the nursing management of patients requiring mechanical ventilation: a randomized, controlled trial. *American Journal of Infection Control* 42: 271–276. https://doi.org/10.1016/j.ajic.2013.11.023.

Jansson, M.M., Syrjala, H.P., Ohtonen, P.P. et al. (2016a). Randomized, controlled trial of the effectiveness of simulation education: A 24-month follow-up study in a clinical setting. *American Journal of Infection Control* 44: 387–393. https://doi.org/10.1016/j.ajic.2015.10.035.

Jansson, M.M., Syrjala, H.P., Ohtonen, P.P. et al. (2016b). Simulation education as a single intervention does not improve hand hygiene practices: A randomized controlled follow-up study. *American Journal of Infection Control* 44: 625–630. https://doi.org/10.1016/j.ajic.2015.12.030.

Kalinowski, S., Budnick, A., Kuhnert, R. et al. (2015). Nonpharmacologic pain management interventions in German nursing homes: a cluster randomized trial. *Pain Management Nursing: Official Journal of the American Society of Pain Management Nurses* 16: 464–474. https://doi.org/10.1016/j.pmn.2014.09.002.

Kopke, S., Muhlhauser, I., Gerlach, A. et al. (2012). Effect of a guideline-based multicomponent intervention on use of physical restraints in nursing homes: a randomized controlled trial. *Journal of the American Medical Association* 307: 2177–2184. https://doi.org/10.1001/jama.2012.4517.

Lozano, P., Finkelstein, J.A., Carey, V.J. et al. (2004). A multisite randomized trial of the effects of physician education and organizational change in chronic-asthma care: health outcomes of the Pediatric Asthma Care Patient Outcomes Research Team II Study. *Archives of Pediatrics and Adolescent Medicine* 158: 875–883. https://doi.org/10.1001/archpedi.158.9.875.

Mayou, R.A., Thompson, D.R., Clements, A. et al. (2002). Guideline-based early rehabilitation after myocardial infarction. *A pragmatic randomised controlled trial. Journal of Psychosomatic Research* 52: 89–95. https://doi.org/10.1016/s0022-3999(01)00300-2.

Michie, S., Johnston, M., Francis, J. et al. (2008). From theory to intervention: mapping theoretically derived behavioral determinants to behaviour change techniques. *Applied Psychology* 57: 660–680. https://doi.org/10.1111/j.1464-0597.2008.00341.x.

Moon, K.J. and Lee, S.M. (2015). The effects of a tailored intensive care unit delirium prevention protocol: A randomized controlled trial. *International Journal of Nursing Studies* 52: 1423–1432. https://doi.org/10.1016/j.ijnurstu.2015.04.021.

Murphy, S.L. and Gutman, S.A. (2012). Intervention fidelity: a necessary aspect of intervention effectiveness studies. *American Journal of Occupational Therapy* 66: 387–388. https://doi.org/10.5014/ajot.2010.005405.

Naylor, M.D., Brooten, D.A., Campbell, R.L. et al. (2004). Transitional care of older adults hospitalized with heart failure: a randomized, controlled trial. *Journal of the American Geriatrics Society* 52: 675–684. https://doi.org/10.1111/j.1532-5415.2004.52202.x.

Noome, M., Dijkstra, B.M., van Leeuwen, E., and Vloet, L.C.M. (2017). Effectiveness of supporting intensive care units on implementing the guideline 'End-of-life care in the intensive care unit, nursing care': a cluster randomized controlled trial. *Journal of Advanced Nursing* 73: 1339–1354. https://doi.org/10.1111/jan.13219.

Pagaiya, N. and Garner, P. (2005). Primary care nurses using guidelines in Thailand: a randomized controlled trial. *Tropical Medicine and International Health* 10: 471–477. https://doi.org/10.1111/j.1365-3156.2005.01404.x.

Parker, M.T., Leggett-Frazier, N., Vincent, P.A., and Swanson, M.S. (1995). The impact of an educational program on improving diabetes knowledge and changing behaviors of nurses in long-term care facilities. *The Diabetes Educator* 21: 541–545. https://doi.org/10.1177/014572179502100608.

Pokorny, L.J., Lyle, K., Tyler, M., and Topolski, J. (1988). Introducing a modified nominal group technique for issue identification. *Evaluation Practice* 9: 40–44. https://doi.org/10.1016/S0886-1633(88)80063-1.

Premaratne, U.N., Sterne, J.A., Marks, G.B. et al. (1999). Clustered randomised trial of an intervention to improve the management of asthma: Greenwich asthma study. *BMJ: British Medical Journal / British Medical Association* 318: 1251–1255. https://doi.org/10.1136/bmj.318.7193.1251.

Snelgrove-Clarke, E., Davies, B., Flowerdew, G., and Young, D. (2015). Implementing a fetal health surveillance guideline in clinical practice: a pragmatic randomized controlled trial of action learning. *Worldviews on Evidence-Based Nursing* 12: 281–288. https://doi.org/10.1111/wvn.12117.

Titler, M.G., Herr, K., Brooks, J.M. et al. (2009). Translating research into practice intervention improves management of acute pain in older hip fracture patients. *Health Services Research* 44: 264–287. https://doi.org/10.1111/j.1475-6773.2008.00913.x, https://www.ncbi.nlm.nih.gov/pmc/articles/PMC2669630/.

Vallerand, A.H., Riley-Doucet, C., Hasenau, S.M., and Templin, T. (2004). Improving cancer pain management by homecare nurses. *Oncology Nursing Forum* 31: 809–816. https://doi.org/10.1188/04.ONF.809-816.

van Gaal, B.G., Schoonhoven, L., Mintjes, J.A. et al. (2011a). Fewer adverse events as a result of the SAFE or SORRY? programme in hospitals and nursing homes. part i: primary outcome of a cluster randomised trial. *International Journal of Nursing Studies* 48: 1040–1048. https://doi.org/10.1016/j.ijnurstu.2011.02.017.

van Gaal, B.G., Schoonhoven, L., Mintjes, J.A. et al. (2011b). The SAFE or SORRY? programme. part II: effect on preventive care. *International Journal of Nursing Studies* 48: 1049–1057. https://doi.org/10.1016/j.ijnurstu.2011.02.018.

Van Hoof, T.J. and Meehan, T.P. (2011). Integrating essential components of quality improvement into a new paradigm for continuing education. *The Journal of Continuing Education in the Health Professions* 31: 207–214. https://doi.org/10.1002/chp.20130.

von Lengerke, T., Lutze, B., Krauth, C. et al. (2017). Promoting Hand Hygiene Compliance. *Dtsch Arztebl Int* 114: 29–36. https://doi.org/10.3238/arztebl.2017.0029.

Wright, B., Turner, J.G., and Daffin, P. (1997). Effectiveness of computer-assisted instruction in increasing the rate of universal precautions--related behaviors. *American Journal of Infection Control* 25: 426–429. https://doi.org/10.1016/s0196-6553(97)90093-6.

Zhu, X., Wong, F.K.Y., and Wu, C.L.H. (2018). Development and evaluation of a nurse-led hypertension management model: A randomized controlled trial. *International Journal of Nursing Studies* 77: 171–178. https://doi.org/10.1016/j.ijnurstu.2017.10.006.

12

Field Test, Plan Evaluation, and Prepare to Launch

The last chapter highlighted the importance of targeting implementation strategies to identified barriers and drivers to optimize implementation success. It described tailoring implementation strategies which involves prioritizing the barriers and drivers, mapping implementation strategies to them and then adjusting the selected strategies to be acceptable and deliverable in the local setting. Having tailored the implementation strategies, the group is now nearly ready to do what it has been wanting to do for some time, launch the implementation initiative. There are just three more activities to complete before this should happen: field test the implementation strategies, plan the evaluation, and prepare for the launch. This chapter focuses on this last set of activities related to the Solution Building phase of Roadmap.

Goal: At this stage of Roadmap, the purpose is to ensure that all the final preparations are in place to successfully launch the implementation. Specifically, it involves: (i) field testing the implementation strategies to ensure they can be delivered and are acceptable to potential adopters of the best practice, (ii) designing the plan for how the implementation will be evaluated in terms of uptake of the best practice and impact, and (iii) determining that all the arrangements and plans are in place and that all systems are go for the implementation to be launched.

To guide and assist with activity during this stage here are several pertinent questions to use including:

Field test

- Who will the implementation strategies be tested on?
- What is the timeframe for the field test?
- What are the key field test criteria for success?
- What modifications will be needed before launching the strategies?

Plan Evaluation

- Are all the relevant stakeholders involved in developing the plan?
- What is the purpose(s) of the evaluation?
- What are the evaluation questions?
- What type of evaluation is being planned?

Knowledge Translation in Nursing and Healthcare: A Roadmap to Evidence-informed Practice, First Edition.
Margaret B. Harrison and Ian D. Graham.
© 2021 John Wiley & Sons, Inc. Published 2021 by John Wiley & Sons, Inc.

- What indicators and data sources will be used?
- What is the timeframe for the evaluation?

Prepare Launch

- Has a launch checklist been assembled?
- Are all systems go for the launch? If not, have all remaining/outstanding issues been addressed?

Field Test Implementation Strategies

Although not always required, we do encourage field testing of the implementation strategies before launching an organization-wide or region-wide implementation. Especially if it is a large-scale implementation it is often necessary to test procedures, processes, decision making algorithms, or training information and materials with relevant target users before making significant changes. The field test will give a sense of how the implementation strategies are received in the field and identify potential issues with delivering them that may not have been previously contemplated.

Most importantly, using the results of the field test will guide any modifications to the strategies or how they are delivered before going live. Figuring out and solving the potential glitches can, in the long run, avoid embarrassment, delays and incomplete or ineffective implementation. Furthermore, a false start can undermine confidence in, and the credibility of, the working group. Field testing is also of value should the group underestimate the ease with which an implementation strategy can be implemented. For example, with an educational implementation strategy that needs to involve all staff, timing and scheduling educational sessions and ensuring those on days off or on leave still get the sessions may be more complex than anticipated and a trial run may identify potential challenges. Similarly, a field test may reveal that an expertly planned education session involving for example, role play is a complete flop as participants refuse to role play.

According to the Merriam-Webster dictionary, a field test is defined as a "test (a procedure, a product, etc.) in actual situations reflecting intended use" (Merriam-Webster.com Dictionary 2020). We prefer this term to other similar terms such as feasibility or pilot testing as it emphasizes the test is conducted in the field (real world setting) with potential adopters or users of the best practice that is being implemented. The terms feasibility and pilot testing are sometimes used interchangeably and inconsistently in the literature, often causing confusion (Arain et al. 2010). Both terms are typically used in relation to a subsequent study or research while field testing of implementation strategies may simply be part of implementing best practice and not about preparing to undertake a larger research study or trial of implementation. We agree with Whitehead et al. (2014) who propose that feasibility studies should refer to all preliminary work prior to a subsequent study or implementation and the term pilot be reserved for studies that mimic a definitive trial design, with an intention for further work, and a focus on trial processes (Whitehead et al. 2014). With these definitions, all pilot studies are feasibility studies but not all feasibility studies are pilot studies.

Before discussing field testing it may be useful to briefly discuss the purposes of feasibility and pilot studies and how they differ. It is possible that the working group may decide either of these types of studies would be more appropriate to use. Pilot studies typically evaluate feasibility of recruitment, retention, and implementation of an intervention to be tested in a larger study (Leon et al. 2011). They are "small-scale tests of the methods and procedures to be used on a larger scale" and importantly, are not powered to provide definite answers to effectiveness and should never be used to test effectiveness (National Center for Complementary and Integrative Health 2017). When conducting a pilot study, it is important to determine clear benchmarks for measures by which the pilot is considered feasible for expansion (National Center for Complementary and Integrative Health 2017). For more information on pilot studies and how to conduct them please refer to Smith and Harrison (2009), Leon et al. (2011) and National Center for Complementary and Integrative Health (2017).

In contrast, feasibility studies (the broader concept) are typically not about undertaking a mini trial-run of the future larger study of interest, but rather are more about determining the practicality of a proposed initiative, project or implementation. Bowen et al. (2009) propose eight general areas of focus for feasibility studies: (i) *acceptability* (how do intended recipients – both targets of the intervention and those implementing it – react to the intervention), (ii) *demand for the intervention*, (iii) *implementation* (the extent, likelihood, and manner in which an intervention can be implemented as proposed), (iv) *practicality* (extent to which the intervention can be delivered with the given time, resources, and commitments), (v) *adaptation* (describe modifications that are made to the intervention), (vi) *integration* (assesses the level of system change needed to integrate the intervention, including documentation of changes within the organization that occur as a result of the implementation), (vii) *expansion* (examines the potential for success of an already successful intervention with a different population or setting), and (viii) *limited-efficacy testing* (feasibility studies designed to test an intervention in a limited way, e.g. convenience samples and shorter time frames). The Bowen et al. (2009) paper is a good resource on developing feasibility studies. In our field tests we seldom assess all these areas and what is key is for the working group and relevant stakeholders to consider and prioritize the areas the field test should cover.

Turning to our concept of field testing, we borrow elements from both feasibility and pilot studies. Field tests can be considered a form of feasibility study but are not a pilot test using the definitions above. The purposes of field testing we have undertaken are primarily to: (i) determine whether the implementation strategies can be delivered with fidelity, (ii) collect preliminary data on whether the strategies are working as expected, and (iii) assess acceptance of (and satisfaction with) the strategies to the potential adopters of best practice and other stakeholders. We have also used them to determine whether the selected indicators of knowledge use and impact to evaluate implementation can be collected as anticipated. Our approach is also akin to a formative evaluation which is used to ensure that a program or implementation strategy is feasible, appropriate, and acceptable before it is fully implemented (Centers for Disease Control and Prevention 2007).

Criteria for determining whether the field test is successful must be identified prior to conducting the field test. If the predetermined field test "success criteria" are met, then the implementation strategies would be deemed ready for launch. If some or all of the success criteria are not met, then the group must consider what changes need to be made to the implementation strategies or their delivery methods before being ready to launch. If major modifications are required, the group may decide it is necessary to conduct a second field test of the revised strategies before proceeding. If the modifications are considered minor then there may not be a need to re-field test.

Typically, implementation strategies are field tested on convenience or purposefully selected samples (rather than random samples), as the intent is to produce an understanding of the issues rather than necessarily generalizable findings. The purpose is to determine whether the implementation strategies are being deployed as expected and whether the implementation is occurring as anticipated. This general feedback on the implementation process is also very similar to what is done with usability testing (Wikipedia contributors 2020). For example, for an education implementation strategy, the goal would be to have a group of potential adopters of the best practice take the educational sessions. The audience or learners for the sessions could be staff from a particular unit, or a team, or several purposefully selected healthcare providers (e.g. novices through to expert practitioners). Having diversity in the sample can enrich the test findings. The intent would be to run the participants through the entire educational process (which might involve participating in multiple sessions, role playing, practicing, etc.). Assessment could include both the participants' acceptance of the education sessions as well as satisfaction with it. Measuring changes in conceptual knowledge use following the sessions could also be done to get a sense of what participants learned from the sessions. Also, the fidelity with which the educational sessions were delivered could be assessed. Use the measures/indicators of fidelity the group decided on (see the previous chapter). All the findings from the field test are then used to determine whether the educational sessions require any modifications or whether the way they were delivered needs adjusting. Criteria for determining the field test success might be something like, at least 75% of intended participants attended >90% of the sessions, mean scores on knowledge tests were >75%, >80 of participants were satisfied with the sessions and found them useful, and/or educators covered >90% of the syllabus for each session.

If the implementation strategy was more a barriers' management strategy (i.e. an organizational strategy) such as audit and feedback, the field test would involve running the audit and feedback process for some period of time with a sample of potential end users. This would be done to determine whether the auditing data can be captured and processed as anticipated, whether the feedback process as it was designed works as it should, whether the health care providers and their supervisors are happy with the feedback process and will be able to and inclined to use it. Criteria for determining the success of the audit and feedback field test could be things like, >95% of the audit data is retrieved and synthesized, the feedback reports are 100% accurate, > 90% of supervisors and staff find the feedback reports and the entire audit and feedback process acceptable and satisfactory.

Box 12.1 Are you ready to go?

With one project, part of the implementation strategy involved running a wound care clinic. One of the a priori criteria for determining when the clinic was fully functional was wait times for appointments being less than 15 minutes. As part of the field test, several patients were given clinic appointments. The waiting times were longer than 15 minutes so more patients were scheduled until the average wait time was less than 15 minutes. At this point the clinic was ready to be officially opened. The field test revealed the clinic staff needed a few weeks to get the clinic operating efficiently which is not uncommon when activating complex implementation strategies.

Plan the Evaluation

Conducting an evaluation of the initiative is critical for understanding how the implementation is happening (or not), to be able to make any course adjustments informed by evaluation data, to explain how implementation strategies work, and to be able to make judgments about the success or failure of the implementation. Planning the evaluation is therefore an essential component of the Solutions Building phase of Roadmap. It goes without saying that an evaluation plan needs to be developed prior to the launch, and for transparency, needs to take the form of a written document that stakeholders can review and comment on. If the working group does not have members with adequate methodological expertise (or could simply benefit from more such expertise – many hands make light work), now is the time to bring in methodologists, epidemiologists, biostatisticians, qualitative researchers as well as individuals from the quality improvement department to help with evaluation planning.

Guiding questions for planning an evaluation include:

- What is the purpose(s) of the evaluation?
- Who are the intended users of the evaluation? Who needs to be involved in evaluation planning? Is there stakeholder consensus on the evaluation plan? What are their evaluation questions?
- What is the evaluation design?
- What indicators, data sources and data collection methods will be used?
- What is the timeline for the evaluation?
- Have adequate resources been obtained for the evaluation?
- Have the relevant authorities signed off on the evaluation plan?

In this section, our intent is to provide a high-level overview of what should be considered in an evaluation plan, not to describe all the methods and nuances of conducting the evaluation. For details on conducting evaluations please refer to Appendix 12.A and 12.B.

We see five main purposes for undertaking an evaluation (Centers for Disease Control and Prevention 2007): (i) to ensure that an implementation program/initiative is feasible, appropriate, and acceptable before it is fully implemented and to improve it before it is launched (this is a formative evaluation and is what we consider the purpose of the field test), (ii) to determine whether the implementation strategies have been implemented as intended and to understand the implementation process (process or implementation evaluation), (iii) to measure the effects of the implementation program and to determine whether it has achieved its objectives – uptake of the best practices (outcome/effectiveness evaluation – sometimes referred to as summative evaluation), (iv) to determine impact of the implementation on health and other outcomes of interest (impact evaluation, sometimes referred to as summative evaluation) (Centers for Disease Control and Prevention 2007; Bowen 2012), and (v) to assess costs relative to effects (economic evaluation) (Quinn and Ward 2013; Cidav et al. 2020; Severens et al. 2020).

In recent years, process/implementation evaluation has also been advanced as a means of understanding how complex interventions work in the field of implementation science (Gale et al. 2019a, b; Holdsworth et al. 2020; Moore et al. 2015; Limbani et al. 2019). Thinking back to the elements of the Knowledge to Action Framework of monitor knowledge use and evaluate outcomes (impact) there are a couple of points to mention. Monitoring knowledge use or measuring adherence to best practice would fall under the concept of outcomes/effectiveness evaluation of the implementation strategies as this information is used to determine if the tailored implementation strategies are producing the uptake of the best practice in your setting. If practice is not changing to come in line with the best practice recommendations, it means the implementation strategies are not working (are not effective) and need to be intensified, modified, or changed and/or additional ones adopted that better address the identified barriers. In other words, the information from the outcomes/effectiveness evaluation is used to inform changes to the implementation plan. Measuring impact of the implementation initiative provides information on which to judge the ultimate value of the initiative, i.e. the extent to which implementing best practice has improved (or not) health, healthcare provider or health system outcomes of interest. Thinking about the goal of each type of evaluation and what information is needed for the initiative will help determine the scope of the evaluation.

Often evaluation of implementation projects is seen as a quality improvement exercise to provide information to guide local decisions, while at other times the evaluation is designed and conducted as research with the additional purpose of generating generalizable knowledge. This is not to say that doing an evaluation under the rubric of quality improvement cannot also adopt experimental or quasi experimental evaluation designs (Cook and Campbell 1979). Many of the evaluations we have conducted have been framed as research and published (Harrison et al. 2002, 2005), but this was largely because of our roles as academics and expectations that we conduct research. Being able to apply for research funding to undertake the evaluations was also another motivation for framing the evaluations as research. The grants provided additional resources to allow us and the settings to conduct more comprehensive evaluations and to build the implementation science knowledge base.

A number of steps in evaluation planning that the group should consider following is below (Bowen 2012).

Box 12.2   Don't let perfection be the enemy of progress

Our advice in a nutshell – use the most relevant evaluation design and methods and make the evaluation as rigorous as it needs to be to achieve its purpose. When the evaluation is done as research rather than as quality improvement, institutional research ethics approval should be obtained. When in doubt about whether the evaluation requires ethics approval or not, it is always best to confer with the research ethics board before proceeding.

Consider the Purpose(s) of the Evaluation

An evaluation plan should start with defining the purpose of the evaluation. The group needs to discuss all the purposes and prioritize them. Some members of the group may be more interested in implementation process, others with whether adherence with best practice has changed, still others may be more interested in impact. What is critical to know?

What are the available resources for the evaluation? What can be achieved in the time available? These are all important issues the group needs to grapple with as they scope out the evaluation. Defining the purpose or purposes will help determine whether a process, outcome/effectiveness, or impact evaluation, or some combination of them is most appropriate and doable in your setting.

Identify Intended Users of the Evaluation and Their Evaluation Questions

As with every aspect of Roadmap, being attentive to who needs to be involved and involving them can have implications for the success of the evaluation but also and very importantly, the use of the results coming from the evaluation. The group overseeing the evaluation may be the working group, or another group assembled specifically to plan the evaluation. Another option is to create an evaluation steering committee to support the working group with this task. During the planning, there is value in engaging managers as this is one group that has access to resources and has an interest in evidence-informed practice. Knowing their issues and concerns means it is possible to ensure the evaluation addresses their questions. For example, if they are preoccupied with costs related to implementation and return on investment, the evaluation can collect data on these issues and provide evidence of whether the implementation is affordable or good value for money. Similarly, patients may be particularly interested in the impact of implementation on them so this could be built into the evaluation. Thinking about who will use the evaluation findings and for what purposes allows the group to build the evaluation to address the end users' need for data. This is what Michael Quinn Patton refers to as "Utilization Focused Evaluation" (Patton 2008), a concept many have built further on, and one that is very relevant to Roadmap. We always make this a foundation as we assist with evaluations. For example, will the implementors want to use evaluation findings to improve implementation? Will managers want information to decide on whether to continue resourcing implementation strategies? Will the hospital board want information from the evaluation to show how care is meeting best practice benchmarks? Will administrators want to use information for accreditation purposes? The group will need to consider all the evaluation questions and information needs, prioritize the questions, and reach consensus on what is critical for the evaluation to focus on taking into consideration feasibility and practicality issues. As we know, a useful strategy for bridging the gap between research and practice is to build commitment to (and "ownership of") the evaluation findings by those in a position to act on them (Cargo and Mercer 2008).

Decide on Evaluation Design

The group will initially need to decide whether the evaluation falls more along the lines of quality improvement or research. Table 12.1 illustrates some of the similarities and differences. The nature of the evaluation also figures into design considerations since process/implementation evaluations are typically about following and understanding what is happening in real time (or trying to understand what was happening during the implementation period) where outcome/effectiveness and impact evaluations can use experimental and quasi research designs but can also be done with observational study

Table 12.1 Illustrating differences in approach and emphasis between quality improvement and implementation research.

Quality Improvement	Implementation Research
Process outcomes	Process and Impact outcomes
Error reduction	Effective care/outcomes improvement
Variation reduction	Adoption of best practice, for consistency, improved care, and outcomes
Short turn around	Intermediate, longer timeframe
QI team	Investigator team, organization members (end users)
Institutional Ethics approval may or may not be required	Institutional Ethics review and approval required
Internally funded	Internal and/or externally funded
Industry or clinical standards	Scientific standards

designs. An observational design is a descriptive or correlation study that investigates a phenomenon without trying to change anything (e.g. a cross-sectional study design without a control or a qualitative study) while an experimental or quasi-experimental design (such as randomized controlled trial, cluster randomized controlled trial, interrupted time series, etc.) manipulates exposure to an intervention (or implementation strategy in our case). For each evaluation purpose and evaluation question the group will need to make decisions about the most appropriate evaluation design to use – will it use an observational or experimental or quasi-experimental design, or will it focus on adherence to the best practice (outcome/effectiveness evaluation) or impact (impact evaluation)? (Shadish et al. 2001; Lu 2009; Rezigalla 2020).

Select Indicators, Data Sources and Collection Methods

Thinking about past stages of Roadmap, the group has already made many decisions about what data to collect and how. For example, when the group was selecting and customizing the best practice to implement, it also identified indicators of how to measure adherence or uptake which can be used in the outcome/effectiveness evaluation. The group has also already identified measures of fidelity of implementation strategy delivery that can be used as part of the process evaluation. The group has determined indicators of conceptual and instrumental knowledge use (best practice adherence) that can be used for an outcome/effectiveness evaluation as well as impact indicators that can be used for an impact evaluation. In the previous stages, when these measures were considered and selected, the group also discussed data sources and how to collect the data (using the electronic health record, chart audit or other administrative databases, or primary data collection [surveys, interviews, etc.] or by observation, for example). Now the group may need to carefully (re) consider the data sources and data collection methods to ensure they remain feasible, appropriate, and affordable.

Evaluation Timeline, Resources, and Sign Off

Thinking through the timeline for the evaluation can be a useful exercise. For a process evaluation, the intent is often to collect data during the implementation period which means being ready to collect data as soon as the implementation is launched or even earlier if pre- or baseline data are needed. For outcomes/effectiveness and impact evaluations, in addition to any baseline data collection, data need to be collected post implementation. Thought needs to go into how long to wait to collect the post implementation data. Sufficient time must be given for potential adopters to start using the best practice and even longer is usually needed to be able to capture impact data.

During every step of the evaluation planning process, the group must also be attentive to evaluation costs and the availability of resources to undertake the evaluation. Conducting evaluations involves resources and expenditures for collecting data (e.g. if there is a fee to access health record data or if someone is needed to audit charts), providing the data (e.g. staff time to complete surveys or participate in interviews), and for analyzing the data. These resource implications can also affect decisions about the nature and type of evaluation that the group is able to conduct. The evaluation is a critical component of the implementation initiative as described above as it may provide data on the value of the initiative and therefore should be resourced accordingly. Regrettably, evaluation is often an after-thought and inadequately resourced because the bulk of available funding goes into creating and delivering the implementation strategies. Use the evaluation plan to raise the importance and profile of the evaluation with key stakeholders and to build the case for the need for adequate resources to undertake it. See Table 12.2 for a sample evaluation planning and reporting template suggested by Sarah Bowen (Bowen 2012). This can be used to plan and report on the evaluation.

Finally, the group should seek the sign off for the evaluation plan from the relevant authorities or stakeholders. This step ensures there is consensus on the evaluation questions and methods and that nothing has been left out of the evaluation that is important to the key stakeholders. It also means, the authorities are aware of the cost involved and have signed off on those as well.

As mentioned, our approach to evaluation has been greatly influenced by Patton's utilization focused evaluation (Better Evaluation). This type of evaluation is specifically designed to generate information that stakeholders can use in their decision-making about the program or implementation. Utilization focused evaluations emphasize early and meaningful engagement with key stakeholders and build in strategies to promote "buy in" and use of the evaluation findings (Bowen 2012). Bowen has observed that there are

Table 12.2 Sample evaluation planning and reporting template.

A) Background: Summary of initiative

B) Evaluation Purpose: Why is evaluation being undertaken?

C) Intended Use of Evaluation: How will results be used?

D) Intended Users: Who are intended users of the evaluation? What other stakeholders should be involved in some way?

E) Evaluation Focus

F) Evaluation Methods (can include Table 12.3 evaluation matrix)

---

similarities in principle and approach between integrated knowledge translation and utilization-focused evaluation. Namely that both keep utilization (of evaluation results or research findings) prominent through all phases of the process, promote research and evaluation conducted in response to stakeholder identified needs, promote early and meaningful involvement of the intended users of the research or evaluation activity and view the evaluator/researcher as a member of a collaborative team.

We have found it useful when working with groups, to develop an evaluation planning matrix that lays out the key elements of the evaluation and how the components of the evaluation line up (Table 12.3). The matrix we use was inspired by one initially developed by Bowen (2012).

Before moving on to preparing for the launch, we are going to quickly review a common implementation evaluation framework and describe some implementation study designs.

Table 12.3 Example evaluation planning matrix.

Purpose of evaluation	Evaluation questions	Evaluation design and methods	Indicators	Data sources	Data collection methods	Evaluation timeframe	Responsibility/ resources
Process/implementation evaluation							
Outcome/effectiveness evaluation							
Impact evaluation							

RE-AIM

RE-AIM is a common implementation planning and evaluation framework. RE-AIM stands for Reach, Efficacy, Adoption, Implementation, Maintenance. It was initially published in 1999 to evaluate public health interventions and has become a widely used evaluation framework (Glasgow et al. 1999; Harden et al. 2015, 2020; Kwan et al. 2019, 2020; RE-AIM 2020; Shelton et al. 2020).

The elements of the framework are:

- Reach – Who is the intended audience for the implementation strategies, and did we reach them?
- Effectiveness/efficacy – What was the impact of the best practices on outcomes?

- Adoption – What and how many settings have made use of the best practices?
- Implementation – What is the extent to which the desired behavior (the clinical intervention) has been used?
- Maintenance – To what extent has the best practices continued to be used over time?

The RE-AIM website (http://www.re-aim.org) describes the framework and maintains a repository of tools, measures, related publications, other resources, and online training. The framework is particularly useful when implementing public health interventions.

Implementation Science Study Designs

There is growing literature on implementation study designs (Brown et al. 2017; Mazzucca et al. 2018) and if the group is interested in these, it should ensure it has access to the appropriate methodological expertise. Within the field of implementation science there is growing interest in what are known as hybrid study designs. There are essentially three hybrid study types:

- Type 1 are used to test the effects of a clinical intervention on relevant outcomes while observing and gathering information on implementation
- Type 2 simultaneously test clinical and implementation strategies
- Type 3 test an implementation strategy while observing and gathering information on the clinical intervention's impact on relevant outcomes (Curran et al. 2012; Bernet et al. 2013; Landes et al. 2019)

Others have expanded the combination and permutations of these three hybrid designs (Kemp et al. 2019) illustrating how many dozens of hybrid study designs are available and why a methodologist may need to be consulted.

Another study design that has become popular is stepped wedge cluster randomized trial (Brown and Lilford 2006; Beard et al. 2015; Copas et al. 2015). This study design involves sequentially rolling-out of a clinical intervention or implementation strategy to practices, units, organizations (cluster). The timing of when the clusters receive the intervention/strategy is randomly selected. The advantage of this study design is that each cluster serves as its own control so by the end of the study all clusters have received the intervention/strategy.

If the group is interested in more complex evaluation designs, there are a number of slide presentations on the web that provide basic information about these types of study designs. See, for example, *Innovative Study Designs for Implementation Research* (Curran 2017) and *Designs for Dissemination and Implementation Research for Small Populations* (Kilbourne n.d.).

Prepare to Launch

After months of preparation and planning that is part of Phase 2 of Roadmap, the working group will be eager to start implementing the best practice. By now the group has field tested the implementation strategies that were tailored to the local context, made any necessary modifications to the strategies or how they are delivered, and if required, undertaken another field test. The group has also developed an evaluation plan. At this point the working group essentially needs to develop a launch checklist and then go through it to determine if all systems are go for launch of the implementation strategies. Questions guiding this stage include:

- Have managers and leaders in the organization endorsed the implementation plan?
- Is stakeholder support in place and critical relationships with key players established?
- Are the necessary facilities, equipment and resources secured and in place?
- Have all the relevant adopters been trained?
- Is the evaluation plan sorted out and in place?

Although by this point there is usually a general feeling that everything is ready to launch, we have found it prudent to have the working group pause and systematically assess launch readiness. The group should consider all the relevant launch issues (what is required for successful implementation) and develop a launch checklist that it will systematically use to determine if everything is truly in order and ready for implementation. The concept of the implementation launch checklist is like the checklists that airplane pilots go through just prior to take off to make sure that all system are go. It is always prudent to do one last check to make sure every implementation detail has been attended to and nothing has been missed in the haste to implement. The critical factors that need to be in place prior to widespread implementation will depend on the nature of the best practice being implemented, the implementation strategies being deployed and the nature of the local context. For example, is it something simple that health care providers can easily implement? or does it require more complex changes within the organization? It also relates to the nature of the implementation strategies (and their complexity). The size and clinical diversity of the group (various levels of nursing or interprofessional team) whose practice is to change also plays into this. The more people who need to adopt the best practice, the longer it will take adoption to occur as each one will need to learn about the best practice and start using it.

Things to include in a launch checklist include criteria related to all the components of the implementation strategies which need to be in place (e.g. have changes in the documentation system been made and are working, is the needed equipment in place, etc.).

Table 12.4 presents a rudimentary launch checklist classified by the Ottawa Model of Research Use (OMRU) barriers categories that can be adapted by the working group.

After the group has developed the launch checklist, it should be included in the written implementation plan. Responsible people should be nominated to carry out the check.

Before moving to the launch, complete the Action Map with the activities undertaken and decisions about the evaluation made in this pre-launch phase. Table 12.5 continues with the wound care example. It would be prudent to update your Implementation Plan to consider resources and expenditures required for the launch and evaluation process.

Table 12.4 Example of launch checklist.

Barriers management

• Managers and leaders are on board and committed to the best practice and the implementation plan	Yes	No
• Stakeholders on are board (staff, patients, partners have endorsed the best practice)	Yes	No
• Necessary resources have been acquired to deliver the best practice	Yes	No
• Necessary space/infrastructure/equipment have been acquired	Yes	No
• Evaluation plan has been signed off	Yes	No
• Communications with all staff, patients, partners about the implementation has been approved and disseminated (e.g. all members of interdisciplinary teams have been made aware of the best practice and its potential impact on the team/their discipline)	Yes	No

Knowledge transfer strategies

• The field test was successful	Yes	No
• Modifications to the implementation strategies, or their delivery have been complete	Yes	No
• Educational implementation strategies are ready for implementation	Yes	No
• Staff delivering the educational strategies are prepared to deliver the program	Yes	No
• Practice reminder accessories (e.g. unit poster, pocket cards) are in place	Yes	No

Maintenance strategies

• Resources and process are in place to update best practices as new evidence evolves	Yes	No
• Data collection process needed for indicators of uptake and impact are in place and operational	Yes	No
• Contingency plans are ready if key champions leave, retire (e.g. a process for grooming people is in place)	Yes	No
• Resources and process are in place to continue to deliver the educational strategies following initial implementation to keep people trained up	Yes	No

Summary

With the field test completed, the evaluation plan in place, and the launch checklist gone through, the group is now ready to move on to Phase 3 of Roadmap and put all the Solution Building preparation and planning into action. The next chapter offers advice on the action stages of launch and evaluate.

Table 12.5 Phase 2: ACTION MAP for solution building (*with Wound Example*).

Customized best practice recommendations	Barriers and facilitating factors (drivers)	Implementation Strategies and Field Testing
1. Evening shift RN to daily conduct head to toe skin assessment during HS care and document in flow chart	Factors related to each recommendation, potential adopters, or context. *What would aid or prevent implementation?*	Implementation strategies are mapped, tailored and field tested.
	Most nurses familiar with head-to-toe skin assessment	On unit education briefing during evening shifts to ensure all staff are aware of best practice
	Not in orientation for new staff	Add best practice to Staff Orientation
	HS routine happens with every patient so will be incremental extra	Chart audit for assessment. Indicator: 90% of patients should be assessed on evening shift
2. Braden Risk assessment conducted with head to toe skin assessment by attending RN on evening shift daily and documented in nursing notes	Staff on several units not familiar with risk assessment scale (6 sub-scales), questioning total score, perceived as a lot of work	On-unit education in identified areas plus handout materials (flyer, pocket cards). Clinical shadowing with someone trained
	Not in orientation for new staff	Add education module to Staff Orientation
		Hold consultation on how to make it even more easy to chart and use subscale deficit(s) and to decide on clinical interventions to address patient deficits identified by subscales
		Chart audit for assessment. Indicator: 90% of patients should be assessed on evening shift
3. etc.		
Sustainability thinking continues here. . .	Barriers assessment conducted such that it can be redone in future, if necessary.	Implementation strategies selected in part based on being able to continue them in future.
	Target implementation strategies to known barriers and drivers to improve the uptake and ongoing maintenance.	Use all data and info for ongoing maintenance, planning and evaluation.
Chapter 8	Chapters 8 and 9	Chapters 10 (+ appendix), 11, 12

Appendices: Conceptual and Measurement Issues Related to Implementation Evaluation

Appendix 12.A: Some Background Information About Evaluation

Evaluation is a critical component of Roadmap in that the results of evaluation are used to determine the success of the implementation and to guide efforts to maintain or sustain implementation success. In Roadmap, planning for evaluation takes place during Phase 2 – Build Solutions and Field Test them while the actual evaluation occurs in Phase 3 after the implementation strategies are launched. Furthermore, elements of evaluation are part of multiple stages of Phase 2. For example, selecting knowledge use (adherence/outcomes) and impact indicators or measures to be used may initially occur early when determining the evidence-practice gap. During the stage of customization of best practice to the local context, we advise selecting or developing indicators of knowledge use and impact related to each best practice recommendation. This is to know what to measure in future and help hone the measures. This comes up as well when customizing the best practice recommendations to be more actionable and measurable. The exercise of creating indicators for best practice recommendations encourages more careful thought about the wording of the recommendations so that the recommended behaviors are precisely stated and measurable. Finally, measuring knowledge use and impact is critical to the stage that involves planning the evaluation of implementation. It is at this stage that the group should be determining what and how to measure the future extent of best practice use as well as the impact it may be having at relevant levels (individual/family, provider, organization, health system).

What follows is a discussion of some of the conceptual and methodological issues related to monitoring best practice use, measuring impact of best practice, and issues related to developing indicators of knowledge use and impact. This information is foundational and is useful when the group is making decisions during Phases 1 and 2 of Roadmap. By its very nature, the content of this Appendix is more theoretical, but the core concepts are important to know about as they will facilitate planning and carrying out the evaluation.

Knowledge Use and Impact

Conceptual and Methodical Issues with Measuring Best Practice

The following discussion draws heavily on two book chapters we have written (Straus et al. 2009; Graham et al. 2010). Evidence-informed practice (best practice) is a type of knowledge use, with the knowledge being used in this case (best practice), derived from research. Recall the Knowledge to Action (K2A) Framework (Graham et al. 2006), there are two stages related to measurement: monitor knowledge use (use or adherence of best practice that ultimately relates to individuals' decision making and behavior) and evaluate impact (originally labeled as outcomes in the K2A framework) of best practice use. Impact is what results from use of the best practice, i.e. patient health outcomes, provider outcomes (e.g. satisfaction with work), and organization or system outcomes (e.g. improved, more efficient and cost-effective delivery of care).

Knowledge Use

In the literature, knowledge use is sometimes referred to as adherence to the best practice or process measures. It is only through measuring knowledge use that it is possible to know the extent to which a best practice has been adopted (cognitively accepted) and is used (put into practice). Best practice uptake is typically complex and relates to knowing about the best practice, having skills to perform it, acquiring positive attitudes and perceptions about it, its integration into decision making and practice, followed hopefully by, the best practice being applied in practice. All these factors can influence the success of implementation.

Stages of Change

Some time ago, Grol and Wensing (2005) reviewed 10 models and theories of stages or steps in the change process originating from different disciplines. This analysis revealed how remarkably similar they all were. All the stages of change models differentiate between conceptual knowledge use (becoming aware of the innovation e.g. stages labeled: awareness, comprehension, seeking information), increasing one's knowledge (stages labeled: knowledge, understanding, skills), forming positive attitudes (stages labeled: attitude formation, attitude change, agreement, positive attitude), developing intentions to use (stages labeled: decision, intention to change) and instrumental use (initial and ongoing use labeled: initial implementation, behavior change, change of practice and sustained implementation, consolidation, maintenance of change, routine adherence). Grol and Wensing's own model of the process of change for care providers and teams consists of orientation (promote awareness, stimulate interest), insight (create understanding), acceptance (develop positive attitudes, a motivation for change, create positive intentions or decision to change), change (promote actual adoption into practice), and maintenance (integrate new practice into routines) (Grol and Wensing 2004). All of these models illustrate how knowledge use can be conceptualized as a continuum running from awareness, understanding, attitudes and decision making/intentions (conceptual use) through to practice and policy change (instrumental use) (Figure 12.A.1).

Monitoring knowledge use, especially in real time during the implementation phase, can help identify when implementation is sub-optimal and cue the group that they should further explore the barriers and supports to best practice uptake and take action to refine the implementation strategies to overcome the barriers and strengthen the drivers. Measuring and determining knowledge use is still in its infancy so there is no one tried and true

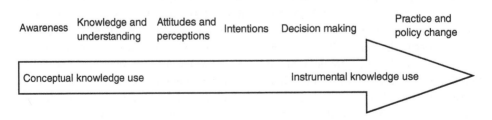

Figure 12.A.1 Phases of Knowledge Use.

Box 12.A.1   Unanticipated barriers

With one nursing guideline implementation initiative, educational strategies were deployed and appeared to be working (the nurses knew the best practice and were positive about it) yet adherence to the guideline was not improving. On further investigation it became evident that physicians following a medical guideline, rendered patients ineligible for the nursing best practice. Discussions between nursing and medicine helped to identify when each guideline should be most appropriately applied to patients. Monitoring adherence rates alerted the implementation group to an unanticipated emergent barrier to adoption of the new guideline that they were then able to develop an implementation strategy for.

---

approach. As is often the case, the definition of knowledge use depends on what one considers the "knowledge" of interest and how one defines "use," and these are both in the eye of the implementor and potential adopter.

In our chapter entitled, Measuring Outcomes of Evidence-based Practice: Distinguishing Between Knowledge Use and its Impact (Graham et al. 2010), we describe several models or classifications of knowledge use that have grouped knowledge use as either: conceptual (indirect), instrumental (direct), or symbolic (persuasive or strategic) use (Weiss 1979; Larsen 1980; Beyer and Harrison 1982; Dunn 1983; Estabrooks 1999). We have found this classification useful in deciding about implementation strategies as well as in determining evaluation approaches.

Conceptual or indirect knowledge use refers to knowledge that informs or influences the way people (e.g. health care providers or patients) think about or conceptualize issues (this includes the notion of enlightenment). Conceptual knowledge only occurs at a cognitive (thinking) level and precedes behavior although it can influence behavior. Measures of conceptual use of knowledge include comprehension, attitudes, changes in decision making and intentions to follow best practice.

Instrumental or behavioral knowledge use is about knowledge that influences action or behavior (i.e. direct use of best practice as revealed by behavior or practice changes). Adherence to best practice as determined by process of care indicators is a measure of instrumental knowledge use.

Symbolic (persuasive or strategic) knowledge use involves using research as a political or persuasive tool to legitimize and sustain predetermined positions. When it is about using the evidence that underpins a best practice to persuade others to accept the best practice (conceptual knowledge use) and use it (instrumental knowledge use) it can be considered "good" symbolic knowledge use. In fact, symbolic knowledge use is actually an implementation strategy that should be used in learning health organizations striving to be evidence-informed. However, the reason that symbolic knowledge use has not always been seen in a positive light, is that symbolic knowledge use has, more often than not, been invoked to bring about a specific change, when the evidence cited to persuade is incomplete or taken out of context. In other words, selective research evidence is deliberately used to persuade others to change (when the totality of the evidence does not actually support the alleged best practice). Symbolic knowledge use when used in this way is akin to propaganda and is manipulative and antithetical to evidence-informed practice.

We find it useful to differentiate conceptual, instrumental and symbolic knowledge use when planning and implementing best practice. As described above, conceptual use of knowledge implies changes in understanding, attitudes, decision making, and intentions. Knowing about best practice could change thinking and be considered in decision making but not result in practice or policy change for a number for reasons. Reasons for this include the change is simply not prudent to make at this time (competing priorities), the required equipment or infrastructure electronic health record is not available to support doing the best practice, or the chaotic healthcare environment causes motivated providers to simply forget to apply the best practice to name a few. From an evidence-informed practice perspective, the aim would be to have conceptual knowledge use become the impetus for instrumental use. For example, a practitioner becomes knowledgeable about a best practice, understands the supporting evidence and believes it, develops both positive attitudes toward it and intentions to want to do it which in turn motivates action (instrumental use). It is also important to remember that use of best practice (instrumental knowledge use) can also occur in the absence of conceptual use of the best practice (positive attitudes toward it or intentions to use it). For example, staff can be pressured to use a best practice and may comply even if they do not believe in the best practice or would rather not do it. This is more likely to occur when there are strong incentives to adopt an evidence-based practice (or disincentives to carry on with current practice), even when a provider may be skeptical or unaware of the underlying evidence for the practice or believe that it will not accrue its expected benefits. Our view is that this sort of approach can be counter-productive as evidence-informed practice should be premised on individuals making decisions based on the evidence which they accept, not on being coerced or inappropriately incentivized to follow it.

Instrumental knowledge use is the application of knowledge in practice. An example of instrumental knowledge use is when knowledge that has been transformed into a usable form such as a best practice is applied. An example of instrument knowledge use would be nurses using the Braden Scale to assess risk for pressure injury.

Complete or Partial Knowledge Use

There is one more issue to consider, regardless of whether it is conceptual or instrumental; knowledge use may be complete or partial. For example, best practice may consist of multiple recommendations, providers may be aware of all of them or only some, they may know how to do all of them or only some of them, they may view all of them positively or view only some of positively, they may use all of them in decision making or only consider some of them, and they may apply all the recommendations in practice or only some of them. It is further complicated when thinking about instrumental knowledge use (doing the best practice). All best practice recommendations can be applied all the time or some of them can be used all the time or some recommendations can be used some of the time. In other words, conceptual and instrumental knowledge use can be partial or complete and with the same best practice, some recommendations might result in conceptual use of some recommendations and instrumental use of others. While the goal is usually complete instrumental knowledge use, in reality it usually only ends with partial instrument knowledge use (often for very legitimate reasons, e.g. patient preferences, differences in the nature of health conditions between patients, etc.). Furthermore, instrumental use of the same best practice might involve intentionally disregarding some recommendations while adhering to others. A practitioner's approach to recommendations in the same guideline could range from conceptual use of some of them (they understand the recommendation but do not adhere with it), partial instrumental use of some of them (they follow some of the recommendation but not all of it, or are not able to follow all of it because of the circumstances of their practice setting) and complete instrumental use of others (they follow the recommendation to the letter).

Measuring Knowledge Use

When thinking about measuring best practice the working group needs to consider indicators or measures from several perspectives: definitional, approach to measurement, and selection of measures and tools. The operational definition of the indictor is a first step. This involves determining whether the group is interested in measuring knowledge use (and within this broad concept – conceptual, instrumental or symbolic use) or measuring impact (and at what level) or both (measuring knowledge use and impact).

Measurement of indicators can be direct or indirect. Direct measures would be ones where the indicator can be directly observed or measured, such as observing who performs hand hygiene and how adherent they are to the hand hygiene best practice recommendations. Indirect or surrogate measures are ones that only report on the outcome such as documentation in charts of the provision of care. Measures can also be subjective or objective. Subjective reports such as those based on self-reports by providers, patients or families often suffer from recall bias. Measures often considered more objective in nature (i.e. less susceptible to recall bias) would include observation and those derived from administrative databases of health records (e.g. the existence of test results indicating that a test was in fact performed). However, measures derived from documents are only as reliable as the quality and thoroughness of the original documentation. Indeed, health care providers may be engaged in providing the best practice but not documenting it. Methods for collecting indicators of knowledge use typically include audit, surveys, interviews, and observation.

Selection of knowledge use indicators should be guided by considerations such as scientific merit as well as pragmatic issues such as resource requirements to collect the data as well as the potential burden of administration. Issues related to scientific merit require assessment of the available measures as to their reliability, validity, and clinical sensitivity. Meaningful and sensitive measurement requires purposeful consideration of these factors in consultation with the stakeholders.

As has been revealed above, knowledge use is a continuous and complex process rather than a single discrete event occurring at one point in time. Measuring knowledge use can therefore be complex requiring a multidimensional, iterative and systematic approach. Squires et al. (2011) conducted a systematic review of self-reported research utilization measures (including their psychometric properties). They identified 60 measures but only seven were used in more than one study. Most measures targeted provider use of knowledge. A main conclusion from this review is that little is known about the validity of measures of knowledge use. In our work, we first look for existing measures that may be useful but often have had to develop measures or indicators specific to the project. When looking for measures of knowledge use, the National Coordinating Centre for Methods and Tools', Registry of Knowledge Translation Methods and Tools in Public Health is a good place to start (National Collaborating Centre for Methods and Tools 2020). This register is a collection of knowledge use (and other) measures and includes information on their validity and reliability. A limitation with this registry is that the focus is on public health, however, many of the included measures can be used to measure knowledge use in other practice settings.

Conceptual knowledge use can be measured by tests of knowledge/understanding (e.g. the extent to which clinicians acquire the knowledge and skills taught during training sessions) which is why surveys of attitudes and intentions (e.g. measures of attitudes toward a specific practice, perceptions of self-efficacy performing the practice, or intentions to perform them) are common outcome measures in implementation studies or studies of evidence-based practice (Godin et al. 2008).

In recent years, measures of instrumental knowledge use have been used and reported more frequently (Estabrooks et al. 2003). For example, in upwards of 89% of practice guideline implementation studies in medicine and allied health professionals studies report measures of instrumental knowledge use (i.e. guideline adherence) (Grimshaw et al. 2004; Hakkennes and Green 2006; Harrison et al. 2009). Given instrumental knowledge use is measured by determining uptake of, or adherence to, best practices and best practice recommendations, they are typically specific to the clinical focus of the best practice. It is therefore not surprising that there are few generic measures of instrumental knowledge. Each indicator needs to be tailored to the desired behavior of interest. Quality indicators is a good place to look for measures of instrumental knowledge use as they are usually designed to measure practice in specific clinical areas. Increasingly, scholars are focusing on implementation outcome measures (Weiner et al. 2017; Lewis et al. 2018; Shepherd et al. 2019).

Who Is the Focus of the Knowledge Use?

In addition to considering the type of knowledge use, the group should also be clear about who they want to use the knowledge (i.e. point of care providers, individuals/families, the public, managers/administrators, policy makers, etc.). Different target audiences may require different strategies for monitoring knowledge use. When assessing knowledge use by nurses, the working group could consider measuring awareness of the existence of best practice, knowledge of the content of the best practice recommendations, intentions to use the recommendations and actual application of best practice (either by observation, documentation in the health record, self-report, or by asking patients about the care they received). When assessing knowledge use by individuals and families it is important to consider a couple of extra aspects such as stage of life (ability to communicate, memory, etc.) their age, abilities and degree of illness. If the target is policy makers, a decision to adopt or endorse a particular best practice for their jurisdiction (conceptual knowledge use) enables instrumental use when the policy takes effect. Assessing use of knowledge by policy makers may require strategies such as interviews and document analysis (Hanney et al. 2003).

How Much Knowledge Use Is Enough?

When implementing best practice, it is also important for the group to consider the degree of knowledge use that they are aiming for. This should be based on discussions with all the relevant knowledge users and stakeholders including consideration of what is acceptable and feasible, whether there is a minimum level that is required or whether a ceiling effect may exist. After launch of the best practice, if the level of knowledge use is found to be adequate (i.e. meeting a predefined level – for example the group may decide that if at least 90% of individuals receive the best practice assessment on admission, this is successful implementation as there may be legitimate reasons why achieving 100% adherence to the best practices would not be feasible). Strategies for monitoring ongoing (sustained) knowledge use should also be considered with predetermined levels of what is adequate knowledge use (e.g. assessment on admission should continue to occur with not less than 90% of patients). If the level of knowledge use is less than expected or desired, this information can be used by the group to trigger reassessing barriers to knowledge use. For example, key informants could be asked about their intentions (or lack of intentions) to use the knowledge or factors affecting their ability to adhere to the best practice. This exploration may uncover new barriers that may need to be addressed with another round of implementation strategies or reveal more of the same implementation strategies are required.

Evaluating the Impact of Knowledge Use

While the level of knowledge use is important to know (i.e. the extent to which best practice is applied), the goal of evidence-informed practice is ultimately improved individual health, e.g. (wound healed), health care provider (e.g. satisfaction with professional practice), agency (e.g. efficient use of resources) and system (and potentially societal) outcomes (e.g. reduced wait times allowing more people to be cared for). Ultimately the goals of evidence-informed practice are improved health status and quality of care. However, in some cases the group may decide it is not necessary or even possible to measure impacts on health. For example, it may take years for the health impacts related to use of a best practice to materialize as is often the case with prevention best practices. In these cases, demonstrating that the preventive measures were being used may be sufficient to determine the success of the implementation initiative.

As advised by Straus et al. (2009), evaluation of impact should start with formulating the question of interest. Using the PICOT framework (described in Chapter 6) can be very useful for this task. As you will recall, using this framework, the "P" refers to the population of interest which could be the public, patients/family caregivers, health care providers or policy makers. The "I" refers to the implementation strategy which was deployed, and which might be compared to another group ("C"). The "O" refers to the outcome of interest (impact) which in this situation refers to health, provider or system/organizational outcomes. In this case the outcomes are actually the impacts of using the best practice. The "T" refers to the time period for the evaluation.

Types of Impacts Resulting from Implementing Best Practice

Hakkennes and Green (2006) conducted a systematic review of methods used to measure change in outcomes following an implementation or knowledge translation intervention. They grouped measures into three main categories which we have modified to focus on impact of knowledge use:

1) Individual level
   - measures of an actual change in health status such as mortality, morbidity, signs and symptoms, functional status, quality of life, adverse events, etc.
   - other measures of impact on the patient unrelated to health status such as satisfaction with care.
2) Health care provider level
   - measures of provider satisfaction. Note that changes in provider behavior are not considered an impact measure of implementation but rather are a measure of instrumental knowledge use. Impact for this and the other categories should be thought of as: when providers use best practice what is the effect or outcome (impact).
3) Health system level (including organizational and societal level when appropriate)
   - measures of change in the health care system (e.g. wait-time, length of stay, health care visits, readmissions) or expenditures and in some cases changes that affect society (e.g. productivity levels, work presentism or absenteeism, employment rates, expenditures on health and social care).

Impact measures are used less frequently than instrumental use outcomes. In our systematic review of guideline implementation in nursing, about two thirds of studies included measures of impact compared with about half of studies in medicine or rehabilitation (Grimshaw et al. 2004; Hakkennes and Green 2006). Of guideline implementation studies in medicine, just over 20% included measures of patient health status while under 40% included measures of system impact (Grimshaw et al. 2004; Hakkennes and Green 2006).

Table 12.A.1 describes examples of measures of knowledge use and impact, strategies for data collection and possible sources of data. A key implementation evaluation decision is when to measure knowledge use and when to measure the impact of knowledge use. In cases where the implementation intervention targets a behavior for which there is a strong evidence of benefit, it may be appropriate to focus on measuring instrumental knowledge use (whether the behavior has occurred) rather than measuring impact (whether a change in patient/client health status outcomes has occurred).

Measuring Impact

Similar to measuring knowledge use, it is important to be selective and have a good rationale for selecting each measure. There are several key considerations related to evaluating the impact of best practice implementation:

- What types of impacts are of particular interest (individual, provider, organization, system outcomes)?

Table 12.A.1 Measures of knowledge use and impact.

Construct	Description	Examples of Measures	Strategy for Data Collection	Source of data
		Knowledge use		
• Conceptual (patient or provider)	Changes in knowledge levels, understanding, attitudes, intentions	Knowledge; attitudes; intentions to adopt practice	Self report	Questionnaires, interviews with patients or providers
• Instrumental (patient or provider)	Changes in behaviour or practice	Adherence to recommendations (e.g. adoption of a new nursing practice or abandonment of existing practice; change in prescribing or test ordering)	Audit, observation, self-report	Administrative database or clinical database, observations of patients-provider encounters, Questionnaires, interviews with patients about provider behaviour, questionnaires, interviews with providers
		Impact		
• Patient impact	Impact on patients of using/ applying the knowledge	Health status (morbidity or mortality, signs, symptoms, pain, depression); health related quality of life; function Satisfaction with care	Audit, Self-report	Administrative database, clinical database, questionnaires, interviews
• Provider impact	Impact on providers of using/ applying the knowledge	Satisfaction with practice; time taken to do new practice	Self-report, observation	Questionnaires, interviews
• System/ Organization impact	Impact on the health system of using/applying the knowledge	Length of stay; wait times, readmissions; expenditures and resource use; hospitalizations	Audit, self- report	Administrative database, clinical database, questionnaires, interviews with patients or providers

Source: Reprinted with permission from Straus et al. (2013).

- What specific impact measures will be used?
- How will the measure be operationalized (what is the numerator and what is the denominator)?
- Criteria to consider when selecting impact measures are: how easily can the data be collected? How reliable and valid are the data?
- What is essential to know? Will the information be used to inform the implementation process and prompt course corrections or is information being collected because it would be nice to know because people are curious?

Finally, there is the issue of how long after implementation should you wait for measuring impact? Usually it takes time for practice changes to translate into impacts. If you measure too soon, little impact will be observed leading to the wrong conclusion that the implementation strategies did not work rather than insufficient time has elapsed to have impact. How often should impact be measured? Every six months? Month 6, 12, and then annually? Or at some other time intervals? And finally, how much impact is enough? For example, if thinking about healing rates as a health outcome, what percent of patients should be healed by three months to declare success? 70%, 80%, 90%, >95%. Perhaps it is not about meeting a certain healing rate but simply about improving the rate over time. The decision about how much impact is enough is always an arbitrary one as all sorts of factors affect healing rates in addition to best practice. What is important is that the group work through the issues and has a rationale for its decisions.

Box 12.A.2   It takes time to change

With one implementation project, the team trained all the staff on the new best practice. They came back two months later and started to collect data on use of pain best practice (assessing and managing pain i.e. instrumental knowledge use) and impact (pain scores). There was no increase in assessing or managing pain and the mean patient pain score remained unchanged. The team was very discouraged that the implementation project had failed. Deciding to figure out why the training had apparently not worked, they had discussions with some staff. They found the staff were very keen on implementing the pain best practice and clearly understood the best practice (conceptual knowledge). When asked why there had been no changes, the staff reported they were waiting for the documentation system to change to allow easier charting that the best practice recommendations had been performed. Implementation takes time and sometimes the implementation team think it can happen quicker than is realistic in the real world. It is also important to remember, like a contagion, the bigger the target audience for the change, the longer it takes to get everyone doing it. The moral of this story is to have realistic expectations about how long it will take to implement best practice and how long it may be necessary to then wait to allow impact to materialize before attempting to measure impact.

General Advice on Selecting and Developing Indicators or Measures of Knowledge Use or Impact

As described above, best practice indicators measure process (i.e. the care activities fulfilling the essence of the recommendations) or impact (i.e. what results from using the recommendations). At their simplest, indicators are measures. They always need a numerator (e.g. the number of people receiving the recommended practice or having the outcome of interest) and a denominator (e.g. the total number of people for whom the recommendation is appropriate). Indicators are typically presented as a proportion, ranging from 0% (for example, no one received the best practice) to 100% (all eligible patients received the best practice). To calculate this proportion, the numerator (number receiving the best practice or having the condition) is divided by the denominator (total eligible for the best practice or the relevant population) and multiplied by 100%. For example, if the recommendation was that all patients with venous leg ulcers should be offered high compression bandaging, the indicator for this recommendation would be: (the number of people with venous leg ulcers receiving compression therapy / the total number of people with venous leg ulcers for whom compression therapy is indicated) x 100%. The group might also want an indicator of inappropriate use of compression therapy (the number of individuals with non-venous leg ulcers receiving compression therapy / the total number of individuals with non-venous leg ulcers) × 100%. When the numerator is based on the best practice recommendation, then the data collected will directly speak to the gap between current practice and best practice.

To be accepted in a setting, the relevant stakeholders should agree upon what is included in both the numerator and denominator. For instance, achieving 100% may not be possible if there are factors in the setting at play beyond the uptake of evidence. For example, a patient with a venous leg ulcer may have edema that prevents the use of compression therapy until the edema is resolved, so they are eligible for compression therapy because they have a venous leg ulcer, but the treatment is not possible at the moment. The indicator could be modified so that the denominator is adjusted to exclude cases where compression therapy might be contra-indicated to give a more precise measure of adherence of compression therapy.

When deciding to measure best practice adherence (knowledge use) or impact, the working group should agree on key indicator selection criteria as well as the process they plan to use to in selecting or developing indicators. As with all the phases of Roadmap, it is critical that the group be inclusive of all the relevant stakeholders and hear the perspectives of the participants on the criteria.

When contemplating best practice indicators, start by checking practice guidelines to see if they offer indicators. When there are no relevant guidelines or when a guideline does not provide best practice indicators, and before developing new best practice indicators, the group should consider whether existing indicators might be relevant. Perform a scoping review of the literature to identify potentially relevant indicators. Studies of practice variation can be good sources of indicators and advice on measurement. If no potentially relevant indicators can be found, then the group will need to create them. Practice guideline recommendations can be used to generate indicators for them. There are several methods for developing indicators (mostly quality indicators) ranging from quite methodologically sophisticated approaches to more practical and intuitive approaches.

For a detailed description of methods for developing quality indicators see Stelfox and colleagues' approach (Bobrovitz et al. 2013; Stelfox and Straus 2013a, b; Santana et al. 2014). Another approach that has been used to develop quality indicators is the Delphi technique. This involves a group anonymously rating the appropriateness of proposed indicators, the ratings get fed back to the group for discussion and then another round of voting followed by more discussion and voting until the group reaches consensus about the indicator (Shekelle 2004).

It is important to approach indicator selection or development with a sense of pragmatism – creating the perfect indicator is not going to be helpful if you cannot reasonably collect data for either the numerator or denominator. At the same time do not feel you have to restrict the indicators to only data that may be available in the electronic health record or administrative databases. Be prepared to collect the relevant data if it is currently not being captured in your databases. If this should be an important indicator for the organization, engage the relevant data custodians to begin routinely collecting the required data. Convince them of the value and need for these data in order to determine what best practices and outcomes are occurring in the organization, to determine evidence-practice gaps, and to monitor ongoing use of best practice measures.

There are several criteria we have found useful to guide discussions about what indicators will be most useful for the purpose at hand. These include:

- How clinically important the indicator is to stakeholders? This relates to whether the indicator reflects an issue that is relevant to stakeholders. For example, is the indicator important to patients and their carers, to health care providers, managers, policy makers, etc.? Is there solid evidence available to support the indicator (i.e. is it a reliable indicator)?
- How reliable and valid is the indicator? Does it measure what it is supposed to measure accurately? Does the indicator have clear and interpretable cutoff points? Are the results of the indicator easy to understand?
- Are the data needed to calculate the indicator readily available? Are they easy to collect? Are they high quality (valid, reliable, and timely)?
- How amenable to action is the indicator? This is about whether the behavior or outcome the indicator reflects is amenable to change (for example, is it within the power of healthcare providers or patients to change).

For more information about criteria for selecting indicators, please see Janakiraman and Ecker (2010) and Hermann and Palmer (2002).

We have had success in having the group select/develop indicators using informal discussion. We have taken best practice recommendations and then proposed indicators (numerators and denominators) and encouraged the group to then review the selection criteria with each indicator and discuss whether it meets the criteria or not.

One example of developing best practice indicators comes from Valery Fiset, one of our doctoral students, who conducted a study as part of her PhD to examine the evidence-practice gap in the use of pain best practices at a tertiary hospital. To be able to do the chart audit, Val had to identify pain best practices from existing guidelines, identify relevant recommendations and then develop indicators she could use in the chart audit. She described the process in her thesis which was published as a paper (Fiset et al. 2019).

Val adapted the indicator development process described by Kotter et al. (2012) which consists of six steps for developing guideline-based quality indicators: (i) topic selection; (ii) guideline selection; (iii) extraction of recommendations; (iv) quality indicator selection; (v) practice test; and (vi) implementation. The first three steps are very similar to the Roadmap stages of determining the evidence-practice gap and customizing best practice for local use. The step of selecting the indicators involved following Nothacker et al. (2016) suggestions to use relevance, scientific soundness and feasibility when deciding on which recommendations for which to develop indicators (very similar to the criteria we suggested above). In Val's case, the choice of indicators involved an advisory committee considering the outcomes of each of the candidate guideline recommendations (best practices) that would contribute most to improvements in patient care plus considering how measurable they would be (i.e. considering whether the data needed to create the indicator was available or accessible). Using these criteria, all the potentially relevant candidate guideline recommendations were reduced into a shorter list of recommendations that could have feasible and measurable indicators.

The working group, as it works its way through this process may find that many recommendations may not lend themselves to the creation of indicators. This is sometimes because the recommendations are poorly specified (e.g. are vague or involve multiple behaviors making it difficult to measure). Kotter et al. (2012) step 5 involves using the developed indicators and doing a practice test to see how easy (or challenging) it is to collect the data, how reliable the data is that are being collected, and how meaningful the indicators actually are. Doing this can reveal that what was thought to be measurable or easy to retrieve may not be the case. Val did not do the final step in the Kotter et al. (2012) process which is implementing or institutionalizing the indicator as a measure of quality care. We strongly encourage working groups before embarking on indicator development, to review the Fiset paper for advice on how to do this but also for some of the conceptual, methodological, and pragmatic challenges related to developing best practice indicators.

Keep in mind that the evaluation might serve as a testing ground to provide data on the ongoing use of indicators. For example, in one implementation, the group preferred time to healing with a chronic wound, however, they discovered that in practice, a monthly population healing rate was more feasible and meaningful to the team and their organization. It is vital to make decisions about what is essential to measure versus what would be nice to measure. Measuring takes time and resources and can burden those who must provide the data, if not automatically collected. When selecting and using indicators, it is usually best to keep it pragmatic and simple by remembering, measurement should be seen as a means of supporting implementation not a goal in and of itself.

Box 12.A.3   Getting everyone on board

We have also had experience with a more structured approach to develop indicators for a clinical dashboard. The process used by Dunn et al. (2020) started with brainstorming, consulting with clinical experts, and scanning the literature to identify potential key performance indicators that reflected healthcare quality domains (i.e. appropriate and effective care) that were clinically meaningful, feasible to measure and actionable at the point of care. The process also included doing a modified Delphi survey with deliberative dialogue, consensus building, and priority setting with all team members to select the final list of indicators and set evidence-based benchmarks.

Appendix 12.B: Resources for Conducting Evaluations

Utilization-Focused Evaluation:

Better Evaluation Utilization-Focused Evaluation. [Online], Available: https://www.betterevaluation.org/en/plan/approach/utilization_focused_evaluation.

A Developmental Evaluation Primer:

Gamble, J. A. A. (2008). *A Developmental Evaluation Primer*. Montreal, Quebec, Canada: The J.W. McConnell Family Foundation.

Developmental evaluation: applying complexity concepts to enhance innovation and use:

Patton, M. Q. (2011). *Developmental evaluation: applying complexity concepts to enhance innovation and use*. Guilford Press: New York, NY. https://www.guilford.com/books/Developmental-Evaluation/Michael-Quinn-Patton/9781606238721

Gordis Epidemiology:

Celentano, D. D. and Szklo, M. (2019). *Gordis Epidemiology* 6e. Philidelphia, PA: Elsevier. https://www.elsevier.com/books/gordis-epidemiology/celentano/978-0-323-55229-5

Improving Patient Care: The Implementation of Change in Health Care Chapters 20–23:

Wensing, M. and Grimshaw, J. (2020a). Chapter 20: Experimental Designs for Evaluation of Implementation Strategies. In: *Improving Patient Care: The Implementation of Change in Health Care* 3e (eds. M. Wensing, R. Grol and J. Grimshaw): Wiley Blackwell. https://onlinelibrary.wiley.com/doi/10.1002/9781119488620.ch20

Wensing, M. and Grimshaw, J. (2020b). Chapter 21: observational evaluation of implementation strategies. In: *Improving Patient Care: The Implementation of Change in Health Care* 3e (eds. M. Wensing, R. Grol and J. Grimshaw): Wiley Blackwell. https://onlinelibrary.wiley.com/doi/10.1002/9781119488620.ch21

Hulscher, M. and Wensing, M. (2020). Chapter 22: Process evaluation of implementation strategies In: *Improving Patient Care: The Implementation of Change in Health Care* 3e (eds. M. Wensing, R. Grol and J. Grimshaw): Wiley Blackwell. https://onlinelibrary.wiley.com/doi/10.1002/9781119488620.ch22

Severens, J. L., Hoomans, T., Adang, E. and Wensing, M. (2020). Chapter 23: Economic evaluation of implementation strategies In: *Improving Patient Care: The Implementation of Change in Health Care* 3e (eds. M. Wensing, R. Grol and J. Grimshaw): Wiley Blackwell. https://onlinelibrary.wiley.com/doi/10.1002/9781119488620.ch23

Knowledge Translation in Health Care: Moving from Evidence to Practice Chapters 5.1 and 5.2:

Bhattacharyya, O., Hayden, L. and Zwarenstein, M. (2013). Chapter 5.1: methodologies to evaluate effectiveness of knowledge translation interventions In: *Knowledge Translation in Health Care. Moving From Evidence to Practice*. 2e (eds. S. Straus, J. Tetroe and I.D. Graham). Chichester, pp. 331–348: Wiley Blackwell. https://www.wiley.com/en-ca/Knowledge+Translation+in+Health+Care%3A+Moving+from+Evidence+to+Practice%2C+2nd+Edition-p-9781118413548

Quinn, E., Mitton, C. and Ward, J. (2013). Chapter 5.2: Economic evaluation of KTI In: *Knowledge Translation in Health Care. Moving From Evidence to Practice* 2e (eds. S. Straus, J. Tetroe and I.D. Graham), pp. 349–360. Chichester: Wiley Blackwell. https://www.wiley.

com/en-ca/Knowledge+Translation+in+Health+Care%3A+Moving+from+Evidence+to
+Practice%2C+2nd+Edition-p-9781118413548

Types of Evaluation:

Centers for Disease Control and Prevention (2007). *Types of Evaluation*. Available at: https://www.cdc.gov/std/Program/pupestd/Types of Evaluation.pdf.

Experimental and quasi-experimental designs for research:

Campbell, D. and Stanley, J. (1963). *Experimental and Quasi-Experimental Designs for Research*. Chicago, IL: Rand-McNally.

Quasi-experimentation: Design and analysis issues for field settings:

Cook, T. D. and Campbell, D. T. (1979). *Quasi-experimentation: Design and Analysis Issues for Field Settings*. Boston, MA: Houghton Mifflin Company.

References

Arain, M., Campbell, M.J., Cooper, C.L., and Lancaster, G.A. (2010). What is a pilot or feasibility study? A review of current practice and editorial policy. *BMC Medical Research Methodology* 10 https://doi.org/10.1186/1471-2288-10-67.

Beard, E., Lewis, J.J., Copas, A. et al. (2015). Stepped wedge randomised controlled trials: systematic review of studies published between 2010 and 2014. *Trials* 16 https://doi.org/10.1186/s13063-015-0839-2.

Bernet, A.C., Willens, D.E., and Bauer, M.S. (2013). Effectiveness-implementation hybrid designs: implications for quality improvement science. *Implementation Science* 8 https://doi.org/10.1186/1748-5908-8-S1-S2.

Better Evaluation *Utilization-Focused Evaluation*, [Online], Available: https://www.betterevaluation.org/en/plan/approach/utilization_focused_evaluation [Accessed May 29, 2020].

Beyer, J.M. and Harrison, M.T. (1982). The utilization process: a conceptual framework and synthesis of empirical findings. *Administrative Science Quarterly* 27: 591–622. https://doi.org/10.2307/2392533.

Bobrovitz, N., Parrilla, J.S., Santana, M. et al. (2013). A qualitative analysis of a consensus process to develop quality indicators of injury care. *Implementation Science* 8: 45. https://doi.org/10.1186/1748-5908-8-45.

Bowen, S. (2012). *A Guide to Evaluation in Health Research*: Canadian Institutes of Health Research. Available at: https://cihr-irsc.gc.ca/e/documents/kt_lm_guide_evhr-en.pdf.

Bowen, D.J., Kreuter, M., Spring, B. et al. (2009). How we design feasibility studies. *American Journal of Preventive Medicine* 36: 452–457. https://doi.org/10.1016/j.amepre.2009.02.002.

Brown, C.A. and Lilford, R.J. (2006). The stepped wedge trial design: a systematic review. *BMC Medical Research Methodology* 6 https://doi.org/10.1186/1471-2288-6-54.

Brown, C.H., Curran, G., Palinkas, L.A. et al. (2017). An overview of research and evaluation designs for dissemination and implementation. *Annual Review of Public Health* 38: 1–22. https://doi.org/10.1146/annurev-publhealth-031816-044215.

Cargo, M. and Mercer, S.L. (2008). The value and challenges of participatory research: strengthening its practice. *Annual Review of Public Health* 29: 325–350. https://doi.org/10.1146/annurev.publhealth.29.091307.083824.

Centers for Disease Control and Prevention (2007). *Types of Evaluation*. Available at: https://www.cdc.gov/std/Program/pupestd/Types of Evaluation.pdf.

Cidav, Z., Mandell, D., Pyne, J. et al. (2020). A pragmatic method for costing implementation strategies using time-driven activity-based costing. *Implementation Science* 15: 28. https://doi.org/10.1186/s13012-020-00993-1.

Cook, T.D. and Campbell, D.T. (1979). *Quasi-Experimentation: Design and Analysis Issues for Field Settings*. Boston, MA: Houghton Mifflin Company.

Copas, A.J., Lewis, J.J., Thompson, J.A. et al. (2015). Designing a stepped wedge trial: three main designs, carry-over effects and randomisation approaches. *Trials* 16 https://doi.org/10.1186/s13063-015-0842-7.

Curran, G. M. (2017). *Innovative Study Designs for Implementation Research*, [Online], Available: https://www.slideshare.net/HopkinsCFAR/innovative-study-designs-for-implementation-research [Accessed May 29, 2020].

Curran, G.M., Bauer, M., Mittman, B. et al. (2012). Effectiveness-implementation hybrid designs: combining elements of clinical effectiveness and implementation research to enhance public health impact. *Medical Care* 50: 217–226. https://doi.org/10.1097/MLR.0b013e3182408812.

Dunn, W.N. (1983). Measuring knowledge use. *Knowledge* 5: 120–133. https://doi.org/10.1177/107554708300500107.

Dunn, S., Reszel, J., Weiss, D. et al. (2020). The experience of using an integrated knowledge translation approach to develop, implement and evaluate an audit and feedback system in Ontario maternal-newborn hospitals. In: *How We Work Together: The Integrated Knowledge Translation Research Network Casebook* (eds. A. Kothari, C. McCutcheon, L. Boland and I.D. Graham), 2–6. Ottawa: Integrated Knowledge Translation Research Network https://iktrn.ohri.ca/projects/casebook.

Estabrooks, C.A. (1999). The conceptual structure of research utilization. *Research in Nursing & Health* 22: 203–216. https://doi.org/10.1002/(sici)1098-240x(199906)22:3<203::aid-nur3>3.0.co;2-9.

Estabrooks, C.A., Floyd, J.A., Scott-Findlay, S. et al. (2003). Individual determinants of research utilization: a systematic review. *Journal of Advanced Nursing* 43: 506–520. https://doi.org/10.1046/j.1365-2648.2003.02748.x.

Fiset, V.J., Davies, B.L., Graham, I.D. et al. (2019). Developing guideline-based quality indicators: assessing gaps in pain management practice. *International Journal of Evidence-Based Healthcare* 17: 92–105. https://doi.org/10.1097/XEB.0000000000000160.

Gale, R.C., Wu, J., Erhardt, T. et al. (2019a). Comparison of rapid vs in-depth qualitative analytic methods from a process evaluation of academic detailing in the Veterans Health Administration. *Implementation Science* 14 https://doi.org/10.1186/s13012-019-0853-y.

Gale, R.C., Wu, J., Erhardt, T. et al. (2019b). Comparison of rapid vs in-depth qualitative analytic methods from a process evaluation of academic detailing in the Veterans Health Administration. *Implementation Science* 14: 11. https://doi.org/10.1186/s13012-019-0853-y.

Glasgow, R.E., Vogt, T.M., and Boles, S.M. (1999). Evaluating the public health impact of health promotion interventions: the RE-AIM framework. *American Journal of Public Health* 89: 1322–1327. https://doi.org/10.2105/ajph.89.9.1322.

Godin, G., Belanger-Gravel, A., Eccles, M., and Grimshaw, J. (2008). Healthcare professionals' intentions and behaviours: a systematic review of studies based on social cognitive theories. *Implementation Science* 3: 36. https://doi.org/10.1186/1748-5908-3-36.

Graham, I.D., Logan, J., Harrison, M.B. et al. (2006). Lost in knowledge translation: time for a map? *The Journal of Continuing Education in the Health Professions* 26: 13–24. https://doi.org/10.1002/chp.47.

Graham, I.D., Bick, D., Tetroe, J. et al. (2010). Measuring outcomes of evidence-based practice: distinguishing between knowledge use and its impact. In: *Evaluating the Impact of Implementing Evidence-Based Practice* (eds. D. Bick and I.D. Graham), 18–37. Oxford: Wiley Blackwell.

Grimshaw, J.M., Thomas, R.E., Maclennan, G. et al. (2004). Effectiveness and efficiency of guideline dissemination and implementation strategies. *Health Technology Assessment* 8: iii–72. https://doi.org/10.3310/hta8060.

Grol, R. and Wensing, M. (2004). What drives change? Barriers to and incentives for achieving evidence-based practice. *The Medical Journal of Australia* 180: S57–S60. https://doi.org/10.5694/j.1326-5377.2004.tb05948.x.

Grol, R. and Wensing, M. (2005). Effective implementation: a model. In: *Improving Patient Care* (eds. R. Grol, M. Wensing and M. Eccles), 41–57. Edinburgh: Elsevier.

Hakkennes, S. and Green, S. (2006). Measures for assessing practice change in medical practitioners. *Implementation Science* 1: 29. https://doi.org/10.1186/1748-5908-1-29.

Hanney, S.R., Gonzalez-Block, M.A., Buxton, M.J., and Kogan, M. (2003). The utilisation of health research in policy-making: concepts, examples and methods of assessment. *Health Research Policy and Systems* 1: –2. https://doi.org/10.1186/1478-4505-1-2.

Harden, S.M., Gaglio, B., Shoup, J.A. et al. (2015). Fidelity to and comparative results across behavioral interventions evaluated through the RE-AIM framework: a systematic review. *Systematic Reviews* 4 https://doi.org/10.1186/s13643-015-0141-0.

Harden, S.M., Strayer, T.E. III., Smith, M.L. et al. (2020). National Working Group on the RE-AIM planning and evaluation framework: goals, resources, and future directions. *Frontiers in Public Health* 7 https://doi.org/10.3389/fpubh.2019.00390.

Harrison, M.B., Browne, G.B., Roberts, J. et al. (2002). Quality of life of individuals with heart failure: a randomized trial of the effectiveness of two models of hospital-to-home transition. *Medical Care* 40: 271–282. https://doi.org/10.1097/00005650-200204000-00003.

Harrison, M.B., Graham, I.D., Lorimer, K. et al. (2005). Leg-ulcer care in the community, before and after implementation of an evidence-based service. *Canadian Medical Association Journal* 172: 1447–1452. https://doi.org/10.1503/cmaj.1041441.

Harrison, M.B., Graham, I.D., Godfrey, C.M. et al. (2009). *Guideline Dissemination and Implementation Strategies for Nursing and Allied Health Professions*. Cochrane Library.

Hermann, R.C. and Palmer, R.H. (2002). Common ground: a framework for selecting core quality measures for mental health and substance abuse care. *Psychiatric Services* 53: 281–287. https://doi.org/10.1176/appi.ps.53.3.281.

Holdsworth, L.M., Safaeinili, N., Winget, M. et al. (2020). Adapting rapid assessment procedures for implementation research using a team-based approach to analysis: a case example of patient quality and safety interventions in the ICU. *Implementation Science* 15: 12. https://doi.org/10.1186/s13012-020-0972-5.

Janakiraman, V. and Ecker, J. (2010). Quality in obstetric care: measuring what matters. *Obstetrics & Gynecology* 116: 728–732. https://doi.org/10.1097/AOG.0b013e3181ea4d4f.

Kemp, C.G., Wagenaar, B.H., and Haroz, E.E. (2019). Expanding hybrid studies for implementation research: intervention, implementation strategy, and context. *Frontiers in Public Health* 7 https://doi.org/10.3389/fpubh.2019.00325.

Kilbourne, A.M. (n.d.). *Designs for Dissemination and Implementation Research for Small Populations*: Department of Psychiatry, University of Michigan, VA Quality Enhancement Research Initiative (QUERI). Available at: https://sites.nationalacademies.org/cs/groups/dbassesite/documents/webpage/dbasse_184763.pdf.

King, D.K., Shoup, J.A., Raebel, M.A. et al. (2020). Planning for implementation success using RE-AIM and CFIR frameworks: a qualitative study. *Frontiers in Public Health* 8 https://doi.org/10.3389/fpubh.2020.00059.

Kotter, T., Blozik, E., and Scherer, M. (2012). Methods for the guideline-based development of quality indicators--a systematic review. *Implementation Science* 7: 21. https://doi.org/10.1186/1748-5908-7-21.

Kwan, B.M., McGinnes, H.L., Ory, M.G. et al. (2019). RE-AIM in the real world: use of the RE-AIM framework for program planning and evaluation in clinical and community settings. *Frontiers in Public Health* 7 https://doi.org/10.3389/fpubh.2019.00345.

Landes, S.J., McBain, S.A., and Curran, G.M. (2019). An introduction to effectiveness-implementation hybrid designs. *Psychiatry Research* 280: 112630. https://doi.org/10.1016/j.psychres.2019.112513.

Larsen, J.K. (1980). Review essay: knowledge utilization: what is it? *Knowledge* 1: 421–442. https://doi.org/10.1177/107554708000100305.

Leon, A.C., Davis, L.L., and Kraemer, H.C. (2011). The role and interpretation of pilot studies in clinical research. *Journal of Psychiatric Research* 45: 626–629.

Lewis, C.C., Mettert, K.D., Dorsey, C.N. et al. (2018). An updated protocol for a systematic review of implementation-related measures. *Systematic Reviews* 7: 66. https://doi.org/10.1186/s13643-018-0728-3.

Limbani, F., Goudge, J., Joshi, R. et al. (2019). Process evaluation in the field: global learnings from seven implementation research hypertension projects in low-and middle-income countries. *BMC Public Health* 19 https://doi.org/10.1186/s12889-019-7261-8.

Lu, C.Y. (2009). Observational studies: a review of study designs, challenges and strategies to reduce confounding. *The International Journal of Clinical Practice* 63: 691–697. https://doi.org/10.1111/j.1742-1241.2009.02056.x.

Mazzucca, S., Tabak, R.G., Pilar, M. et al. (2018). Variation in research designs used to test the effectiveness of dissemination and implementation strategies: a review. *Frontiers in Public Health* 6: 32. https://doi.org/10.3389/fpubh.2018.00032.

Merriam-Webster.com Dictionary (2020). *"Field-test"*, [Online], Available: https://www.merriam-webster.com/dictionary/field-test [Accessed May 29, 2020].

Moore, G.F., Audrey, S., Barker, M. et al. (2015). Process evaluation of complex interventions: Medical Research Council guidance. *BMJ* 350 https://doi.org/10.1136/bmj.h1258.

National Center for Complementary and Integrative Health (2017). *Pilot Studies: Common Uses and Misuses*, [Online], Available: https://www.nccih.nih.gov/grants/pilot-studies-common-uses-and-misuses [Accessed May 29, 2020].

National Collaborating Centre for Methods and Tools (2020). *Registry: Knowledge Translation Methods and Tools for Public Health*, [Online], Available: https://www.nccmt.ca/knowledge-repositories/search [Accessed June 18, 2020].

Nothacker, M., Stokes, T., Shaw, B. et al. (2016). Reporting standards for guideline-based performance measures. *Implementation Science* 11: 6. https://doi.org/10.1186/s13012-015-0369-z.

Patton, M.Q. (2008). *Utilization-Focused Evaluation*, 4e. Thousand Oaks, CA: Sage.

Quinn, E., Mitton, C., and Ward, J. (2013). Chapter 5.2: economic evaluation of KTI. In: *Knowledge Translation in Health Care. Moving from Evidence to Practice*, 2e (eds. S. Straus, J. Tetroe and I.D. Graham), 349–360. Chichester: Wiley-Blackwell.

RE-AIM (2020). *Welcome to RE-AIM.org! http://RE-AIM.org!*, [Online], Available: http://www. re-aim.org [Accessed May 31, 2020].

Rezigalla, A.A. (2020). Observational study designs: synopsis for selecting an appropriate study design. *Cureus* 12: e6692. https://doi.org/10.7759/cureus.6692.

Santana, M.J., Stelfox, H.T., and Trauma Quality Indicator Consensus, P (2014). Development and evaluation of evidence-informed quality indicators for adult injury care. *Annals of Surgery* 259: 186–192. https://doi.org/10.1097/SLA.0b013e31828df98e.

Severens, J.L., Hoomans, T., Adang, E., and Wensing, M. (2020). Chapter 23: economic evaluation of implementation strategies. In: *Improving Patient Care: The Implementation of Change in Health Care*, 3e (eds. M. Wensing, R. Grol and J. Grimshaw). Wiley Blackwell https://doi.org/10.1002/9781119488620.ch23.

Shadish, W.R., Cook, T.D., and Campbell, D.T. (2001). *Experimental and Quasi-Experimental Designs for Generalized Causal Inference*, 2e. Wadsworth Publishing.

Shekelle, P. (2004). The appropriateness method. *Medical Decision Making* 24: 228–231. https://doi.org/10.1177%2F0272989X04264212.

Shelton, R.C., Chambers, D.A., and Glasgow, R.E. (2020). An extension of RE-AIM to enhance sustainability: addressing dynamic context and promoting health equity over time. *Frontiers in Public Health* 8: 134. https://doi.org/10.3389/fpubh.2020.00134.

Shepherd, H.L., Geerligs, L., Butow, P. et al. (2019). The elusive search for success: defining and measuring implementation outcomes in a real-world hospital trial. *Frontiers in Public Health* 7: 293. https://doi.org/10.3389/fpubh.2019.00293.

Smith, L.J. and Harrison, M.B. (2009). Framework for planning and conducting pilot studies. *Ostomy/Wound Management* 55: 34–48. https://www.o-wm.com/content/ framework-planning-and-conducting-pilot-studies.

Squires, J.E., Estabrooks, C.A., O'Rourke, H.M. et al. (2011). A systematic review of the psychometric properties of self-report research utilization measures used in healthcare. *Implementation Science* 6: 83. https://doi.org/10.1186/1748-5908-6-83.

Stelfox, H.T. and Straus, S.E. (2013a). Measuring quality of care: considering conceptual approaches to quality indicator development and evaluation. *Journal of Clinical Epidemiology* 66: 1328–1337. https://doi.org/10.1016/j.jclinepi.2013.05.017.

Stelfox, H.T. and Straus, S.E. (2013b). Measuring quality of care: considering measurement frameworks and needs assessment to guide quality indicator development. *Journal of Clinical Epidemiology* 66: 1320–1327. https://doi.org/10.1016/j.jclinepi.2013.05.018.

Straus, S., Tetroe, J., Graham, I.D. et al. (2009). Monitoring knowledge use and evaluating outcomes. In: *Knowledge Translation in Health Care. Moving from Evidence to Practice* (eds. S. Straus, J. Tetroe and I.D. Graham), 227–236. Wiley Blackwell.

Straus, S.E., Tetroe, J., Bhattacharry, O. et al. (2013). "Chapter 3.5 Monitoring knowledge use and evaluating outcomes" (Table 3.5.1). In: *Knowledge Translation in Health Care. Moving From Evidence to Practice*, 2e (eds. S. Straus, J. Tetroe and I.D. Graham), 227–236. Chichester: Wiley Blackwell.

Weiner, B.J., Lewis, C.C., Stanick, C. et al. (2017). Psychometric assessment of three newly developed implementation outcome measures. *Implementation Science* 12: 108. https://doi. org/10.1186/s13012-017-0635-3.

Weiss, C.H. (1979). The many meanings of research utilization. *Public Administration Review* (5): 426–431. https://doi.org/10.2307/3109916.

Whitehead, A.L., Sully, B.G.O., and Campbell, M.J. (2014). Pilot and feasibility studies: is there a difference from each other and from a randomised controlled trial? *Contemporary Clinical Trials* 38: 130–133. https://doi.org/10.1016/j.cct.2014.04.001.

Wikipedia contributors (2020). *"Usability testing"*, [Online], https://en.wikipedia.org/wiki/Usability_testing [Accessed May 29, 2020].

Part 3

Phase III: Implement, Evaluate, and Sustain

13

Launch and Evaluate

Introduction

Nearly there! After the months of preparation and planning that is Phase 2 of Roadmap, the working group will be eager to start implementing the customized best practice. By this point, you have field tested the implementation strategies tailored to your context and made any necessary modifications. If required, the group has undertaken another field test of the revised strategies. The group should also have received the endorsement of managers and leaders in the organization to begin implementing. With stakeholder support in place, critical relationships with key players established, the necessary facilities and equipment secured, the trainers for the potential adopters prepared and the evaluation plan sorted out, everything is in place for successful implementation.

This chapter focuses on the actual launch – "going live" and carrying out the planned evaluation. This signals the beginning of Phase 3 of Roadmap which is Launch, Evaluate and Sustain. In the last chapter the focus was on all the final preparations to successfully launch the implementation which included field testing the implementation strategies to ensure they can be delivered and are acceptable to potential adopters of the best practice, designing the evaluation plan for the implementation in terms of the uptake of the best practice and impact, and lastly, developing the checklist of all the arrangements and plans that are in place that would signal that all systems are go for the implementation to be launched.

Goal: In this final Phase of Roadmap, the purpose is to ensure that a successful launch is accomplished in your setting, there is confidence that the processes are in place, and then to measure the process outcomes and the effectiveness and impact evaluations as planned.

All your work and planning will now be put to the test and again there are several pertinent questions to use as a guide:

- Is everything in place for the launch? How will you activate and mark the launch officially? Are any needed approvals in place?
- What is the oversight process for the evaluation? Who will be responsible for the oversight process of the evaluation?

Knowledge Translation in Nursing and Healthcare: A Roadmap to Evidence-informed Practice, First Edition. Margaret B. Harrison and Ian D. Graham.
© 2021 John Wiley & Sons, Inc. Published 2021 by John Wiley & Sons, Inc.

- How will results from the process evaluation be used in real time to manage changes in the implementation plan?
- How will results from the summative evaluation be managed in relation to:
  - Making course corrections based on best practice adherence data.
  - Impact data collected at the end of the evaluation period.
  - Sharing "good news" that the best practice is successfully being implemented as expected.
  - Sharing "bad news" that the best practice is not being implemented as expected or occurrence of unexpected events, e.g. adverse event.

Launch

Run Through Launch Checklist

Using the launch checklist described in the last chapter, the working group should go through the checklist to ensure that all the relevant launch issues required for successful implementation are in place. If everything is in place, then it is time to launch. If there is any hesitation that some aspect of the plan may not be completely organized, it is important to investigate the issues and address them. As we have already mentioned, it is better to delay the launch and get it right than to rush to launch when some implementation issues or supports are not in place.

Activate the Launch

It is important to clearly and visibly kick off the launch of the best practice to ensure that everyone knows that the planning is complete, and implementation is now officially underway. The working group might consider organizing a celebratory event to publicly mark the implementation launch. This is a valuable opportunity to formally recognize and thank all the stakeholders who contributed time, effort, and resources toward bringing about the use of the best practice.

Acknowledging everyone in getting to this point demonstrates the working group's efforts have been essential and appreciated. This is also an opportunity to signal to the organization and stakeholders that the best practice is embraced by the organization and that there is a strong expectation that it be used. The line is drawn in the sand now – things are going forward with the new best practices. This is a major milestone to be applauded. Celebrations could include bringing the unit or organization together for refreshments and treats, hosting an open house, and/or issuing a news release internally through usual communication channels (e.g. emails, newsletters). If the implementation is of interest beyond the institution, a press release or press conference could be held, or a public meeting could be organized. Celebrating the project milestones not only recognizes the work done to this point, it can also help build awareness and maintain momentum which is important to sustain the adoption of the best practice.

During the early days following the launch, the working group should regularly monitor progress (the process evaluation). Doing walkabouts is an easy way to get a sense of how things are going at the point of care. Informal chats with staff and managers can also alert the group to potential issues with the implementation. Continuously ask how the implementation is going and whether anything can be done to make it smoother. Being present allows the working group to see what is happening. Also, the members of the working group being seen asking about the implementation can bring reassurance to those adopting the new best practice by signaling what they are doing is valued. Do not be surprised if there are small hiccups or glitches during the launch. Try to identify them quickly and deal with them promptly. Small issues can become big ones if they are not dealt with. Transparency in dealing with implementation glitches is usually the best policy. If something is not working as planned, the working group should acknowledge it and indicate how they are working to resolve the issue. Thank people for bringing problems to the attention of the working group. Not being transparent when things are not working well, can undermine trust in the working group and further negatively impact potential adopters' intentions to implement. Continue to acknowledge and celebrate uptake of the best practice which not only reminds people what they are doing is important but also reveals the working group is paying attention to what they are doing.

Oversee the Implementation and Evaluation

As you begin, it will be vital to have a person or small group responsible for managing and oversight of the evaluation. This can be a member of the working group, the whole working group or someone or group outside the working group. In nominating a person (or small group) for this, there are a few considerations:

- What knowledge characteristics and skills should overseers have?
- If they are not members of the working group, how should they be linked into the working group?
- Who are they responsible to? (need to be clear about lines of accountability/authority-who do they report to)

To oversee the implementation and evaluation you may decide to choose a member or a small group from your working group. Alternatively, it may seem time to engage new people, for instance having individuals from each practice area (e.g. unit or clinic or outpatient team) be overseers to promote and advocate for the best practice and monitor the evaluation. We have often used this approach and termed these individuals as the unit or team champion. A reporting mechanism should be established with the working group (e.g. weekly debriefing sessions, or brief progress surveys by email). Sessions could be one-on-one with the working group (usually a small number of designated members) or with the champions as a group. A positive aspect of the group approach is that they raise issues with the implementation or evaluation that others may have not faced yet and the group can then problem solve together. We have found this approach exceptionally helpful with implementations especially if the implementation strategies are complex and involve a series of tasks. For example, once a pressure ulcer risk is noted using a scale, the nurse must document and then action a clinical intervention (e.g. pressure relieving surface, turning schedule) based on the level of risk. A referral may also be necessary. All these steps must be tracked and in place for the process evaluation data to measure. In this case, the champions together came up with reminder strategies that they used for documenting, mentoring, and supporting the nurses' direct care.

Gaining as Much as Possible from the Evaluation

Your chosen approach will be either a process, and or summative evaluation (outcomes and impact). With both approaches, the working group will gain information not only about the success of the implementation process, outcomes and impact, but detail about how to improve it and make it more efficient in your setting. This is where taking field notes comes in handy for details that might otherwise be lost. A field notebook is simply a lined note pad or book (like a journaling book) in which a designated person keeps rough notes of what is happening. It can be minimally structured to gather information, e.g. date, timing, issues arising, observations and thoughts for improvements and other open-ended space. An easy way to do this is have the person(s) overseeing the evaluation regularly connect with a "champion" in each area involved. This is about having ears on the ground and conducting informal reconnaissance. When the working group is visiting the implementation settings and chatting with staff about how the implementation is going, their observations can be entered into the journal. All these data become part of the process evaluation and can be particularly valuable in trying to fully understand any difficulties with implementing or uptake of specific recommendations that emerge in different areas of the organization. It also helps to reveal what is going well and what should be shared with other units.

Use Process Evaluation Results to Manage the Implementation

The process evaluation is intended to determine if things are in place (the implementation strategies are working as they should). It is vital to ensure this before proceeding with the outcomes and impact evaluations or the results will not capture the true value of using evidence informed practice.

If things are not going as well as expected (i.e. in terms of adherence rates), it is important to use information gathered from the process evaluation as well as to gather information from potential adopters about what is making it hard to do the best practice. Could it be due to a lack of knowledge that is not addressed by the educational strategy? Not having the right equipment or support? Or that practitioners are too busy and forget? Also, determine if the leadership remains committed to the best practice and that the best practice is important and expected to be used in the organization. You may find there is a need for another barrier's assessment. The implementation strategies may need to be adjusted or tweaked. Maybe boosters are needed, for example pocket cards as reminders. It may also be, that different strategies are needed as different barriers have emerged with more people trying to use the best practice and as potential adopters gain experience with the best practice.

Box 13.1   Running into an unexpected road block

In one project, everything was set for the implementation. Patients required a systematic assessment on admission to the service. The nursing agency and home care authority had agreed upon the elements of the assessment. Unfortunately, no one realized that the assessment would take an hour until they started doing them. The pre-existing contract between the nursing agency and the homecare authority indicated that the nursing agency could charge 30 minutes for an assessment on admission. When the nursing agency started charging for assessments that took 60 minutes, the homecare authority declined to pay for the extra 30 minutes. This problem only became known several months into the initiative when the finance department realized the nursing agency was not receiving the full reimbursement they were expecting. More negotiations between the two parties took place with the research team and an agreeable solution to the funding issue was found and the implementation trajectory was back on track.

Box 13.2   Fidelity Clarified

With our leg ulcer example, there were many challenges to assure both types of fidelity. Community nurses required education to take on the two main recommendations: a comprehensive assessment including an ABPI and, the bandaging techniques if a venous etiology was found with the wound.

The implementation strategy fidelity: knowledge was tested after a theory and practical program. Post tests were conducted for knowledge and clinical acumen was evaluated in a clinic setting by an expert.

Evidence implementation fidelity: the process of delivering the comprehensive assessment and bandaging was evaluated in the practice setting with a buddy system whereby the novice was shadowed by an experienced practitioner. This involved the complete process of care from admission, assessment, bandaging and evidence-informed documentation and follow-up.

Manage Summative Evaluation (Outcomes and Impacts) Results

One of the major challenges the group may encounter during the implementation period relates to how to respond to slow uptake of the best practice as revealed by adherence indicators. Waiting for the rates to be calculated and watching them over time can be painful for the working group who are keen to see the best practice in use. The conundrum is about whether to act quickly when the adherence rates are not moving upward as expected or, to wait. It is easy to act prematurely based on early data. But remember, change takes time and the larger the group the longer it takes. On the other hand, waiting too long to intervene can also be detrimental as it may be harder to course correct as more time passes. There is no right answer about when to intervene. But we do have some advice on how to manage the decision to intervene: monitor indicators regularly, use information gathering and feedback to supplement what is really happening out there, debrief with the potential adopters often and try to be patient. It is critical to do these things in real time to be able to make prompt decisions.

When uptake is not happening or not happening quickly, it is also important to keep an eye out for new barriers that may emerge with more people trying to use the best practice and as potential adopters gain experience with the best practice. These emergent barriers are usually not things that could be foreseen when the initial barriers assessment was asking about perceived or hypothetical barriers to using the best practice. When individuals start trying the best practice, barriers they never thought of might start occurring. For these reasons, it is essential to analyze the evaluation data as it is coming in so that it is possible to use the information to act on implementation problems and as they arise.

Sharing Good News and Breaking Bad News

Always keep everyone informed of progress. Communicating about what is happening and with what effect is a way to keep the implementation at top of mind, especially during the early days. Those adopting the best practice like hearing about how well uptake is going. Also, the working group and other stakeholders can be anxious to learn the evaluation results and see how the implementation is going or the impact using the best practice is having. Take every opportunity to celebrate and widely share good news about the implementation. Good news stories can motivate ongoing use of the best practice.

When the results are less positive, it may be useful to share them with mangers and organizational leaders before widely disseminating, so they can prepare how to respond to them. It is generally a good idea to give managers time to think about how to respond to less positive (as well as positive) evaluation results. Similarly, the working group may need to decide based on the evaluation results, whether more time is needed for implementation to occur, or whether modifications to the implementation plan are needed, including changing the implementation strategies or the doses of them. And finally, as we suggested with the launch, use the evaluation data to celebrate advances in the use of evidence-informed practice every chance you get.

At this point it is wise to complete the Action Map (Table 13.1) with information that might be lost in the excitement of finishing the implementation and evaluation. This information will be vital if the group is required to complete a report for the organization. It will also be helpful to support reflection about how to sustain the changes made.

Summary

This chapter concludes the implementation phase of the Roadmap journey. The activity during the implementation period is the culmination of all your efforts. It may also lead to recognition of other areas for best practice implementation. The next chapter provides a focus on sustaining the gains you have made with the implementation.

Table 13.1   Phase 3: ACTION MAP for implementing, evaluating and sustaining (*with Wound Example*).

Customized best practice recommendations	Deploy and monitor implementation strategies *(conduct Process Evaluation)*	Measure outcomes. What is adherence to the best practice? *(Outcomes Evaluation of knowledge use indicators)*	Measure impact *(Impact Evaluation)*
	Full implementation of field-tested strategies. Make adjustments to strategies as needed.	Monitor uptake/adherence of the best practices.	Analyze impact over set period (Impact Evaluation). Develop a report and seek endorsement for ongoing use of best practice.
1. Evening shift RN to conduct daily head to toe skin assessment during HS care and document in flow chart	Process evaluation results: all staff informed or oriented to evening routine with head-to-toe skin assessment and documentation requirement. Orientation, training on-unit completed, 100% attendance. Adjustment to the flow chart completed	Outcome evaluation: 88% receiving head-to-toe assessment daily (nearly at target: 90%) 100% documentation on assessed cases.	Impact goal: 25% reduction in incidence of pressure injuries from baseline. Occurrence of new pressure injuries documented, tallied by unit, 3 mos. Report to evaluation team. At hospital level, 25% reduction met. 2 units did not meet the goal and are being followed up for debriefing to understand issues. Impact data to be collected quarterly by quality program to measure risk and occurrence (prevalence and incidence). Next steps integrate ulcer staging.
2. Braden Risk assessment conducted with head to toe skin assessment by attending RN on evening shift daily and document in flow chart	Process evaluation: 98% of unit staff received Braden Scale training and handout materials. 100% new staff orientated. Clinical shadowing for accuracy of assessment of risks ongoing, 15% completed	Outcome evaluation: 86% patients risk assessed the evening of admission (reasons why not documented on the 4%). 100% documentation on assessed cases.	Risk assessment identified at individual and population level to pinpoint higher risk units and patients needing further intervention

(Continued)

Table 13.1 (Continued)

Customized best practice recommendations	Deploy and monitor implementation strategies *(conduct Process Evaluation)*	Measure outcomes. What is adherence to the best practice? *(Outcomes Evaluation of knowledge use indicators)*	Measure impact *(Impact Evaluation)*
3. Etc. Sustainability thinking continues here. . .	Use process evaluation data to make changes to strategies if needed. Partial implementation may be a threat to sustainability. Ensure implementation strategies continue to be useful and deployable Chapters 13 and 14	Outcome/adherence indicators selected because they can continue to be used in future. Skin and risk assessment proved useful as care benchmarks hospital wide and unit specific data assisted in unit-based QI Chapters 13 and 14	Use impact data to demonstrate the value of best practice on patient and system outcomes, to motivate ongoing use of best practice and justify the ongoing use of resources. Fit/align indicators with quality portfolio. Chapters 13 and 14

14

Sustain the Gains

Introduction

You made it! You followed Roadmap through the implementation of your best practices and now the attention turns to maintaining those gains. This chapter on sustainment focuses on the last aspect of Roadmap Phase 3: Launch, Evaluate and Sustain. Although you have been 'thinking sustaining' throughout it is now time to reflect and plan to ensure that the evidence-informed practice stays in place.

The last chapter described the activities related to launching the implementation strategies and activating the evaluation. This chapter focuses on planning for, nurturing, and sustaining best practice following its implementation. Sustaining a change in practice requires ongoing monitoring of both process and outcomes, including attention to the guideline renewal plan referred to in Chapter 6. At this stage, the working group needs to be vigilant about monitoring adherence to best practice and be prepared to intervene when adherence rates fail to rise to desired levels or if they are climbing, begin prematurely leveling off or even start to slip to pre-implementation levels. It is important to continue to integrate changes into system routines while at the same time remaining alert to: (i) emerging new evidence, (ii) any differences in the adopters and potential adopters, and (iii) changes in the practice environment which occur over time. Ideally, this monitoring is happening throughout the process evaluation and/or the effectiveness/outcomes evaluation and aligned with established quality improvement approaches in the setting.

Sustainability of best practice is a major concern as Ament et al. (2015) have quantified. In their study of professionals' adherence to a clinical practice guideline in medical care, they found that a year after implementation, adherence had decreased in half the studies they reviewed. Following initial uptake of a customized or "new" best practice, there may be a natural tendency for health care providers (and patients) to fall back into usual routines and return to the way they used to do things "pre" best practice. When the uptake of best practice fails to occur or when there is uptake that subsequently falls off, the implications are the same – all the time, effort, and resources that went into implementation planning and execution have not produced a return on investment and have been wasted. Hence, maintaining or sustaining the gains in the use of the best practice is essential for long term success of evidence informed practice and better health outcomes. Continued investment

Knowledge Translation in Nursing and Healthcare: A Roadmap to Evidence-informed Practice, First Edition. Margaret B. Harrison and Ian D. Graham.
© 2021 John Wiley & Sons, Inc. Published 2021 by John Wiley & Sons, Inc.

in sustaining best practice use is always required if the return on the investment in implementation is to be realized.

The goal of the Sustain stage of Roadmap is to: (i) plan for sustainability, (ii) monitor ongoing uptake of best practice (adherence), and (iii) act on the incoming information about adherence rates by reinvestigating ongoing or emerging barriers to change and taking appropriate measures (e.g. undertaking booster implementation strategies or activating new sustainability strategies to deal with newly emergent barriers).

Pertinent questions the working group can use to guide its sustainability activities include:

- Has the sustainability plan been drafted?
- Have all the relevant stakeholders been involved in the planning?
- Who is responsible for monitoring adherence rates and what are the criteria that should trigger investigating slow or declining rates?
- What are the plans for redoing the barriers assessment and for mapping implementation strategies to what are now actual (ongoing or emerging) barriers?
- When will sustainability strategies be activated?

What Is Sustainability

Davies and Edwards (2013) in their chapter on sustaining knowledge use, identify inter-related terms and concepts and the confusion caused by authors sometimes using the terms interchangeably. In summary these terms related to sustainability include:

- Routinization: when an innovation becomes entrenched into regular activities and loses distinct identity (Rogers 2005).
- Institutionalization: the "staying power" or relative endurance of change in an organization (Goodman and Steckler 1989). The change becomes part of everyday activities or normal practices in an organization.
- Re-Invention: Adapting the innovation to fit with a local situation or the degree of modification by the adopters (Rogers 2005).
- Spread: "The process through which new working methods developed in one setting are adopted, perhaps with appropriate modifications, in other organizational contexts" (Buchanan et al. 2007).
- Expanded: In addition to sustaining knowledge use over time, there is a broader implementation to transcend disciplines, organizational units of care, health care sectors, and/or communities (e.g. service, academic) (Davies et al. 2008).
- Scalability: "the ability of a health intervention shown to be efficacious on a small scale and or under controlled conditions to be expanded under real world conditions to reach a greater proportion of the eligible population, while retaining effectiveness" (Milat et al. 2013).

Terms for lack of sustainability include:

- Improvement evaporation, initiative decay or erosion: Decreased application of the innovation over time (Buchanan et al. 2007).
- Discontinuance: A decision to de-adopt or stop the implementation of an innovation (Rogers 2005).
- Relapse: Reverting to previous ways of operating (Bowman et al. 2008).

Turning to the definition of sustainability, early on, Rogers defined it as "the degree to which an innovation continues to be used after initial efforts to secure adoption are complete" (Rogers 2005, p. 429). In 2017, Julia Moore and colleagues conducted a review of the literature to identify definitions of sustainability and then conducted essentially a content analysis of the retrieved definitions (Moore et al. 2017). They identified four published knowledge syntheses of sustainability that included 209 relevant articles which yielded 24 definitions. Based on their analysis they crafted a definition of sustainability that encompassed five key constructs that emerged from the literature: (i) after a defined period of time; (ii) the program, clinical intervention, and/or implementation strategies continue to be delivered; and/or (iii) individual behavior change (i.e. clinician, patient) is maintained; (iv) the program and individual behavior change may evolve or adapt; while (v) continuing to produce benefits for individuals/systems. All 24 definitions were remapped to the comprehensive definition. Of the 24 definitions, 17 described the continued delivery of a program (70.8%), 17 mentioned continued outcomes (70.8%), 13 mentioned time (54.2%), 8 addressed the individual maintenance of a behavior change (33.3%), and 6 described the evolution or adaptation (25.0%). Recently, Nadalin Penno et al. (2019) have identified an additional two constructs related to sustainability. They emerged during their theory analysis of sustainability frameworks – namely defining sustainability as a "process," or as a "stage/phase of ongoing use" after implementation. While all these papers contribute to defining the concept of sustainability and increase conceptual clarity, the challenge remains that the definition by Moore et al. (2017) has yet to be universally adopted or used. This means it is essential when reading the literature on sustainability to identify the definition being used in each paper and interpret the findings of the paper in relation to the definition used. For a selective review of some of the sustainability literature, including sustainability factors and resources, please refer to Appendix 14.A.

While there is no widely agreed upon criteria for determining when the implementation period turns into the sustaining period, two years post implementation seems to be a common benchmark in the literature, although many studies of sustainability occur at one-year post implementation. No doubt the relatively short follow-up time periods for studying sustainability relates to how grants are funded, i.e. they fund implementation studies but not the follow-up period. Another sustainability consideration is that, like implementation, sustainability is not an all or nothing phenomenon. Pluye et al. (2004) identify four degrees of program sustainability in organizations which we have modified to relate to evidence implementation. Their four degrees of sustainability are:

1) Absence of sustainability. The best practice is not sustained, there is no ongoing use of it.
2) Precarious sustainability. The best practice is sustained, but its ongoing use is uncertain. Potential adopters make some use of the best practice, but ongoing use depends entirely on the initiative of the potential adopters.
3) Weak sustainability. The best practice is sustained but is not completely entrenched as the new way of doing things. Major changes in potential adopters or the context can pose a considerable threat to ongoing use of the best practice.
4) Sustainability through routinization. The best practice is sustained and has become routinized as the way things should be done, organizational processes and structures support ongoing use.

Further, we know that sustainability or routinization can be demonstrated in several ways including, the investment in and commitment of organizational resources needed to support the use of best practice such as equipment or staff turnover; the technical or practical compatibility of the behaviors comprising best practice with those of the organization (vs. disruption of the operating workflow); the integration of best practice into organizational policies and guidelines; and fit with and/or addressing organizational mission, priorities and objectives.

Planning for Sustained Use of Best Practice

Like the need for an evaluation plan, the group should also develop a plan to sustain the use of the best practice. Anticipating sustainability issues should occur from the very beginning of the Roadmap journey and sustainability issues be considered at every phase and stage of the journey – sustainability of Roadmap processes as well as sustainability of best practice. For example, when selecting the best practices to customize, the group should consider whether there are any reasons to think that they cannot be sustained over the long term or what would make them sustainable. The group also needs to ensure they have a sustainable process for keeping the customized best practices up to date. When selecting implementation strategies, considering strategies that are easily sustainable is wise. When thinking about the evaluation, the group ought to select indications and data approaches that are also sustainable.

Turning to Phase 3, the post implementation period, the group must turn its attention to sustainability strategies (Shelton et al. 2018). We use the term implementation strategy to refer to those activities or interventions to encourage the initial uptake of best practice and the term sustainability strategy for activities that occur post-implementation directed at encouraging the ongoing use of best practice. In both cases, the strategies are intended to overcome barriers to, or nurture drivers of change and encourage use of best practice. Implementation and sustainability strategies may be the same. The labels simply denote the timing of the use of them – at the time of implementation or sometime after implementation.

Davies and Edwards (2013) have some useful advice about developing sustainability plans and suggest considering six factors in development of a sustainability plan. These factors are derived from the literature and their experience resonates with our experience as well. Here are their questions related to each factor. In some cases, we have adapted their questions or embellished them (Davies and Edwards 2013).

Health needs and expected benefits:

- Is there a well-defined need and a priority for the best practice that is being implemented and sustained?
- Is there consensus about what knowledge needs to be sustained and the related benefits across inter-professional and stakeholder groups and most importantly the patients or communities themselves?

The whole Roadmap process is premised on addressing evidence-practice/policy gaps that are deemed to be sufficiently important to address by a local group. As we have noted earlier, aligning the need for best practice with organizational missions and priorities is a strategic approach to implementation and remains a useful strategy during the sustainability stage. The value of engaging all the relevant stakeholders and building consensus on the need for action was examined in the Call to Action stage of Roadmap (Chapter 5). If the perceived need for the best practice declines over time, the ability to sustain the use of best practice will become more difficult. Demonstrating the impact on health outcomes or health system outcomes can be used to persuade potential adopters to continue using the best practice and managers to continue supporting staff's use of best practice. Nothing breeds success like demonstrating success.

Stakeholder support:

- How might the power and support of the original stakeholders and knowledge users be maintained and leveraged over the long term?
- Have new stakeholders emerged since implementation that need to be engaged?

Reviewing (or reconducting) the stakeholder analysis undertaken as part of the stage of discovering barriers and drivers of best practice implementation (Chapter 9) is a systematic way to get answers to these questions. Remember this includes the knowledge users and leaders (see next factor which is exclusively about leaders). Knowledge users are those adopting and performing the best practice and are ultimately the ones who determine whether the best practice will continue to be used or not. Without the ongoing support of all stakeholders and knowledge users, the use of best practices can easily drop off. The appreciation of the value of engaging patients and their carers as key stakeholders and knowledge users has grown in recent years. They can exert considerable influence on health care providers and policy makers for evidence-informed practice and should not be overlooked during the sustainability stage.

Multi-level and collective leadership:

- What actions might senior leaders, clinical leaders, and champions take to support the sustainability of the new best practice and ongoing knowledge use?
- Are there champions for the change at various system levels (health care provider peer mentors, team leaders, senior management)?
- Who is responsible for continued implementation of the best practice and making modifications as new knowledge or contextual changes in the setting occur?
- Who will be accountable for the monitoring process to ensure that progress toward the relevant outcomes is being assessed and acted upon?

As we have already described (Chapter 4 Appendix 4.A), leaders have the legitimate authority to set and enforce performance expectations of staff, can role model the value of using best practices, and also have the ability to allocate resources that can support ongoing best practice use. Without their ongoing support for the use of the best practice, especially when resources are essential to being able to do the best practice, sustainability can be greatly threatened. During the sustainability stage it is critical to keep supportive leaders on side and cultivate support from leaders who may be new or previously ambivalent or resistant.

Financial and human resources:

- What funding is required to sustain the use of the best practice?
- Are efficiencies gained through sustaining use of the best practice?
- Can lower-cost yet effective strategies be used in the future to maintain the core elements of the best practice?
- Are human resources and staffing systems supportive for ongoing use of the best practice for the long term?

Both implementing and sustaining use of best practice come with a cost. These include the time to learn and do the best practice, expenses related to developing and delivering implementation and sustainability strategies, and expenditures for acquiring necessary equipment or infrastructure (monitoring systems). It is also important to consider opportunity costs. Given resources are typically scarce in health care it means the use of resources in one way prevents their use in other ways (Palmer and Raftery 1999). Are there things that will not be done because the funding and human resources are being allocated to implement and sustain the new best practice? Without ongoing human resources, the best practice is unlikely to be sustained.

Effectiveness of the system to monitor progress:

- Is there an evaluation system that will be sustained to provide ongoing quantitative and qualitative data to inform formative learning and determine evidence of outcomes and impact?
- Have interactive feedback processes with potential knowledge users been put in place?
- Are communication systems available to inform patients, staff, the organization and the community about indicators and outcomes?

As we have explained, the evaluation of the implementation, as well as the sustainability time-frame provides critical information for making course corrections. The evaluation data also demonstrates the value of the initiative in terms of the process of care indicators and impact on individuals and the health system. The latter can then be used to justify the ongoing outlay of support and resources for the best practice, if that continues to be required. Using indicators of adherence and impact, and data collection processes that make collecting these data easy, automatic, and routine, means that evaluation data will be timelier, more complete and therefore, more useful for decision making.

As with all stages of Roadmap, there should always be feedback loops where initial phases inform subsequent phases (e.g. implementation strategies are mapped to identified barriers and subsequent phases re-inform past phases; declining adherence rates trigger the need for more assessment of barriers). Throughout all stages of the Roadmap, strong and effective communication with stakeholders and, the knowledge users are critical for obtaining and maintaining buy-in. This is particularly true in the sustainability stage when the benefits (value) of using the best practice become quantified. For health care providers, seeing the benefits of using best practice provides strong reinforcement and motivation to continue following the best practice protocol. For example learning that as a result of their using the best practice protocol they developed, the three month leg ulcer healing rates rose from 23 to 56% – in addition to clinically seeing improved healing and getting positive patient feedback, nurses were motivated to want to continue using the protocol (Harrison et al. 2005). Similarly, for managers, seeing the "numbers" (e.g. expenditures for supplies drop, improved efficiency of nursing visits) can have the same effect. Of course, the anticipated benefits of implementing the best practice may be less than expected and therefore have less effect on motivating sustained change, but regardless having these data always permits more evidence-informed decisions.

Box 14.1   Interpreting the Impact

With one group, the implementation of best practice was a success in terms of high adherence rates to the new practice guideline. However, when the summative evaluation was conducted, the health benefits were not as high as the group had expected based on the clinical trial findings related to the recommendations. When the group discussed this apparently disappointing finding with management, management agreed that they would have liked to have seen a larger impact on patient health outcomes. But, they still considered the implementation (and its sustainability) a huge success as there was now data to show that the organization was delivering high quality evidence-informed care. They continued to support the ongoing use of the best practice.

Adaptability and alignment of the improved process:

- Will the improved process resulting from the ongoing use of the best practice be adaptable as other organizational or socio-political changes occur over the long term?
- What management decision making processes need to be considered when determining how to align the ongoing use with other current and future best practices?

This factor relates to potential adopters and organizations needing to be able to adapt best practices (or the innovations) as well as the implementation and sustainability strategies over time to align with changes in context. These changes can be related to internal changes such as organizational restructuring, or changes in external context such as new laws, regulations, accreditation standards, etc. Similar to the concept of customization of best practice to the local context (chapter 8), over time the best practice needs to continue to be customized to the changing context. This can be related to changes in the evidence supporting the best practice – as the source recommendations are updated based on new evidence. Adjustments may also need to be made to the customized best practice over time. For example, if the composition of the patient population at a facility changes as admission criteria are altered over a period of months or years, there may be a need to modify how a particular best practice assessment is conducted by increasing the use of personal service workers. This is essentially another customization of the best practice which initially had Registered Nurses conducting all the assessments. The Roadmap implementation process is sufficiently flexible and builds in many opportunities for adaptation and alignment that can continue in the post implementation stage.

Our Approach to Sustainability

We have come to think of the post implementation period as a time when the processes of the Building Solutions phase of Roadmap may need to be re-visited (feedback loops). The ongoing monitoring of indicators of process and impact during and post implementation period, provide the data to re-assess the evidence-practice gap (which hopefully is closing). If the evidence-practice gap is not closing as anticipated, the working group can use this information to trigger the decision to re-examine barriers to implementation or ongoing use of the best practice (is the problem that implementation was not successful or is something happening during the post implementation period that is affecting adherence rates).

Our re-consideration of barriers has typically taken the form of informal discussions with point of care staff, patients, managers, and other key stakeholders. We asked how implementation is going and what things are inhibiting even greater use of the best practice and what factors they see as driving the ongoing use. Sometimes we have first asked key informants how well they think the implementation is going and why, and then provided the evaluation data to them. If there is a lack of concordance between how well they think implementation is going and the verified adherence rates, we ask them to think about what might explain the divergence. Sometimes, the key informants do not accept the evaluation data which leads to a discussion of why the adherence indicators may not be reliable or accurate. It is important to determine if there is a measurement problem or a perception problem. How to tackle each of these is different. Ruling out a measurement issue is sometimes easier to deal with. The data can be rerun, data quality issues addressed, or more data collected. When the evaluation data are correct and stakeholders accept this, then the challenge becomes how to persuade knowledge users that they are not actually using the best practice as often as they think. That discussion can explore why they think they are using the best practice more than the data indicate and what could be done to support their even greater use of it. It remains essential to conduct these discussions in a tactful, supportive and positive way and never to blame or shame knowledge users for failure to adhere to the best practice. The focus must always be on improving quality of care not blaming or punishing knowledge users. Always acknowledge and praise any uptake, no matter how small it is and concede that change can be hard but working collectively it can be achieved.

Box 14.2   Be wary of blockers

In one situation, uptake of nursing recommendations was not occurring despite nurses and managers believing it was. After describing how the indicator was calculated and how the data were collected and analyzed, the nurses conceded the data were probably right. We then explored what might be affecting uptake of the recommendations. It was soon learned that the concurrent use of a medical guideline essentially meant the nursing recommendations could not be implemented (the story of competing guidelines). We also learned that on evening shift one of the coordinators essentially discouraged nurses from following the recommendations as the coordinator did not believe the recommendations were beneficial despite the evidence upon which they were developed. Implementation strategies to deal with these new barriers (neither of which were anticipated or suggested in the initial barriers assessment) were to convene a meeting of medical and nursing departments to discuss the two guidelines and how to navigate when each should be applied. The evening coordinator was taken aside to have a one-on-one discussion about the recommendations, her views on them, the evidence supporting the benefits of the recommendations and management's expectations about supporting their use.

In another instance an unexpected driver was a clinical leader who had recently completed a KT course in a master's program and soon became a clinical lead in the unit. The message being, that not all barriers or drivers can be anticipated until an implementation begins.

Distinguishing between initially identified barriers and new emergent ones is important. As the solution to the first may be increasing the dose of the implementation strategies already being used (implementation strategy boosters) or considering supplementary strategies. When the barriers are ones that have emerged since the implementation process began (previously unidentified barriers), it usually means doing another mapping of (what is now sustainability) strategies to the newly identified barriers (Chapter 11). Paying attention to the drivers of change during the post implementation period and leveraging them is always useful. You will recall from the discussion of the Ottawa Model of Research in Chapter 3 (Graham and Logan 2004), that the maintenance or follow-up implementation strategies refers to the need to potentially adjust and apply more or new strategies to support ongoing use. The more formal barriers assessment approaches described in Chapter 9 can be used again to increase insight into sustainability factors.

Finally, the data continuing to be collected by the process evaluation on the delivery and use of the existing strategies, and what have become the new sustainability strategies, can help the group to determine whether the changes to the implementation and sustainability plans are having the desired effect. And if not, then the implementation and sustaining cycle continues until the group determines the adherence rates meet their expectations and they can focus on another evidence-practice gap.

Spread and Scaling

There are two complementary concepts to sustain; spread and scale. As with the concept of sustainability, there are no commonly accepted definitions of spread and scale. Cote-Boileau et al. (2019) recently conducted a scoping review of spreading, sustaining and scaling healthcare innovations. They note that "spread is commonly defined as both passive and deliberate efforts to communicate and implement an innovation, and usually involves adapting an innovation to a new setting" (Hempel et al. 2019). They further observe that, "scale-up commonly refers to the process in which the coverage and impact of an innovation are expanded to reach all potential beneficiaries" (Hempel et al. 2019). They define the terms this way:

- Spread-The process through which new working methods developed in one setting are adapted, perhaps with appropriate modifications, in other organizational contexts.
- Scale-The ambition or process of expanding the coverage of health interventions, but can also refer to increasing the financial, human, and capital resources required to expand coverage.

From their scoping review, they identified four mechanisms that are consistently related to 3S (spreading, sustaining, scaling). These were substance – characteristics of the innovation, how it is perceived by potential adopters in terms of need and value; processes – the dynamics underpinning the 3S (e.g. frequent monitoring and feedback, collective learning, institutionalization of new values, beliefs, norms and organizational practices); stakeholders – working across interprofessional and interorganizational boundaries; and context – unpredictable and influences 3S. They also identify seven enabling factors: adaptable innovations (substance), distributed leadership, reciprocal accountability, absorptive context, iterative timing and pace of change, empowering management support and decentralized governance. Based on their findings, they proposed the following framework of actionable guidance for 3S (see Figure 14.1). The Roadmap approach strongly aligns with this framework and focuses on:

- The why: the Call to Action is about stakeholders exploring why they and their organization(s) are interested in the problem and value best practice. Assembling the Local Evidence is about being explicit about why there is a need to address the evidence-practice gap and exploring why to commit to the best practice.
- Perceived value and feasibility: customizing best practice is about identifying the value in guideline recommendations and determining the feasibility of adopting them.
- What people do rather than what they should do: all the phases and stages of Roadmap orient toward stakeholders and in particular knowledge users adapting and customizing best practice to their context and co-creating solutions through collective action and learning as they go.
- Creating a dialogue between policy and delivery: Roadmap work is essentially relational and provides guidance for stakeholders to negotiate a way to move from the problem (an evidence-practice gap that is important to them) to co-creating a solution and implementation plan that is grounded in their values, interests and context. The stages of Roadmap are designed to enable dialogue and problem solving to achieve agreed upon common goals.
- Inclusivity and capacity building: at every stage of Roadmap, a critical element is ensuring that all the relevant stakeholders are involved with specific focus on including the entire range of interdisciplinary healthcare providers, managers and patients and their carers. A hallmark of the process is capacity building and mutual learning at each stage of the journey (e.g. from using critical appraisal skills, to conducting barriers assessment, to implementation strategy mapping, to evaluation).

In our work, we have not focused on scaling up but have had some experience with studying spread. In one project, a leg ulcer protocol that was developed (following the process described in chapter 8) by one group, was shared with three other geographically dispersed sites in the province. The three new sites were encouraged to consider implementing the protocol in their setting. Two of the sites used a participatory approach to mobilize stakeholders in assembling local data about their own evidence-practice gaps and current

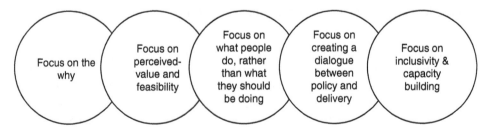

Figure 14.1 Framework of actionable guidance for 3S across five key focus areas. *Source:* Reprinted with permission under the terms of the Creative Commons Attribution 4.0 International License (http://creativecommons.org/licenses/by/4.0) from Cote-Boileau et al. (2019).

practice and further customizing the protocol to their own context. They selected and launched implementation strategies (education being a core strategy but also other strategies such as using an interdisciplinary team approach). In both cases adherence to the protocol was high and healing rates improved. These findings suggested that groups may not need to develop customized best practices from scratch if there are trusted source guidelines and protocols and they are able to customize them for their setting. With the third site, the group did not see the need to engage relevant stakeholders, chose not to collect any local data of current practice or the problem, and unilaterally decided that all that was needed was to provide education to a small number of community nurses. Implementation of the protocol failed to occur in site 3.

For more information on spread and scale, please refer to appendix 14.C for a selective list of references.

Integrating Roadmap with Organizational Quality Improvement Approaches

Finally, there is one grand implementation (and sustainability) strategy we would like to discuss – the use of existing quality improvement strategies. Roadmap phases and stages are complementary to many quality improvement approaches. Table 14.1, maps Roadmap stages to three of the most common quality improvement frameworks. Many of the Roadmap stages are already part of these frameworks. Differences however, include Roadmap's greater emphasis on implementing evidence-informed practice, focusing implementation on reducing the evidence-practice gap, systematically customizing the best practice to the local context, emphasizing the use of effective implementation strategies, and historically, greater reliance on implementation science. The advantages of integrating Roadmap efforts with quality improvement processes are that: the improvement processes already exist (and making use of them may save duplication of efforts), stakeholders are familiar and experienced with these processes, they are supported by existing resources (human and financial) and infrastructure, and the quality improvement portfolio often reports to the board. In fact, in some jurisdictions it is actually a compulsory requirement.

Furthermore, many quality improvement techniques are complementary or alternative ways of collecting data suggested by Roadmap. Common quality improvement data collection techniques include:

- Cause and Effect or Fishbone diagrams which are a tool to explore cause to a single effect (or event) through brainstorming.
- Flow charts are used to diagram the processes or process steps to understand their flow.
- Pareto charts, also known as the 80:20 principle, is a bar chart showing the frequencies of different causes or factors in descending order to reveal the most significant factors.
- Histograms are bar charts used to understand the nature of data.
- Check sheets are used for data collection.
- Scatter plots visually depict the relationships between two variables.
- Control charts are used to check whether process data remains under control (e.g. adherence rates remain within target levels).

Table 14.1 Comparison of Roadmap stages with three commonly used frameworks for quality improvement work.

Roadmap	Issues clarification	Find best practice	Assemble evidence and determine evidence-practice gap	Customize best practice to local context	Discover barriers/drivers to implementation	Tailor implementation strategies	Field test, Implement, Evaluate	Sustain
Model for Improvement (Deming 2000; Langley et al. 2009; East London NHS Foundation Trust: Quality Improvement 2020)	What are we trying to accomplish?		How will we know that a change is an improvement? Outcomes, process, balance			What changes can we make that could result in improvement? Gather ideas of how improvement can be driven. What are the possible solutions?	How do we test the solutions?	How do we sustain and standardize what we have achieved? What changes need to be made next?
	Forming the team. Setting aims		Establishing measures			Selecting changes	Establishing measures. Testing changes. Implementing changes	Spreading changes
PDSA cycle				Plan			Do-Study	Study-Act
Six Sigma (DMAIC) (Rastogi 2018)	Define the problem and objective	Improve. Determine potential solutions	Measure what we need to improve and what we can measure. Analyze gaps between actual and goal performance		Analyze the process, define the factors of influence. Find root cause of business inefficiencies.	Improve. Determine potential solutions, ways to implement them, test and implement them for improvement. Control. Post implementation results are evaluated. Progress ascertained.	Do-Study	Control. Assure that improvements will sustain by generating a solution monitoring plan.
Lean (5 principles) (planview 2020; Quality-One International 2020)	1. Identify costumers and what they value.	3. Create flow	2. Map steps in value stream	2. Map value stream	3. Create flow. Eliminate waste and variation at the root cause.		4. Establish pull. Transform approach	5. Seek perfection. Standardize flow, sustain, continuously improve

Box 14.3   A Tip from experts
Formulating an action plan based on the best available scientific evidence with clearly defined and measurable outcomes is an essential component of a quality improvement initiative. Institutional leadership, support, and staff accountability are critical factors that enhance the implementation process and promote the sustainability of quality improvement initiatives. The healthcare provider of the twenty-first century should possess a variety of skills and strategies essential to be the catalyst for quality improvement (Clutter et al. 2009, p. 283).

Each of these techniques can be used as part of the Roadmap stage of assembling local evidence on context and current practice, to examine and understand the evidence-practice gap. Some can also be used in evaluation efforts.

Summary

This chapter has reviewed some of the promising practices related to sustaining best practice that should be included in a sustainability plan. It has also described how the Roadmap journey incorporates many of the elements believed to nurture and support sustainability of evidence-informed practice. In the final chapter, we reflect on the challenges and benefits of Roadmap and pursuing a journey to evidence-informed practice.

Appendix 14.A: Sustainability

This appendix provides a selective review of sustainability factors and useful resources.

While interest in understanding sustainability and how to ensure best practices are maintained is relatively recent, the literature in this area growing. Over the past few years there have been several reviews or syntheses on aspects of sustainability. For example, there are at least six scoping or systematic reviews of sustainability studies (Gruen et al. 2008; Wiltsey Stirman et al. 2012; Ament et al. 2015; Lennox et al. 2018), strategies (Iwelunmor et al. 2016; Tricco et al. 2016) or frameworks and models (Gruen et al. 2008; Lennox et al. 2018; Nadalin Penno et al. 2019) as well as another ongoing systematic review of sustainability interventions for chronic disease management in older adults (Nadalin Penno et al. 2019). Many of these reviews cataloged sustainability studies or frameworks and analyzed the components of sustainability. The expectation is that by knowing what key ingredients are needed to sustain best practice, the critical ingredients can be built into sustainability planning and support ongoing use of the best practice.

In 2018, Lennox and colleagues undertook a systematic review of sustainability approaches in healthcare. The review identified 62 publications identifying a sustainability approach (32 frameworks, 16 models, 8 tools, 4 strategies, 1 checklist, and 1 process). Comparison of the constructs across the approaches revealed 40 individual constructs of sustainability which they summarized and called a consolidated framework for sustainability constructs in healthcare. The constructs are organized under six emergent themes: the initiative design and delivery, negotiating initiative processes, the people involved, resources, the external environment and the organizational setting. The analysis revealed that none of the approaches included the same combination of constructs, however, six constructs were included in over 75% of the approaches, these being: general resources (90%), demonstrating effectiveness (89%), monitoring progress over time (84%), stakeholder participation (79%), integration with existing programs and policies (79%), and training and capacity building (76%). Of note is that the consistency of constructs with the approaches was independent of proposed interventions, settings, or application types. This paper is a good resource for finding sustainability frameworks or sustainability constructs. Table 14.A.1 presents the 40 constructs

Table 14.A.1 Consolidated framework for sustainability constructs in healthcare.

The initiative design and delivery	Negotiating initiative processes	The people involved	Resources	The organizational setting	The external environment
• Demonstrating effectiveness 89%	• Belief in the initiative 63%	• Stakeholder participation 79%	• General resources 90%	• Integration with existing programs and policies 79%	• Socioeconomic and political considerations 63%
• Monitoring progress over time 84%	• Accountability of roles and responsibilities 56%	• Leadership and champions 73%	• Funding 68%	• Intervention adaptation and receptivity 73%	• Awareness and raising the profile 45%
• Training and capacity building 76%	• Defining aims and shared vision 53%	• Relationships and collaboration and networks 65%	• Infrastructure 26%	• Organizational values and culture 71%	• Urgency 5%
• Evidence base for the initiative 52%	• Incentives 31%	• Community participation 56%	• Resource_ Staff 26%	• Organizational readiness and capacity 56%	• Spread to other organizations 5%
• Expertise 23%	• Workload 27%	• Staff involvement 42%	• Resource_ Time 6%	• Support available 40%	
• The problem 15%	• Complexity 24%	• Ownership 26%		• Opposition 5%	
• Project duration 8%	• Job requirements 19%	• Power 18%			
• Improvement methods 6%		• Patient involvement 16%			
• Project type 2%		• Satisfaction 11%			

under Lennox and colleagues' six themes. The percentages in the Table refer to the number of approaches that included each construct (there were in total 62 approaches included in the analysis).

Specifically in terms of implementation frameworks, there are a number of them that either include sustainability as an element of the implementation process or focus exclusively on sustainability. For example, our own synthesis of planned action models that gave rise to the Knowledge to Action Cycle framework, revealed that of the 31 frameworks reviewed, 11 included a separate phase following initial implementation that was labeled maintain the change or sustain ongoing knowledge use (Graham et al. 2013). This suggests that for these frameworks, sustainability is considered part of the implementation life cycle as opposed to a process that occurs independently of it.

Nadalin Penno et al. (2019) systematic review and theory analysis of selected sustainability theories, frameworks or models (TFM) found eight TFM of sustainability of best practice in acute care or an unspecified healthcare organization/setting (they excluded frameworks related to public or community health). The theory analysis revealed 152 sustainability factors that were reduced to 37 *core factors*, which were further grouped into 7 *themes*: (i) characteristics of the *innovation*/evidence informed practices, (ii) *adopter/user* factors influencing sustained use, (iii) *leadership and management* influences/factors, (iv) *inner context* (practice setting/organization) factors where the evidence informed practices are delivered; (v) *inner processes*/infrastructure factors that support the evidence informed practices (e.g. processes, methods, systems, structures, or strategies); (vi) *outer context* or broader system factors; and (vii) *outcomes* descriptions without defined factors. When examining the occurrence of the core factors across the 8 frameworks, 16 were classified as common factors as they appeared in half or more of the frameworks. Table 14.A.2 lists the factors in each framework and permits comparison between frameworks. Note the similarity of factors/constructs between this and the Lennox paper. Consider how many of these factors have been ones we have already discussed in relation to planning for implementation. Most of them are things that might be first assessed or come up during the barriers assessment stage. What these papers are suggesting to us is that these factors may need to be re-assessed during the implementation and sustainability stages and if they are appearing as barriers will need to be dealt with. If they are driving (facilitating) best practice use, they will need to be nurtured. If following implementation these factors emerge as ongoing or new barriers, then this may call for another mapping of implementation strategies to the barriers.

For the most part, sustainability frameworks have yet to be empirically tested with the exception of the Mayer and colleagues' UK National Health Service (NHS) Sustainability Model (Mayer et al. 2010). Most frameworks also do not come with tools or measures with the exception of the NHS Sustainability Model and the Slaghuis and colleagues' framework for sustainability of work practices in long-term care (Slaghuis et al. 2011). Other potentially useful tools are the Program Sustainability Assessment Tool (Center for Public Health Systems Science 2020b) for public health programs and the Clinical Sustainability Assessment Tool (Center for Public Health Systems Science 2020a) developed by researchers at the Center for Public Health Systems Science at the Washington University, St Louis MO. The website includes the tools and the scoring systems for them. For a review of program sustainability tools see Hutchinson (2010).

Table 14.A.2 Synthesis of themes and factors found in sustainability frameworks/models/theories for acute care (n = 8).

Theme/concept	Core factors	Unspecified setting Frameworks					Acute care Frameworks		
		1	2	3	5	6	4	7	8
Innovation (defined as: new process/change/product/practice or program, innovation, intervention)	[a]Relevance/consistent with competitive strategy	✓	✓			✓		✓	✓
	[a]Characteristics (scale, shape and form, age, nature, type, integrity)	✓	✓		✓	✓		✓	✓
	[a]Perceived centrality to organizational performance/platform/services	✓	✓		✓	✓		✓	✓
	Fit with org's vision/mission, procedures/strategies	✓		✓				✓	✓
	Adaptability of innovation			✓		✓		✓	
	[a]Benefits to patient, staff, organization (cost-effective, efficiency and quality of care)	✓		✓	✓	✓		✓	
	Barrier identification					✓			
Adopters (defined as staff, stakeholder, user, adopter, actor, and or individual)	Human resources – recruitment, processes, succession and leave planning (staffing)				✓	✓			
	[a]Individual commitment to innovation	✓	✓			✓		✓	
	[a]Individual competency (skill knowledge, absorptive capacity) to perform innovation	✓	✓		✓		✓	✓	✓
	Internal cohesion between individual and commitment within the organization/stakeholder engagement leads to increased performance		✓					✓	
	Stakeholder commitment to innovation						✓		
	Stakeholder beliefs, attitude, perceptions, emotions, expectations toward innovation	✓		✓		✓		✓	
	Champion presence and involvement			✓					✓
Leadership and management (defined as style, approach, behaviors, engagement support, or feedback)	[a]Management approach and engagement	✓	✓	✓	✓	✓		✓	✓
	[a]Senior leadership involvement and actions	✓	✓	✓				✓	

Dimension	Factor	1	2	3	4	5	6	7	8
Inner context (defined as context, practice setting or organization)	[a]Infrastructure support – policies and procedures based on innovation	✓	✓				✓	✓	✓
	Infrastructure support for innovation in the job description with the mechanism for recognizing achievement	✓	✓			✓	✓	✓	
	[a]Infrastructure support-equipment and supplies for innovation	✓		✓			✓	✓	✓
	Organization—absorptive capacity for innovation						✓	✓	✓
	Cultural—beliefs, values, and perceptions to innov	✓					✓	✓	
	[a]Cultural – climate	✓		✓			✓	✓	
	Cultural—innovation integrated into Norms (documents, protocols, manuals)	✓						✓	
	Political internal stakeholder coalition, power, influence	✓			✓		✓	✓	
	Financial performance budgeting and measurement	✓			✓		✓	✓	
	Financial-internal funds and other non-financial resources of innovation				✓	✓	✓	✓	
Inner processes (defined as processes, methods, systems, structures, or strategies)	[a]Education and training processes	✓	✓		✓	✓	✓	✓	
	Processual—planning, method, and timing of embedding innovation	✓	✓		✓	✓	✓	✓	
	[a]Processual – project structure and system to monitor/manage innovation	✓	✓		✓	✓	✓	✓	
	[a]Organization – communication capacity for monitoring (exchange and feedback)	✓	✓	✓	✓	✓	✓	✓	
	Behavioral change strategies								
Outer context (defined as external condition, context, system, or environment)	Socio-economic political threats, stability	✓	✓		✓	✓	✓	✓	
	[a]External conditions, compatibility for innovation	✓	✓		✓	✓	✓	✓	
	Connection to broader external context	✓	✓			✓	✓		
	External support for innovation from stakeholders	✓	✓		✓	✓	✓	✓	

Appendix 14.B: Selective List of Sustainability References

Ament, S.M., de Groot, J.J., Maessen, J.M. et al. (2015). Sustainability of professionals' adherence to clinical practice guidelines in medical care: a systematic review. *BMJ Open* 5: e008073. https://doi.org/10.1136/bmjopen-2015-008073.

Center for Public Health Systems Science (2020a). *Clinical Sustainability Assessment Tool*, [Online], Available: https://cphss.wustl.edu/items/csat.

Center for Public Health Systems Science (2020b). *Program Sustainability Assessment Tool*, [Online], Available: https://www.sustaintool.org/psat.

Graham, I.D., Tetroe, J., and KT Theories Group (2013). Planned action theories. In: *Knowledge Translation in Health Care: Moving from Evidence to Practice* (eds. S.E. Straus, J. Tetroe and I.D. Graham), 277–287. Wiley Blackwell: Oxford, UK.

Gruen, R.L., Elliott, J.H., Nolan, M.L. et al. (2008). Sustainability science: an integrated approach for health-programme planning. *Lancet* 372: 1579–1589.

Hutchinson, K. (2010). *Literature Review of Program Sustainability Assessment Tools*, http://communitysolutions.ca/web/wp-content/uploads/2013/07/Review-of-Sustainability-Tools-2010.pdf.

Iwelunmor, J., Blackstone, S., Veira, D. et al. (2016). Toward the sustainability of health interventions implemented in sub-Saharan Africa: a systematic review and conceptual framework. *Implementation Science* 11: 43. https://doi.org/10.1186/s13012-016-0392-8.

Lennox, L., Maher, L., and Reed, J. (2018). Navigating the sustainability landscape: a systematic review of sustainability approaches in healthcare. *Implementation Science* 13: 27. https://doi.org/10.1186/s13012-017-0707-4.

Mayer, L., Gustafson, D., and Evans, A. (2010). *Sustainability Model and Guide*, https://webarchive.nationalarchives.gov.uk/20160805122935/http://www.nhsiq.nhs.uk/media/2757778/nhs_sustainability_model_-_february_2010_1_.pdf.

Nadalin Penno, L., Davies, B., Graham, I.D. et al. (2019). Identifying relevant concepts and factors for the sustainability of evidence-based practices within acute care contexts: a systematic review and theory analysis of selected sustainability frameworks. *Implementation Science* 14: 108. https://doi.org/10.1186/s13012-019-0952-9.

Slaghuis, S.S., Strating, M.M., Bal, R.A., and Nieboer, A.P. (2011). A framework and a measurement instrument for sustainability of work practices in long-term care. *BMC Health Services Research* 11: 314. https://doi.org/10.1186/1472-6963-11-314.

Tricco, A.C., Ashoor, H.M., Cardoso, R. et al. (2016). Sustainability of knowledge translation interventions in healthcare decision-making: a scoping review. *Implementation Science* 11: 55. https://doi.org/10.1186/s13012-016-0421-7.

Wiltsey Stirman, S., Kimberly, J., Cook, N. et al. (2012). The sustainability of new programs and innovations: a review of the empirical literature and recommendations for future research. *Implementation Science* 7: 17. https://doi.org/10.1186/1748-5908-7-17.

Appendix 14.C: Selective List of Spread and Scale References

Atkinson, J., Patel, C., Wilson, A. et al. (2013). *Drivers of large-scale change in complex health systems: an Evidence Check rapid review brokered by the Sax Institute* (www.saxinstitute.org.au) *for the NSW Agency for Clinical Innovation.*

Barker, P.M., Reid, A., and Schall, M.W. (2016). A framework for scaling up health interventions: lessons from large-scale improvement initiatives in Africa. *Implementation Science* 11: 12. https://doi.org/10.1186/s13012-016-0374-x.

Ben Charif, A., Zomahoun, H.T.V., LeBlanc, A. et al. (2017). Effective strategies for scaling up evidence-based practices in primary care: a systematic review. *Implementation Science* 12: 139. https://doi.org/10.1186/s13012-017-0672-y.

Gogovor, A., Zomahoun, H.T.V., Ben Charif, A. et al. (2020). Essential items for reporting of scaling studies of health interventions (SUCCEED): protocol for a systematic review and Delphi process. *Systematic Reviews* 9: 11. https://doi.org/10.1186/s13643-019-1258-3.

Greenhalgh, T., Wherton, J., Papoutsi, C. et al. (2017). Beyond adoption: a new framework for theorizing and evaluating nonadoption, abandonment, and challenges to the scale-up, spread, and sustainability of health and care technologies. *Journal of Medical Internet Research* 19: e367. https://doi.org/10.2196/jmir.8775.

Hempel, S., O'Hanlon, C., Lim, Y.W. et al. (2019). Spread tools: a systematic review of components, uptake, and effectiveness of quality improvement toolkits. *Implementation Science* 14: 83. https://doi.org/10.1186/s13012-019-0929-8.

McLean, R. and Gargani, J. (2019). *Scaling Impact: Innovation for the Public Good.* Abingdon, Oxon: Routledge.

Milat, A.J., Bauman, A., and Redman, S. (2015). Narrative review of models and success factors for scaling up public health interventions. *Implementation Science* 10: 113. https://doi.org/10.1186/s13012-015-0301-6.

Milat, A., Lee, K., Conte, K. et al. (2020). Intervention scalability assessment tool: a decision support tool for health policy makers and implementers. *Health Research Policy and Systems* 18: 1. https://doi.org/10.1186/s12961-019-0494-2.

Øvretveit, J., Garofalo, L., and Mittman, B. (2017). Scaling up improvements more quickly and effectively. *International Journal for Quality in Health Care* 29: 1014–1019. https://doi.org/10.1093/intqhc/mzx147.

Price-Kelly, H., van Haeren, L., and McLean, R. (2020). *The Scaling Playbook: A Practical Guide for Researchers.* Ottawa, Canada: International Development Research Centre https://idl-bnc-idrc.dspacedirect.org/bitstream/handle/10625/58780/IDL-58780.pdf?sequence=2&isAllowed=y.

Shaw, J., Shaw, S., Wherton, J. et al. (2017). Studying scale-up and spread as social practice: theoretical introduction and empirical case study. *Journal of Medical Internet Research* 19: e244. https://doi.org/10.2196/jmir.7482.

Slaghuis, S.S. (2016). *Riding the Waves of Quality Improvement: Sustainability and Spread in a Dutch Quality Improvement Program for Long-Term Care.* Erasmus Universiteit Rotterdam https://pdfs.semanticscholar.org/9bd3/bbdfc9bbce9bd8fa82e6972bd06082a7bb06.pdf?_ga=2.103017801.878722381.1599779272-438250037.1599779272.

Sustainable Improvement Team and the Horizons Team (2018). *Leading Large Scale Change: A Practical Guide.* Quarry Hill, Leeds: NHS England https://www.england.nhs.uk/wp-content/uploads/2017/09/practical-guide-large-scale-change-april-2018-smll.pdf.

Wolfenden, L., Albers, B., and Shlonsky, A. (2018). PROTOCOL: strategies for scaling up the implementation of interventions in social welfare: protocol for a systematic review. *Campbell Systematic Reviews* 14: 1–33. https://doi.org/10.1002/CL2.201.

References

Ament, S.M., de Groot, J.J., Maessen, J.M. et al. (2015). Sustainability of professionals' adherence to clinical practice guidelines in medical care: a systematic review. *BMJ Open* 5: e008073. https://doi.org/10.1136/bmjopen-2015-008073.

Bowman, C.C., Sobo, E.J., Asch, S.M. et al. (2008). Measuring persistence of implementation: QUERI Series. *Implementation Science* 3: 21. https://doi.org/10.1186/1748-5908-3-21.

Buchanan, D.A., Fitzgerald, L., and Ketley, D. (eds.) (2007). *The Sustainability and Spread of Organizational Change*. Abingdon: Routledge.

Clutter, P.C., Reed, C., Cornett, P.A., and Parsons, M.L. (2009). Action Planning Strategies to Achieve Quality Outcomes. *Critical Care Nurse* 32: 272–284. https://doi.org/10.1097/CNQ.0b013e3181bad30f.

Cote-Boileau, E., Denis, J.L., Callery, B., and Sabean, M. (2019). The unpredictable journeys of spreading, sustaining and scaling healthcare innovations: a scoping review. *Health Research Policy and Systems* 17: 84. https://doi.org/10.1186/s12961-019-0482-6.

Davies, B. and Edwards, N. (2013). Sustaining knowledge use. In: *Knowledge Translation in Health Care: Moving from Evidence to Practice* (eds. S.E. Straus, J. Tetroe and I.D. Graham), 237–248. Chichester: Wiley Blackwell, BMJ Books.

Davies, B., Edwards, N., Ploeg, J., and Virani, T. (2008). Insights about the process and impact of implementing nursing guidelines on delivery of care in hospitals and community settings. *BMC Health Services Research* 8: 29. https://doi.org/10.1186/1472-6963-8-29.

Deming, W.E. (2000). *The New Economics for Industry, Government, Education*, 2e. Cambridge, Massachusetts, USA: The MIT Press. For more on the development of the PDSA cycle and how it differs from PDCA, see: Moen RD, Norman CL. Circling back: Clearing up myths about the Deming cycle and seeing how it keeps evolving. Quality Progress. November 2010.

East London NHS Foundation Trust: Quality Improvement (2020). The Model for Improvement [Available from: https://qi.elft.nhs.uk/resource/the-model-for-improvement.

Goodman, R.M. and Steckler, A. (1989). A model for the institutionalization of health promotion programs. *Family & Community Health* 11: 63–78.

Graham, I.D. and Logan, J. (2004). Innovations in knowledge transfer and continuity of care. *The Canadian Journal of Nursing Research* 36: 89–103.

Harrison, M.B., Graham, I.D., Lorimer, K. et al. (2005). Leg-ulcer care in the community, before and after implementation of an evidence-based service. *Canadian Medical Association Journal* 172: 1447–1452. https://doi.org/10.1503/cmaj.1041441.

Hempel, S., O'Hanlon, C., Lim, Y.W. et al. (2019). Spread tools: a systematic review of components, uptake, and effectiveness of quality improvement toolkits. *Implementation Science* 14: 83. https://doi.org/10.1186/s13012-019-0929-8.

Langley, G.L., Moen, R., Nolan, K.M. et al. (2009). *The Improvement Guide: A Practical Approach to Enhancing Organizational Performance*, 2e. San Francisco, California, USA: Jossey-Bass Publishers.

Milat, A.J., King, L., Bauman, A.E., and Redman, S. (2013). The concept of scalability: increasing the scale and potential adoption of health promotion interventions into policy and practice. *Health Promotion International* 28: 285–298. https://doi.org/10.1093/heapro/dar097.

Moore, J.E., Mascarenhas, A., Bain, J., and Straus, S.E. (2017). Developing a comprehensive definition of sustainability. *Implementation Science* 12: 110. https://doi.org/10.1186/s13012-017-0637-1.

Nadalin Penno, L., Davies, B., Graham, I.D. et al. (2019). Identifying relevant concepts and factors for the sustainability of evidence-based practices within acute care contexts: a systematic review and theory analysis of selected sustainability frameworks. *Implementation Science* 14: 108. https://doi.org/10.1186/s13012-019-0952-9.

Palmer, S. and Raftery, J. (1999). Economic notes: opportunity cost. *BMJ* 318: 1551–1552.

planview. Lean Methodology 2020 [Available from: https://www.planview.com/resources/articles/lean-methodology.

Pluye, P., Potvin, L., Denis, J.L., and Pelletier, J. (2004). Program sustainability: focus on organizational routines. *Health Promotion International* 19: 489–500. https://doi.org/10.1093/heapro/dah411.

Quality-One International (2020). Lean Methodology [Available from: https://quality-one.com/lean.

Rastogi A. (2018). DMAIC – A Six Sigma Process Improvement Methodology [Available from: https://www.greycampus.com/blog/quality-management/dmaic-a-six-sigma-process-improvement-methodology.

Rogers, E.M. (2005). *Diffusion of Innovations*, 5e. New York: Free Press.

Shelton, R.C., Cooper, B.R., and Stirman, S.W. (2018). The sustainability of evidence-based interventions and practices in public health and health care. *Annual Review of Public Health* 39: 55–76. https://doi.org/10.1146/annurev-publhealth-040617-014731.

15

Reflections

Is It Worth it?

We have come to the end of the implementation journey – we have related our story in developing Roadmap, our learnings and experiences with implementation of best practices in different contexts. We would not be surprised if you are now having second thoughts about undertaking evidence implementation. We cannot lie – the time and effort involved are significant. To understand why and how we kept at it for more than two decades, we need to relate some more stories. Hopefully, these will resonate and motivate you to undertake this journey and consider using Roadmap to guide your way.

As you have probably realized, while the destination of evidence-informed practice is the goal, Roadmap is all about the implementation journey and what you see and do along the way that will contribute to making the trip successful. Roadmap helps chart the general course and identifies stages that should be completed. It does not give all the details, as every setting needs to tailor the implementation process depending on its circumstances. What it does do, however, is guide the planning of the journey and give a sense of where the road is leading, even if it cannot predict what exactly lies ahead and what may happen that will cause a change in plans.

This journey to evidence-informed practice has taken us through the trenches with practitioners, managers, and patients. This is what we thought would be the best way to carve out and navigate our implementation path. Evidence-informed practice does not occur simply from an edict from above, such as a health ministry or by becoming an organizational policy. It is an effort typically requiring an engaged multi-level approach – it requires efforts from the ground-up, top-down, and from those in the middle. The evidence, syntheses, and guidelines may have been developed by researchers and expert panels but the "rubber only hits the road" in the practice setting. We found that point-of-care knowledge and experience is often the missing link in failed implementation and that is why we needed to be doing this work at the point-of-care – not the usual positioning for researchers.

It is not uncommon to hear comments such as, "it is hard to change people's behaviour." It is hard work for sure, but health care providers are devoted to improving the well-being of their patients, and will usually put this objective above all others, even when it means more work for themselves. We have learned repeatedly that nurses, physicians, and others are usually open to changing practice but there must be good evidence for the best practice

Knowledge Translation in Nursing and Healthcare: A Roadmap to Evidence-informed Practice, First Edition.
Margaret B. Harrison and Ian D. Graham.
© 2021 John Wiley & Sons, Inc. Published 2021 by John Wiley & Sons, Inc.

being proposed. Their moto is – "show me the goods!" We have also found that everyone's willingness to change is also related to being authentically involved in selecting the best practice and driving the implementation process. We have also found that organizations that see themselves as learning organizations, easily embrace the principles behind Roadmap and want to support their staff to achieve evidence-informed practice.

We said at the outset, this would be an honest account and there are challenges. Is implementation hard work? Yes. Does it take time to implement? Certainly. Are best practices always implemented completely? Not always. There are clearly challenges and times when you may feel like you are taking two steps forward then one back and sometimes it seems like it is one step forward and two back. Implementation of evidence-informed practice takes time and a great deal of dedicated team effort and persistence. As much work, time, and effort as it takes to develop a quality guideline, this is minimal compared to what it takes to implement it. The practice field has its own "evidence" around context and populations that could make the most well-developed guideline sink into oblivion. Many Roadmap stages highlight the need to generate and use local evidence so that the best practice can be customized to the local context to produce improved care. Gathering and using local data takes time and work and must be done where the implementation is to occur. Unlike guideline panels of experts who have resources (content experts, library scientists, methodologists, etc.), the local hospital or home care authority may not have all of these. However, what we have learned is that they can acquire them, and once in hand, are off and running.

Overwhelming? Yes, at times it can be. This is where the group comes in to support one another during difficult times when they feel like they have hit the wall and want to abandon the journey. Perseverance is always possible with collective support and action. We are reminded of the African proverb that states, "If you want to go fast, go alone. If you want to go far, go together."

But Is It Worth It?

Unequivocally yes! Participating with groups implementing guidelines and other evidence tools, has given us such professional and personal satisfaction. Virtually all our implementations have resulted in a level of improved outcome, as well as better patient and nurse experiences. The "objective" proof is in the research papers we have published, some of which we have shared in this book. When care is guided by best practice, more patients are more likely to receive more effective care and this usually translates into improved health outcomes, health system efficiencies, and at times even cost-savings. For example, with our leg ulcer project, the use of compression bandages (best practice) more than doubled the healing rate. This resulted in cost savings as this effective treatment required less nursing time and fewer supplies than usual care (which involved multiple daily nursing home visits to do dry dressing changes that used lots and lots of gauze and tape). The use of ineffective treatments usually wastes resources (human and financial) and replacing them with effective ones is a win-win for patients, staff, managers, and often the finance department.

More of the impact story, however, comes from those who received or provided the evidence-informed care and it is important to hear from them directly. "This leg has been weeping and smelling for years – now that it is healed my grandson will sit on my knee because I do not smell" (clinic client). "I have had this leg ulcer for 10 years without being healed . . . it has prevented me from going out because I am worried about getting it banged by a shopping cart or something, now I can go out" (home care recipient). "I am so grateful for the booklet (part of evidence-informed practice for congestive heart failure) because I know better when to bring my husband back to emergency" (CHF family member). Similarly, several nurses on the general medical units indicated how grateful they were with the booklet on how to prepare the patients to go home and manage their condition effectively on their own.

There are also other benefits of using Roadmap, some anticipated and others that were not anticipated. Depending on one's perspective, these extremely valuable outcomes, can also be considered as the mechanisms through which Roadmap process results in health and health system impacts. So as you read through the coming list of outcomes, think of them as additional benefits of Roadmap, but also appreciate that taken together, they also represent the mechanisms that we believe, lead to sustained health and health system impacts.

More Consistent, Evidence-Informed Care

Our experience is that following the Roadmap process consistently has led to uptake of best practice. Although the degree of uptake did vary depending on the context and nature of the best practice. Never-the-less, nurses and managers repeatedly told us how, having best practice recommendations to follow, reduced unnecessary practice variation, as they were now all "singing from the same evidence-informed song book." Similarly, a home care manager said the following about the evidence-informed leg ulcer care that was being provided because of the implementation initiative, "It is such a relief to have us all working on the same page . . . there used to be so many different orders and types of dressings and bandages used and so much unnecessary variation in care." The provision of consistent, evidence-informed care means patients receive quality care and quality care impacts health and system outcomes. The reduction in inappropriate practice variation also reduces waste of finite health care resources.

Ownership of Practice Issues and Their Solutions

The participatory and inclusive nature of the Roadmap process supports nurses and other healthcare providers to take ownership of their clinical issues and problems and co-create and implement solutions to them. Roadmap encourages all stakeholders to become involved and have a say about the care they want to deliver in their setting and to drive implementation planning. Many health care providers not only feel alienated because of the volume and pace of work but also because clinical unit cultures may not always actively encourage collective critical thinking or problem solving. Roadmap shines a spotlight on the issues that healthcare providers (and other stakeholders) identify and then provides tools to help them take an evidence-informed approach to get the bottom of the issue, identify evidence-informed solutions, and take an evidence-informed approach to implementing the solutions. Furthermore, taking ownership also means developing solutions that are a perfect, or near perfect fit, for the setting. Similarly, by customizing best practice, they become as useful, useable, and used as they can be. By making evidence-informed practice all about stakeholders at the point-of-care, there is little wonder why the process works as well as it does.

Ownership and buy-in can also take the form of nurses and others embracing the power of using evidence to guide decisions. One nurse leading a community wound initiative put forth the case for eliminating a practice that was not supported by evidence, but physicians consistently ordered it. This nurse summarized and presented the evidence to the working group and the collective decision was to stop the practice. The decision was rightly based on the evidence not the workload. Being armed with the evidence at a decision-making table proved formidable and objective. We were witness to this, many times, and saw the nursing voice strengthened. Another example was when we began seeing nurses questioning sales representatives from wound care supply companies about the evidence behind their products.

In other words, implementing evidence-informed practice works best when there is ownership of the issue and when it is propelled from both the ground up and top down simultaneously. That is not to say a ground swell for change cannot happen at either end to kick off the call to action.

Improved Team Functioning and Interdisciplinary Practice

Another benefit of Roadmap is the inclusive collaborative approach required by the formation of interdisciplinary working groups tasked with identifying and customizing best practice. Through working together on the issue, group members not only develop or improve crucial appraisal skills, working collaboratively sometimes shifts the focus from disciplinary divides to united attention on the evidence and the patient population. This can have a trickledown effect and improves interdisciplinary relations. An example of this was when a group was reviewing leg ulcer guidelines. The physicians were shocked to learn that the medical guidelines they were familiar with failed to meet methodological standards for rigor while the nursing guidelines were much better developed, and they considered them superior. Conversely, the nurses were also surprised (and proud) to learn that the nursing guidelines were of better quality than the medical ones. When selecting specific recommendations to use, this same group experienced an interesting shift in how the specialist physicians and nurses interacted with each other. A senior and respected consultant suggested a consensus-based recommendation be adopted, as collecting the data related to it might make for a publishable paper. As one nurse told us later, prior to this project, the group would have simply gone along with the physician's suggestion, but instead, because of the strong focus on evidence-informed care and being in a safe environment, the nurses felt empowered to question the value of the proposed recommendation as it was not based on empirical evidence. The group discussed the lack of evidence for the recommendation and the operational implications the practice would have on patients and nurses and the physician agreed that following the recommendation might not be the best use of nursing resources. The group had decided at the start to select recommendations based on evidence and the physician withdrew his suggestion to adopt the non-evidence-informed recommendation. The improved interdisciplinary relationships, resulting in part, from working collaboratively in developing the customized best practice and implementing it, could also be seen. In response to a threat to the homecare leg ulcer service, vascular specialists and family physicians came to the aid of the nurses arguing that the leg ulcer care nurses now knew more about effective leg ulcer care than themselves-quite the accolade from physicians.

Capacity Building

Over the years, we have seen impressive capacity building occurring within teams and in members of teams. The process of going through an evidence implementation is educational in and of itself. Working with Roadmap, many skills which are required to support evidence-informed practice are enhanced at the local level. This includes critical appraisal, evidence-practice gap analysis, best practice customization, assessing the barriers and drivers to best practice, selecting and tailoring implementation strategies, evaluation, and sustainability approaches. Following Roadmap for the first time does involve a steep learning curve but getting through the process once also means the skills learned can be reused repeatedly. Indeed, once the Roadmap process is learned, working group members have the knowledge and experience and their decision-making process is changed forever. The question "what's the evidence for that" becomes the new mantra. Knowing how to look for and assess available evidence can become embedded in the local culture. As one administrator told us, this was "their new way of being." Lifelong learning is a personal attribute of effective professionals and Roadmap encourages learning by doing.

Greater Professional Satisfaction

Most of our implementation initiatives were with nurses and to our surprise, many of them became excited about their practice and the opportunity of taking ownership of charting their path to best practices. It seems that Roadmap has the potential to generate professional pride and satisfaction. We had a few nurses who have taken the implementation journey then decide to delay their retirement. This quote comes from a seasoned home care nurse, "I volunteered to work on this (the leg ulcer) project because I wanted to do something different for a little bit before I retired – I was worn out and not happy at work. Being part of this team, has rejuvenated me professionally. I got into nursing to make a difference and doing best practice leg ulcer care, I can see the difference it is making in people's lives. I'm now wanting to stay around a little longer." Other nurses have returned to school to take specialized clinical courses or an advanced degree in an area of interest.

Summary

In summary, over the years, we have identified several key ingredients for successful implementation and Roadmap is designed to leverage and support them.

These ingredients are:

- From the very beginning, stakeholders and knowledge-users decide on the issue of focus and co-create solutions and implementation plans. They will be more likely to act upon the solutions they develop.
- Wisely choosing the issue to focus on.

- Planning for sustainability from the outset.
- Best practice (evidence and research) is accepted as the lynchpin in improving quality and outcomes of healthcare.
- Quality external evidence is the foundation of best practices and provides the benchmark against which current practice can be judged. It also provides leverage for change.
- Maximizing use of best practice requires customizing it to the local context.
- Generating and analyzing local evidence is needed to: clarify the issue/problem, contextualize it, establish current practice, and determine the evidence-practice gap, the barriers/drivers to use of the customized practice, the effectiveness of implementation strategies at increasing uptake of the best practice, and the impact and sustainability of the best practice.
- All external and local evidence should be sufficiently rigorous and pragmatic, while meeting the needs of the project/implementation process and timelines.
- Improving evidence-informed practice is about creating a culture that understands, values, embraces, and applies best practice.
- Culture change takes partnerships, meaningful engagement, common vision, collaborative spirit, leadership, and time.
- Implementation leadership involves coordination and planning, strategies for exchange and to build consensus and trust, monitoring and performance expectations, incentives and rewards, provision of resources (people and financial resources), and sustained effort at the executive, managerial and point-of-care levels.

Box 15.1   Collateral benefits

In a debriefing and final evaluation forum with implementation groups in the Canadian Guideline Implementation Study (Cancer Care), participants offered pertinent insights particularly for those just starting to formally undertake implementation. Steering committee chairs and working group representatives unanimously revealed that by planning for systematic guideline adaptation and implementation, they had achieved significantly greater individual and organizational capacity for providing evidence-informed care. Participants commented on the groundswell of talk, activity, thinking about evidence-informed practice, the synergies, and trickle-down effects on other projects that occurred. Of particular value was a culture change in their organizations along with their educational and professional development outcomes. They learned that a culture dedicated to practice development is integral to the successful adaptation, implementation, and sustainment of evidence-informed practice. Nearly everyone in these groups embarked on subsequent guideline adaptation and implementation initiatives using the skills and tools they received and helped to create over the course of their first implementation.

We would argue that the last critical ingredient, is using a conceptual framework to guide planning and actions/activities. The usefulness of frameworks comes from laying out the big picture and the organization they provide for thinking, planning, for observation, and for interpreting what is seen. They provide a systematic structure and a rationale for actions/activities.

As every book must come to an end, let us end this one on a light note. You have made it through the book because of your motivation to improve practice. Our final words are about what it takes for you (and the working group) to succeed as you work through Roadmap. We have used a graphic (Figure 15.1) with our groups in the early days to warn them about the challenges ahead. It is tongue-in-cheek and jaunty, but below the surface holds many hard truths about what it takes to ensure a successful journey to best practice.

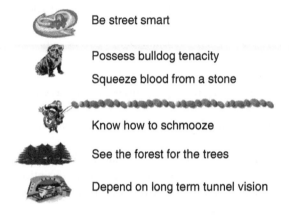

Be street smart

Possess bulldog tenacity

Squeeze blood from a stone

Know how to schmooze

See the forest for the trees

Depend on long term tunnel vision

Figure 15.1   Desirable traits to embark on evidence-informed practice.

It is our genuine hope that this book and Roadmap offers guidance and support to all those working to activate evidence in their practices and in their settings. Stay true to the participatory approach espoused by Roadmap, ensure that the process is inclusive and welcoming of everyone (especially patients and families), focus on aligning the external and local evidence, plan, implement and evaluate and good things will surely result.

Index

Knowledge Translation in Nursing and Healthcare: A Roadmap to Evidence-informed Practice, First Edition.
Margaret B. Harrison and Ian D. Graham.
© 2021 John Wiley & Sons, Inc. Published 2021 by John Wiley & Sons, Inc.